Lonely Children and Adolescents

Malka Margalit

Lonely Children and Adolescents

Self-Perceptions, Social Exclusion, and Hope

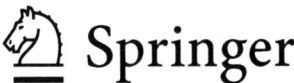 Springer

Malka Margalit
Tel Aviv University
Constantiner School of Education
69978 Tel Aviv
Israel
malka@post.tau.ac.il

ISBN 978-1-4419-6283-6   e-ISBN 978-1-4419-6284-3
DOI 10.1007/978-1-4419-6284-3
Springer New York Dordrecht Heidelberg London

Library of Congress Control Number: 2010928733

Printed on acid-free paper

Springer is part of Springer Science+Business Media (www.springer.com)

To my parents, Hana and Avigdor Gutenberg
my husband, Yoni
my children, Moti and Dubi
and my grandchildren

Preface

Loneliness is a painful and distressful experience. It signals the existence of a failure in the valued area of personal perceptions and interpersonal relationships. It affects children's and adolescents' quality of life and represents a developmental risk for future adjustment. In *Lonely Children and Adolescents: Self-Perceptions, Social Exclusion, and Hope* I seek to synthesize more than 15 years of research with my students. This book addresses the core experience of the emotional and social life of children and adolescents: feeling lonely at home and in school among classmates. Some children keep their loneliness distress to themselves, but many others share their agony and expect to receive support and help from preoccupied and worried parents and teachers. The book proposes a reconceptualization of the children's distress not as a dichotomy model (lonely/not lonely) but as a dynamic multidimensional understanding of movement along continuums between loneliness, connectedness, and solitude within developmental paradigms.

At this time, the constantly growing connectedness opportunities and choices through communication paths such as social networking sites (e.g., Facebook) and cells' oral and written communication, in addition to face-to-face contacts, increase the importance of focusing on children's loneliness. Nowadays, young people keep contacts most of the time with family, friends, classmate peers that they know, as well as "friends of friends," and total strangers. At the same time, they play collaborative games on the computer, update their positions and activities online, send text messages on their mobile, and check who is looking for them on social sites. Social networking is growing in magnitude and importance, enabling diverse routes to challenge social isolation. Yet many youngsters continue to feel alone, even among friends and family members. Parents share anxious concerns when realizing their children's social suffering, feeling helpless and unsure regarding what they can do. Educators express frustrations when they identify children's social exclusion, yet often feel unprepared to provide meaningful help.

The goal of this book is to examine in depth the loneliness experienced by children as related to their individual characteristics and contextual conditions at home and in school. In line with current psychology trends, the book presents loneliness as a risk factor and also discusses protective factors and social-emotional resilience. It concludes in proposing therapeutic implications of the hope theory, empowering strategies for coping with childhood loneliness as well as preventive and intervention approaches.

In this book, loneliness conceptualization as an outcome of a mismatch between children's needs and motivation for connectedness and their perceived social realities is presented. The book is divided into nine chapters that start with clarifying conceptual approaches. Personal characteristics of children are presented, including genetics, psychoanalytic theories of attachment, social learning constructs' self–perceptions, and developmental factors, which may predispose children to the loneliness experiences, or predict their resilience (Chapter 2).

The loneliness construct deals with personal and interpersonal relations within different contextual conditions, and the third chapter discusses the children's first social environment – the family – detailing relations inside the family with parents and siblings, including parenting styles and periods of instability, such as divorce, and their relations to the experience of social isolation. Discussions of the family and school environments as promoting or challenging loneliness and interacting with personal characteristics, including children with special needs, have theoretical importance with educational and parenting implications.

The fourth and the fifth chapters introduce the school environment, including the important roles of teachers and peers for children's connectedness, companionships, and alienation. The sixth chapter presents the Internet environments and the predictive role of virtual connections on children's well-being. Nowadays, children and adolescents feel a strong urge to keep connected most of the time, and the social exclusion as well as their experience of alienation predict a more profound risk to their well-being and development.

The seventh and the eighth chapters display empowering and resilience trends in the discussions of coping with loneliness as an alternative to deficit approaches, with clinical and educational implications. The inclusion of a wide range of classic and innovative therapeutic approaches provides supportive examples to the empowering possibilities. The conclusions and future directions in the last chapter offer future opportunities for research, intervention, and prevention, raising challenges and dilemmas.

In conclusion, I believe that, currently, childhood loneliness is a neglected topic, and I hope that the book meets the unanswered need for a comprehensive updated research-based conceptualization on this significant developmental risk. By proposing the salutogenic (health promotion) paradigm and the hope theory as well as by introducing the possibilities of technological developments, I believe that it has a special value for prevention, counseling, and intervention planning. In the current cultural trends that highlight the significance of social connections and the protective and risk paradigms related to the impacts of friends, I trust that it will extend knowledge that will help bridge social or interpersonal space and empower children, their families, and schools in their struggle with social exclusion and alienation.

Tel-Aviv, Israel   Malka Margalit

Acknowledgments

I would like to express my appreciation to a number of people who encouraged and assisted me in preparing this book. It reflects the insights acquired from studies that I performed during the years with my students. The descriptions of children, families, and teachers that are presented in this book emerged through the work of our research teams, and we changed identifying information to protect privacy. Thanks are expressed to many students, whose creative and inspiring ideas enriched our work, and many institutions that have generously supported my research during the years. There is no way in which I can single each one out for the thanks that are due. Yet I would like especially to express my gratitude to Orly Idan who spent many hours reading and reviewing the manuscript and provided me with thoughtful comments. Finally, to children, parents, and teachers, I voice my deepest gratitude for sharing with me their feelings of loneliness and hope and enable reaching in-depth understanding of their companionship, connectedness, and social isolation.

Contents

Chapter 1
Loneliness Conceptualization

Children's loneliness is a major source of distress, and also a noteworthy developmental problem that can predispose them to immediate and long-term negative consequences. Currently, the importance of this harmful experience is emphasized, bearing in mind the almost unlimited interpersonal connectedness options that have recently been developing, through different paths and modes, such as social networking sites (i.e., Face book), Internet messages (i.e., e-mails) and cells' oral and written communication (i.e., SMS), in addition to face-to-face contacts. Children and adolescents are especially eager to stay "connected" with their friends, along with many classmates, with peers that they know, as well as with "friends of friends" and with people that they meet only on the Internet. Private contents are shared, sometimes in the presence of total strangers (talking on the cells in the streets and buses, disclosing distress in blogs). In this reality, a most surprising and upsetting question is why children and adolescents continue to be lonely regardless of the fact that they stay in contact with others for a large amount of their waking hours. Several modes of connectedness, such as SMS, require the usage of short words and graphic signs promoting the development of "a new language" and enabling individuals to send and receive many messages, sometimes simultaneously, while several children "don't know the language" and feel more excluded and isolated. Social networking is growing and receiving different modes and styles, enabling different routes for challenging the experience of social isolation, yet and maybe even paradoxically because of it, children and adolescents continue to experience elevated loneliness.

Indeed, in our contemporary society, conflicting interpersonal trends are emphasized. On the one hand, there is an increasing and urgent need for constant connectivity (expressed in behaviors such as regular checking of e-mails, frequent contacts with cell phones in public places, sending instant messages) and endless communication. Cell phone companies even adopted these inclinations by announcing "with (name of a cell company) you are never alone" on their commercial advertisements. On the other hand, there is a growing recognition for needs of intensified individualism as expressions of the self, encouraging independent mind-set trends, providing increased opportunities for selective meeting of individual choices of living, working, dressing, and leisure activities. Children and adolescents want to

M. Margalit, *Lonely Children and Adolescents*, DOI 10.1007/978-1-4419-6284-3_1,
© Springer Science+Business Media, LLC 2010

behave and to dress similarly to their friends with whom they want to be connected, and at the same time, paradoxically, they also want to be different, to express their true self, to be themselves in their choice of dresses or music. Indeed our society has often been labeled "The Age of Loneliness" (Moody, 2001) in which the phenomenon of loneliness may be considered almost epidemic and a source of concern in different cultures (Chen & French, 2008). Although many individuals confirm that they are lonely, it was judged as a negative and even an embarrassing condition (Killeen, 1998).

Loneliness may be understood as a structural dimension of existence that may be increased or decreased in various environments (Gierveld & Tilburg, 2006; Nilsson, Lindstrom, & Naden, 2006). Thus, within this ongoing struggle between being connected to others and to staying independent and different in a way that will enable expressing personal uniqueness, it is not surprising that loneliness has become a major issue of concern in our society, emphasizing the in-depth need for the understanding of children's loneliness. The dilemma whether loneliness may be considered an epidemic of our time is not only a theoretical debate. It has practical implications, and parents share their distress and deep worries, feeling helpless when realizing their children's social suffering. Educators express their frustrations and anxiety when they confront children's social exclusion and often feel unprepared to provide meaningful help and support. Surprisingly, the loneliness of adults was widely studied, yet only a few books were devoted to children's loneliness. The goals of this book are first to examine in depth the loneliness experienced by children and adolescents as related to their individual characteristics, including individuals with special educational needs and contextual conditions at home and at school; and second, to identify effective strategies for coping with alienation and successful overcoming or preventing of this social distress. Cultural impacts including the Internet generation culture are discussed. Special attention is devoted to children who are at risk for loneliness, and yet don't feel lonely, in order to identify factors that may empower and inoculate individuals from painful loneliness experiences. At the first stage, there is a need to clarify the meaning of loneliness.

The Meaning of Loneliness

Childhood loneliness is a painful emotional experience that affects the current quality of life and represents a developmental risk for future wellbeing as well. It signals the existence of failure in the valued area of interpersonal relationships. In order to ensure a deeper understanding of the meaning of the loneliness experience within the ecological paradigm, varied aspects of human connections within environments will be described. Stories that were shared with our research group will be presented (with assumed names, in order to protect privacy).

Abby's sad voice expressed her distress. Abby is a single mother who has a 7-year-old son. They recently moved to California. After a few weeks, her son refused to continue going to school. In the mornings he complained about various pains, declaring that he did not feel well enough to sit in class. At first Abby thought that he was catching a cold, and stayed with him at home. However, soon she started realizing that there must be a more profound problem that requested attention. She contacted the school counselor and it became apparent that her son was experiencing social difficulties. He did not initiate contacts with peers at school. The counselor described him as a loner who stayed by himself most of the school hours and inquired if he had similar difficulties at his old school. Abby felt a sudden chill and excitingly denied any prior problems. She blamed the school, the teachers, and the children who did not welcome a newcomer. To me she confided sadly that in his old school he also had few good friends. She was happy to move to the new school, expecting that the new social environment would do him well. However, now, he was all alone at school, even without the few old friends. When she asked him about other boys and girls in his class, he started screaming and yelling. He shared in detail his feelings of loneliness and sadness, when everybody else seemed happy, not wanting him in their group. Abby described their conversation and started crying. She said – "I know well what he is talking about. All my childhood I experienced the agony of loneliness. As a child I was a loner and I don't want him to go through the same agonizing path."

Rene wrote on a parents' e-forum asking what can be done with her daughter's social exclusion: "The friends that Sara, my 10-year-old daughter has, are causing her self-esteem more damage than any of her learning difficulties. She hates school. My husband cannot bear seeing her suffering. It revives his childhood pains and he is angry and sad most of the time. How can I help her? I feel so alone." In reply, she got 86 messages from mothers who had boys and girls at different ages – from preschools to high schools – who wrote empathy letters describing similar experiences of their children and raising their deep concerns. One of the mothers wrote, "when my boy revealed reading problems, I knew how to provide him with a remedial help – but what can I do when children do not want to hang out with him and be his friends?"

It has to be clarified that many parents express their frustrations not only when they, as adults, face the loneliness distress, but when they observe their children experiencing alienation, segregation, and social exclusion. Indeed loneliness is considered a normative segment of human experience. All people, regardless of age or sex, experience loneliness at some periods of their lives. For most people, intense feelings of loneliness are just short lived. For others, loneliness and social alienation are the persistent painful realities of everyday experience. Individual differences exist between people's needs for company. Several individuals have a strong need for social relations and friendship and experience severe distress when their relatedness does not meet personal expectations, while others get tired from intensive social interactions. They need, appreciate, and enjoy times alone and have only a moderate need for networking and social relations. Indeed loneliness is a common distress experience for adults and children and a source of developmental risk to wellbeing. Yet, several people experience more profound and more frequent loneliness. In the past, scientists suggested that children don't experience loneliness. However, research did not confirm this view, clarifying and demonstrating that people feel and report loneliness throughout all of life's stages, from early childhood to old age.

The feelings of alienation and social exclusion were reported and described in philosophical writings, short poetries, and comprehensive novels. In order to establish an in-depth understanding of connectedness, relatedness, closeness – or loneliness, the richness of human relations should be fully acknowledged, exploring the role of these relations in promoting personal and interpersonal perceptions. However, prior to the exploration of interpersonal relations in the family and peer settings and the personal factors characterizing lonely children, the goals of the first chapter are to clarify the significance of loneliness with a special focus on children's loneliness for their current wellbeing and as a risk factor for future development and quality of life, especially in the present when children and adolescents invest continuous effort to stay connected. The study of loneliness is in fact the study of children's interrelations, in all their different forms and variability, including the study of their self-perceptions in terms of how the children view others and themselves, how others view them, and how they feel about these perceptions and conceptions by others. This exploration of children's perceptions, beliefs, conceptions, and feelings may provide valuable information not only on the individual children but also on the social climate in their inherent cultures, social institutions, and natural systems such as schools and families (Rokach, 2008), thus pinpointing breakdowns in social interactions that reflect systemic difficulties originating from gaps between children's expectations and their different environments (Peplau & Perlman, 1982).

Empirical research and theoretical conceptualization will be integrated in this book in order to elucidate the multidimensional construct of children's loneliness, summarizing affective, cognitive, and behavioral aspects within developmental perspectives. Special attention will be given not only on clarifying the loneliness experience, but also on identifying factors that can mediate or buffer personal characteristics and situational variables that may contribute to loneliness (Lavallee & Parker, 2009). The book aims to enhance our awareness of the current life quality of children, highlighting their personal attributes and social contexts and pointing out directions for prevention, empowerment, and intervention. The first chapter first provides a brief overview of the theoretical definitions of loneliness as a multidimensional construct and then touches upon the developmental and contextual frameworks necessary for understanding resilience and empowering approaches.

The fact that loneliness predicts feelings of hopelessness and depressed mood (Page, 1991) even in the early stages of development, emphasizes the importance of early identification and intervention programs for loneliness in order to prevent a later sense of distress and its consequences upon emotional health, adjustment, and development. A rapidly growing trend in social research is currently targeting children with a focus on young children who lack friends or feel lonely and isolated in school. Much of the increased research interest stems from evidence indicating that children who experience poor peer relations and social alienation constitute "at risk" populations who may demonstrate both reduced opportunities for social learning and greater adjustment problems during adulthood (Asher & Paquette, 2003; Asher, Parkhurst, Hymel, & Williams, 1990).

In the first part of this chapter, definitions and theory are presented in order to clarify what is loneliness, and why we feel lonely. Afterward, loneliness is presented as a risk factor within the risk and protective paradigm, and the salutogenic model is applied to focus attention not only on risk factors, but also on protective factors including the Sense of Coherence construct and the hope theory.

Definitions

The classic definition presented by Peplau and Perlman (1982) defined loneliness as an unpleasant experience when individuals perceive a discrepancy between the desired and accomplished patterns of their social networks. This definition considered loneliness as a subjective negative experience, and provided the cause of such an experience – the frustration related to perceptions of the mismatch regarding social relations' domains. Woodward's (1988, p. 4) definition provided an extensive description of the construct, avoiding the proposal of causal explanations: "Loneliness is a feeling of being alone and disconnected or alienated from positive people, places and things." Loneliness is considered a negative feeling – a subjective experience emerging not only from disconnection from desired individuals, but also emerging from disconnections from places or people.

Asher et al. (1990) whose pioneer studies initiated the in-depth examination of children's loneliness, added an important distinction by proposing that the loneliness experience is a global indicator of dissatisfaction from the quality and/or the quantity of individuals' social interrelations. In this definition it is recognized that the negative global feeling can emerge from different sources of social frustration. These definitions clearly differentiated between loneliness as a subjective experience of alienation and the objective situations of social isolation. Two children may be alone, but one child may experience loneliness because he or she desires friends and misses their company, while the other child may not experience loneliness because he or she is reading an interesting book, playing a computer game, or studying for a challenging examination and wishes to stay alone. Children may have many friends, and yet feel lonely. They can be in a large crowd, in a family gathering, or in a jubilant social party, and yet feel alienation from the group. The studies focus on the individual's inner emotional distress, and this feeling is unpleasant, aversive, and painful, and signals a wish for change.

Different Forms of Loneliness

When people say that they are lonely, what do they mean? Do they share the same global experience, or is it possible to differentiate between different dimensions and emphasis in the loneliness experience? There are theoretical disagreements regarding the dilemma if there is a single global experience of loneliness or is it preferable to differentiate between diverse unique subtypes of this distress. In order to figure out this human psychological suffering, and ultimately to develop efficient ways to respond to it, we must first identify its specific nature. Two main approaches were proposed. Loneliness may be considered a global complex construct with interrelated aspects. An alternative approach differentiated between four unique yet interrelated forms of the loneliness experiences:

- Emotional loneliness (Weiss, 1973)
- Social loneliness (Weiss, 1973)
- Existential loneliness (Mayers, Khoo, & Svartberg, 2002)
- Representational loneliness (Bering, 2008).

Weiss (1973) in his classic monograph proposed the bimodal construct of loneliness, differentiating between two types of these emotional distresses: emotional loneliness and social loneliness.

1. *Emotional loneliness*

Emotional loneliness refers to a distress that reflects the lack (or the loss) of intimately close persons (best friends or loved ones). The studies of emotional loneliness were examined within the attachment and the secure-base framework (see Chapter 3 for details), focusing attention on models of early relations between infants and their caregivers, mainly mothers (Mikulincer & Florian, 1998).

Sara's and Adam's stories exemplify this type of loneliness: Sara, a 16-year-old successful student wrote on her Internet blog: "I have many friends and I am often invited to parties, yet yesterday I was sitting with friends, but I felt all alone and I almost started to cry." It should be clarified that Sara was very successful in her studies; she had many friends that she appreciated, yet she felt lonely on that day since she had lost the intimate close relations with her best friend who had moved to another city and with whom she felt very close and attached.

Adam, a 9-year-old boy, told his grandmother when she asked him if he was happy at school (a random question that many adults ask children without expecting an emotional loaded answer): "I hate school! I am so lonely there. Most of the time I play football with several friends, and we hang around during school recesses. However, no one is my true friend."

These examples focused attention on the children's need for close relations and on the presence of other children that does not change this distressed feeling. It is different in quality from social loneliness, but not in the magnitude of the social pain.

2. *Social loneliness*

Social loneliness refers to the distress emerging from the lack (or the loss) of satisfactory connections and belonging to desired social groups such as networks of friends, colleagues, etc. The studies of social loneliness were examined within the conceptualization of peer relations, social status (peer nomination/rejection), and social skills (Asher & Paquette, 2003). The socially lonely individual seeks participation in activities within networks of groups, wishing them to accept him or her as a member. This type of loneliness was best predicted by a lack of reassurance of personal worth and was related to self-identity perceptions in a group. The group's ignoring or even rejecting may prevent gratifications and rewards that can only be mediated by social interchange. Engagement in social activities and enhancement of feelings of belonging, whether based on shared concerns, interests, work, or other activities, may alleviate the feelings of social loneliness and reinforce a reassurance of one's own worth.

Miri's and Gil's stories exemplify this type of loneliness: Miri, a 5-year-old girl, told her sister: "A group of three girls were my friends in the beginning of the year. We used to sit together, laugh and play together. Suddenly, without any reason, they started telling 'secrets' about me, and didn't want me to play with them. Sometimes I saw them laughing and when I come closer they stopped and one of them would say to the others – let's go play in another place." When the sister asked, "so, did you play with other girls in your class"; she said, "indeed many girls asked me to join their play, but I was so sad and I felt so lonely. I don't have any friend and I don't want the other girls to be my friends."

Gil, a successful student, told his girlfriend: "I felt so lonely and disappointed when working teams were established at the laboratory in a science class. I was waiting, expecting the best students to invite me, yet nobody invited me to be in his group." Surprisingly she said – "I don't understand. I heard you talking with some classmates, refusing to join their group." He answered angrily – "I don't want to join any other group." He mentioned names of the most popular students, ignoring many others.

3. Existential loneliness

Existential loneliness has been defined as a self-perception of personal isolation, a primary and inevitable condition of existence, related to feelings of personal meaninglessness, helplessness, isolation, aloneness, and loss of freedom (Mayers, Khoo, & Svartberg, 2002). Since all humans are born into a world where perfect communication with others is impossible, a basic sense of loneliness emerges (Moustakis, 1961). Powerful tragic events, such as death of a close person or separation, trigger the existential loneliness. In addition, unavoidable transitions in life, such as occupational changes, life threatening diseases, and natural calamities may also generate feelings of existential loneliness.

Ronen's and Rivka's stories exemplify this type of loneliness: After a short marriage and a bitter divorce, Ronen felt lonely and isolated. He felt that his life was meaningless, and he was, as a person, worthless. He was convinced that he would never love or be loved again. The sudden death of her close friend left Rivka very lonely and depressed. She missed her companion and felt that her entire life had become meaningless. She felt helpless and socially isolated. Her family expressed their annoyance following her attempts to distance herself from everybody saying that she felt worthless.

4. Representational loneliness

Representational loneliness occurs when the awareness of others comes into conflict with the awareness that the self can never be understood by others in its totality because it can never be experienced by anyone else (Bering, 2008; Humphrey, 2007). This type of loneliness is similar to the existential loneliness due to the loss of positive experience. Yet, unlike the existential loneliness, it is exacerbated by the presence of others. It emerges from the wish to be understood by significant others, the disappointed awareness of the agony that regardless of closeness "people truly will not understand," and the emerging personal distance.

Careen's and Rene's stories exemplify this type of loneliness: Careen, almost 16 years old, was sitting at a party listening to the noisy music and to the girls' laughter and dancing – and she felt very lonely and disconnected. She wished to call them "my best friends," but she looked at their smart dresses and felt ugly and unhappy. She said to herself: "Nobody understands me or truly knows me. Nobody will notice or care if I shall leave." She left the party quietly, not telling anybody – feeling that the happy faces of everybody made her even lonelier.

Rene wrote on the discussion board of parents to children with learning disabilities: "I hate family meetings and reunions. The other mothers talked all the time about their children's achievements, grades and prizes. I cannot see myself telling them how happy I was when, at last, my son was able to read a few words. I felt so lonely knowing that they will never understand my happiness."

Interrelations Between the Loneliness Types

Studies (Dykstra & Fokkema, 2007; Hojat, 1982; Russell, Cutrona, Rose, & Yurko, 1984) supported the distinction between social and emotional isolation, highlighting the multivariate nature of loneliness feelings. Individuals, who reported that their parents had not devoted enough time to them and did not understand them, felt lonely. However, those who recounted that they did not get along with their peers in childhood, experienced loneliness as well (Junttila & Vauras, 2009). Studies reported that social and emotional loneliness shared a high degree of associated common experience, yet indicated their distinctiveness. Both social and emotional isolation were consistently found to be positively related to the quality and quantity of friendships, suggesting the varied functions of friendships for individuals throughout development. Depression was also related to both emotional and social isolation (although the relation was stronger with emotional isolation), whereas anxiety was found to be related mostly to social isolation. The ability to distinguish between aspects of one's loneliness experience may be dependent on developmental stage and cognitive conceptualization. Existential and representational loneliness have similar aspects to emotional loneliness, feeling that the self can never be understood by others in its totality. Yet, the representational loneliness is the only loneliness that is intensified by the presence of others.

The Characteristics of Loneliness

Regardless the unsolved debate between treating loneliness as a global, unified construct with many levels and subtypes or a complex–multivariate index of separate distresses, there are several common acknowledgements of the following loneliness characteristics:

1. *Loneliness is a distressing negative emotional experience.* Similar to negative emotional experiences, such as fear, anxiety, or depression, loneliness is an unpleasant and distressing experience. Individuals who are lonely describe their experience as social pain, unhappiness, and anxiety. Lonely children describe their unhappy moods using words such as "I don't have anything to do, and I am sad" or "I feel sorry for myself." Many times they talk about feeling "bored" in order to describe their loneliness. Staying alone is considered by them an undesired situation.

2. *Loneliness is a subjective experience.* The only way to learn if children are lonely is to ask them. Only self-reports may provide valid information about loneliness. It can be unrelated to objectively measured social connections, or to detailed observations at social interactions. Children can feel lonely while playing in a group, or, alternatively, may remain alone, but do not feel lonely. Children that view themselves as lonely often compare themselves to others. For example, children may say that all of the children they know have many good friends while they remain alone and feel lonely. Thus, no objective measures exist to indicate if loneliness is experienced. In order to confirm that children indeed understand what the loneliness construct means, they were interviewed at different ages and in different cultures. They were asked to provide examples of situations in which they felt lonely. The results clearly showed that even young preschoolers can report these unpleasant subjective experiences (Cassidy & Asher, 1992; Galanaki, 2004).

3. *Loneliness is a complex set of feelings encompassing reactions to unfulfilled social needs.* Loneliness has been considered a response to the absence of or unfulfilled specific individual needs for social interrelations. Within this approach, the unfulfilled developmental need is posited as constituting the cause for later interpersonal difficulties. This need for relatedness to a desired group has been considered a basic psychological need (Patrick, Knee, Canevello, & Lonsbary, 2007), reflecting individual differences. Social needs and interrelation patterns are expressed differently throughout different developmental stages, from the infant's early striving for intimate interrelations, through the young child's attempts to achieve a sense of belonging to a group of peers, and onward to the adolescent's and adult's search for assurance of being acknowledged and appreciated by a significant group of valued persons.

4. *Loneliness is a reaction to unfulfilled intimate needs.* This need for a close and intimate relationship is rooted in the early parent–infant bonding and attachment. It is expressed through different stages of life through the need for feelings of trust and closeness, such as the relations with a good friend with whom the child is ready to share secrets and intimate details and the relations with a trustful teacher (Junttila & Vauras, 2009).

5. Loneliness is *transient* and a temporary state for many individuals, yet a *chronic* state for others. Children may disclose loneliness for short periods as a reaction to social exclusion, but they will be considered a group at risk only if this experience will occur often.

6. *Loneliness "runs" in families.* disclosing the joint impact of genetic and environmental factors, as will be further explained in the second and third chapter.

7. *Loneliness is different from solitude, but it is related to it.* Solitude has been characterized by disengagement from the immediate demands of other peoples, reduced social inhibition, and increased freedom to select and stay uninvolved in mental or physical activities. It may provide time for day dreaming, leisure activities, a restful period after a demanding day, and self-renewal (Larson, 1997). Spending time alone is not necessarily related to negative experiences. In contrast to the consistently negative affect related to loneliness, solitude is often viewed as a pleasant, positive, and sometimes even desirable situation that may promote a creative experience or provide an opportunity for rest from stressful reality and demanding work situations (Marcoen & Goossens, 1990, April). Artists, writers, and scientists often describe solitude as their most creative and productive state. Creativity studies (Csikszentmihalyi, 1996) highlighted the importance of solitude for promoting creativity and reported that adolescents who could not tolerate being alone, often failed to develop their creative talents because such development usually relied on solitary activities, such as practicing one's musical instrument or writing poetry.

Often creativity emerged from the formation of new associations between previously unrelated ideas, and providing expression to those associations in ways that are useful or valuable to the self or others. Solitude could facilitate creativity, since creativity could not occur without a loosening – deconstruction of old connections, and subsequent reconstruction – of new cognitive structures.

Solitude, being different from loneliness, involves a deliberate choice to be alone (Galanaki, 2005; Woodward, 1988). Solitude is typically experienced when a person is alone. However, a person can experience solitude while he or she stays in the presence of others, such as while traveling on a train and the emotional "alone" experience may persist in the physical company of strangers (Long & Averill, 2003). The capacity and the preference to stay engaged in solitary activities may be related to lower levels of loneliness for adults and adolescents. In addition, societies and cultures differ in their views regarding staying alone and the extent to which they encourage and enjoy solitude, or emphasize the important of social connectedness (Seepersad, Choi, & Shin, 2008). The developmental research on solitude is further detailed in Chapter 2, pinpointing attention to developmental dilemmas and educational implications.

Research documented the relations between solitude and self-perceptions of independence and autonomy (Chua & Koestner, 2008). Individual disposition and personality characteristics may also predict individualistic preferences of solitude (Leary, Herbst, & McCrary, 2003), and in addition to individual needs for attachment, affiliation, and social connections, many people also continually seek to spend time in solitude (Long & Averill, 2003). Naturalistic studies have shown that adult humans spend approximately 29% of their waking time alone (Larson, Csikszentmihalyi, & Graef, 1982), and many people wish to have even more time alone. After a demanding working day, many individuals wish to have time alone, since solitude provides relief from the pressures and demands involved in interacting with other people. Many mothers and fathers to young children are looking forward to quite minutes when they can have time alone. They love their children and these wishes don't contradict their emotions. However, their motivation for solitude may stem from their need to rest, the wishes for self-reflection, meditation, or some purposeful activity such as studying or pursuing an interest or hobby.

Solitude provides opportunities not offered by our usual social environment and the freedom to engage in desired activities or thoughts we find intrinsically interesting. We become conscious not only of the other person, but also of ourselves as partners of interactions. Solitude can minimize such intrusive self-consciousness by reducing the immediate demands of experiencing ourselves as the object of another person's thoughts and actions. Storr (1988) suggested that, by extracting ourselves from the customary social and physical contexts (or at least altering our experience of them), solitude facilitates self-examination, re-conceptualization of the self, and coming to terms with changes. People often gain from solitude a new understanding of themselves and their priorities.

8. *Loneliness is different from depressive mood.* Loneliness and depressive mood are correlated, and the strength of their associations often raises questions about their conceptual or functional separation. In many scientific and popular books, the words loneliness and depression (or depressive moods) appear together. Indeed many depressed individuals also feel lonely. However, research demonstrated that they represent distinct constructs based on theoretical and statistical grounds (Cacioppo, Hawkley, et al., 2006). Depression is a disorder of the cognitive representation and of the regulation of mood and emotion (Davidson, Pizzagalli, Nitschke, & Putnam, 2002). The essential feature of depression is either depressed mood or loss of interest or pleasure in nearly all activities. In children and adolescents, the mood may be irritable in addition to sadness. There are also vegetative (e.g., changes in appetite), cognitive (e.g., difficulty concentrating), and emotional (e.g., feelings of guilt and worthlessness) signs (Zahn-Waxler, Shirtcliff, & Marceau, 2008).

Extensive research (Cacioppo & Patrick, 2008) demonstrated that loneliness and depression are closely related and data suggested that they can act in a synergistic effect to reduce wellbeing (Cacioppo, Hughes, Waite, Hawkley, & Thisted, 2006), yet they are conceptualized as two distinct constructs that trigger different constellations of responses. Loneliness promotes a desire to affiliate, together with a feeling of threat. Depression consists of a variety of specific symptoms in addition to negative feelings, such as sadness, including difficulties in making decisions, and in falling asleep. The cognitive processing of depressed people typically indicate automatic (i.e., repetitive, unintended, and not easily controllable) thoughts reflecting themes of loss and revealing negative views of the self, the world, and the future (Haagaa, Dyckb, & Ernstc, 1991). Depression often co-occurs with other emotional and behavioral problems (Hankin, 2008), thus it is not surprising that many individuals complain about depression together with loneliness. However, although both are aversive experiences, in many ways they are different. Loneliness is considered a warning sign to do something in order to alter the aversive condition. Depression doesn't initiate activity – just the opposite. It makes the individual apathetic, hopeless with a negative inferential thinking style. Loneliness is not the cause of depression. Yet, the effects of loneliness and life dissatisfaction on depression are mediated by health. It means that less satisfied and, particularly, lonelier individuals are more likely to report higher levels of depression when they suffer from additional risks such as poorer health (Swami et al., 2007).

Thus, loneliness and depression may often converge, resulting in passive coping styles and self-regulation difficulties. Loneliness represents attempts to approach others, while depression represents a withdrawal to avoid negative feelings. Cacioppo and Patrick (2008) in a comprehensive survey pinpointed attention to the developmental value of the loneliness and depression combinations. In difficult situations, the repeated efforts of the lonely individuals to approach in order to achieve meaningful connectedness may lead not only to feelings of loneliness when meeting social rejection, but also to depressive thinking that will result in passivity. Several studies indicated that loneliness can serve as a central individual difference characteristic, and those changes in loneliness, especially childhood loneliness, can affect a wide range of related attributes ranging from shyness and social skills to self-regulation, optimism, and self-esteem.

In summary, loneliness is a multidimensional yet unique subjective negative feeling that emerges from several unfulfilled needs (i.e., the need for close bonding and/or the need for relatedness). Many times it appears together with additional distressful experiences, but is considered a risk factor only if it is a chronic and prevalent experience. It runs in families, and often appears in early developmental stages, but its transient and temporary nature signals the importance of preventive efforts. In order to fully understand this complicated important construct, there is a need to explore its function.

Why Do We Feel Lonely?

The roots of the loneliness feeling have to be explored within evolutionary perspectives. Popular views proposed that the primary functions of emotions are to start a behavior that will meet important needs (Loewenstein, Weber, Hsee, & Welch, 2001). Emotions were often considered a strong and direct cause of behavior and by identifying someone's emotional state we could understand why the person acted in a certain way. A developmental perspective recognized the importance of the early emotions that children experienced and their impact on current and future behavior (Izard & Ackerman, 2000). Indeed the growing children add continuously new behaviors to the repertoire of a particular emotion, but these new behaviors only complement the earlier ones, remaining functionally similar to them. Many emotions are characterized by heightened bodily arousal, which is generally regarded as mobilizing the body for action. Thus the evolutional goal of loneliness is to initiate social connections. It can be considered a cry for help and an expression of feeling unsafe and unhappy (Cacioppo, Hawkley, & Berntson, 2003). According to the evolutionary model of loneliness, a person who feels lonely also feels unhappy and unsafe; feelings that heighten sensitivity to different threats. This implies that loneliness may influence not only sadness and depressive emotional reactions but also feelings of anxiety and/or anger at those individuals who are responsible for the social exclusion. Fear of negative evaluation may also develop, or maybe (as a reflection of individual differences) a series of positive emotional reactions and activities, such as optimism regarding a positive solution to the current unpleasant social isolation, readiness to activate social skills, and/or to request social support.

Infants are dependent on others for survival and being alone may increase environmental dangers for them. Our ancestors had a selective advantage to survive if they formed social connections that enabled them to communicate and work together in groups, to share food and defense, and even to retaliate together in the face of aggressive threats. In conditions of hardship, individuals who had a genetic disposition to experience social pain when they experienced social separation and alienation (i.e., loneliness) may have been more likely to return to share their food, shelter, or defense with their family and allies in order to reduce the pain of loneliness (Cacioppo, Hawkley, et al., 2006). Individual differences in sensitivity to social pains, in responses to disconnections and also in the positive feelings of reward when those connections were reinstated, are fundamental to the proposed evolutionary model. Thus loneliness can be considered as a risk factor for development, but also as a protective factor, depending on a comprehensive understanding of the varied interrelated personal and contextual factors. In order to fully understand how loneliness can be considered a developmental risk, and when it has positive and resilient impacts, an in-depth understanding of resilient models is required.

Resilience Models

Resilience refers to the dynamic development processes involving interactions between risk and protective processes – internal and external to the individual – that act to modify the effects of adverse life events (Rutter, 1999). Resilience, one of the most intriguing phenomena of human development, has been conceptualized as the individual's capacity for coping successfully and functioning competently despite experiencing chronic stress or adversity or following exposure to prolonged or severe trauma (Luthar, Cicchetti, & Becker, 2000). Stress has been conceptualized as a perceived threat to individuals' development and adjustment, and the experience of chronic stress has been typically associated with deleterious outcomes, such as neurobiological dysfunction, immunological difficulties, and with maladaptation and mental disorder. Yet not all individuals who are exposed to stressful experiences are affected in a uniform fashion at either the biological or psychological level. Multiple converging processes determine such variability in the responses to stressors. Understanding how children develop and function adaptively despite experiencing multitude and chronic stressors offers considerable promise for prevention and intervention and for elucidating developmental theories of coping. Identifying how individuals initiate their coping strategies when confronted with adverse experiences (risk factors) will shed light on the manner in which an organism's active coping strivings influence whether an adaptive or maladaptive developmental pathway will be traversed (Cicchetti & Rogosch, 2009).

Risk factors are defined as the individual's characteristics and especially developmental difficulties or environmental hazards that increase his or her vulnerability to experiencing negative outcomes (Werner & Smith, 1982). Yet, many times, risk factors did not cause maladjustment, and research attempted to identify factors that would alleviate the negative impacts of the risk factors, exploring resiliency. Studies investigated children's difficulties and vulnerabilities as risk factors for future development and showed that a variety of developmental progressions may eventuate in a given disorder, rather than expecting a singular primary pathway to the disorder (Cicchetti & Toth, 2009). Rather than searching for the indicators or predictors of later difficulty, the central focus of resilient models has shifted to investigating and describing the interactive processes that lead to the emergence and course of disturbed behavior. Questions such as "what are the various factors that initiate and maintain individuals on pathways probabilistically associated with a particular challenge such as loneliness?" and "what differentiates those lonely children from those who do not develop maladaptive social connections?" have increasingly challenged understanding with possible educational implications. Although some researchers emphasize one set of initiating and maintaining conditions, whereas other researchers accentuate divergent factors, meaningful answers to questions about risk factors require the utilization of developmental models, with increasing recognition of the dynamic interplay of influences over developmental stages and sensitivity to positive and negative contextual influences (Belsky & Pluess, 2009). It is now widely recognized that neurobiological development and environmental experiences are mutually influencing from very early developmental stages. Rather than adhering to a uni-dimensional belief in the deterministic role that unfolding biology exerts on behavior, it is now widely confirmed that brain function and its subsequent influence on behavior possesses self-organizing functions that can, in fact, be altered by experiences incurred during sensitive periods of development that occur across the life course (Cicchetti & Toth, 2009).

During any given period of development, individuals are expected to engage successfully in multiple domains of functioning. Thus, for example, children in elementary school are expected to do well in learning academic skills, forming and maintaining relationships with peers, and adhering to the standards of conduct for the classroom. Therefore, a child with major problems in any of these domains is not likely to be viewed as developing well. This multiplicity of expectations means that the adaptation of individuals from a developmental task perspective is multidimensional. Because of the multidimensional nature of developmental expectations, children viewed as manifesting resilience in the context of serious adversity would be doing well in multiple domains, successfully engaging or accomplishing multiple key developmental tasks, and resilience consideration usually means that multiple criteria have been met for doing well (Masten, Herbers, Cutuli, & Lafavor, 2008), focusing attention at those factors that protected the adjusted development.

Indeed protective factors play critical roles in children's developmental pathways following stress emerging due to risk factors. Among the array of protective factors that have been identified to promote resilient functioning in development are children's academic engagement, social competencies, average or above average intellectual performance, and the presence of a secure relationship with an adult caregiver (i.e., a father and a mother). Personality characteristics such as an internal locus of control for positive events and higher self-esteem provide further examples of individual characteristics that serve a protective function for developmental stress, mitigating the risk for maladaptive outcomes and potentially enhancing their coping capacities (Cicchetti & Rogosch, 2009).

The trends toward resilience and salutogenic paradigms emerged through the growing realization that many children were able to overcome personal difficulties and familial challenges, reaching successful adjustment regardless of their hardships. Protective factors consisted of inner personal strengths as well as external protective contexts and processes, such as supports provided by families, school systems, and communities (Margalit, 2004). This focus of interest in this line of research – the positive adaptation processes in the context of significant adversity – has a special value for in-depth understanding of children's loneliness. It also provides meaningful guidelines for prevention and intervention programs. Since the two fundamental characteristics of the emerging construct of resilience are (1) the exposure to several significant threats or adversities and (2) individuals' variations in the responses to adversity (Luthar, Cicchetti, & Becker, 2000), recent studies on the relations between varied risk and protective factors to developmental outcomes challenge the classic linear models and suggest alternative dynamic interactive models. The linear model was proposed through the research on cumulative risk and child outcomes. For example, Rutter's investigation of the Isle of Wight sample (Rutter, 1979), demonstrated this linear model, showing that the combined impact of various risk factors was more detrimental than their separate impacts. Following Rutter's early work, numerous investigations reported associations between cumulative risk and more negative developmental outcomes, such as externalizing and internalizing behavior problems (Appleyard, Egeland, Van Dulmen, & Sroufe, 2005). These studies supported the conceptualization of a linear relation between the number of risk factors and children's growth, and more risk factors predicted more unfavorable development outcomes. Gradually, a different approach trend focused attention on different sets of processes. For example, Ackerman and colleagues (1999) reported that maternal positive emotionality attenuated the relation between cumulative risk and child outcomes.

The study of protective predictors in mediating cumulative risks at various developmental age stages challenged the model which proposed that accumulated more or stronger risk factors would predict increased maladjustment (Trentacosta et al., 2008). Simple models failed to provide a comprehensive understanding of interacting situations that conveyed the complexity of the human variability. It also

did not account for inner energy resources of children and how they were combined with external energizing factors (Beasley, Thompson, & Davidson, 2003).
Within this recognition of the complexity of interacting factors, the important role
of peer groups as a protective factor in providing a sense of belonging, socialization, contexts for identity work, and learning skills for life management was widely
recognized, accentuating children's social exclusion and loneliness as a major risk
factor. However, at the same time, peer groups could have a predominant risk when
they were associated with delinquency, antisocial behavior, and educational resistance with various detrimental health and behavioral consequences for individual
members (Bottrell, 2009). Social capital referred to social networks built around
trust and shared norms.

Although the literature on social capital has been associated with resilience in
varying ways, since it was considered a buffer to the adverse effects of disadvantage
contextual conditions (Bottrell, 2009), social networks may also trigger maladjustment, requesting a comprehensive understanding that will attempt to consider the
ongoing processes among the varied factors. People seldom experience an isolated
problem or difficulty. Usually multiple risk factors tend to covary within individuals
and interact in different ways. Often children who experience loneliness have additional developmental difficulties, and the risk research may promote understanding
of the possibly multiple causal paths, some involving complex chains of causal risk
factors leading to disorders. This information can help to decide correctly for whom,
when, and how to intervene to prevent the onset of disorders or to facilitate recovery
(Kraemer, Stice, Kazdin, Offord, & Kupfer, 2001; Rauer, Karney, Garvan, & Hou,
2008). Thus the effects of any single risk factor on adjustment outcomes may depend
on the other risk factors that the individual faces. Individuals who are at risk on one
dimension tend to be at risk on multiple dimensions, and in order to understand the
impact of the risk we need to address the simultaneous interacting effects of multiple
risk factors at once. We need to explore their additive impact, treating the cumulative risk as an exacerbation model, wherein the negative association between an
individual risk factor and developmental outcomes is made worse by the simultaneous presence of other risks. In addition, we have to consider the possibility that risk
factors may interact with protective factors that may reduce their impact. Protective
variables do not act separately or in isolation as well, but they operate in interactive patterns in order to buffer individuals against the effects of risk factors and
stressful situations, thus predicting heterogeneous outcomes (Beasley, Thompson, &
Davidson, 2003). Research proposed several valid models of resilience – and
descriptions will be provided in order to exemplify the complexity of the interactions
and to demonstrate how these factors may operate to alter the trajectory from risk
exposure to negative outcome, disclosing the richness of relations between these factors when several play the role of mediators (intermediate variables) or moderators
(modifiers – increasing or decreasing its effect).

Protective models proposed that assets, personal strengths, and/or resources
moderate or reduce the effects of risk factors on a negative outcome. Luthar and
colleagues (2000), for example, defined a protective model, as factors that help to
neutralize or reduce the effects of risks. Thus, higher levels of risks are associated

with higher levels of negative outcomes when the protective factors are absent. However, there are no or lower relations between the risk and the outcomes when the protective factors are present. Youth whose parents do not provide them with adequate support or monitoring (risk factors), for example those without an adult mentor who is not a family member (a protective resource), may exhibit more delinquent behaviors (as outcomes), whereas those with a non-parental adult mentor may not.

The challenge model presented a different connection between risk factors and outcomes (Garmezy, Masten, & Tellegen, 1984), assuming that the association between them is not linear, but curvilinear. Instead of the belief that exposure to higher levels of a risk factor is associated with more negative outcomes, this model suggested that moderate levels of the risk may be paradoxically related to less negative or to more positive outcomes (Luthar & Zelazo, 2003). A vital point concerning the challenge model is that moderate levels of the risk exposure may be in fact beneficial to development, because they provide children and youth with a chance to practice their coping skills or to experiment employing available resources. In line with this challenge model, the risk exposure must be challenging enough to elicit a coping response, so the adolescent can learn from the process of overcoming the risk. In challenge models, the risk and protective factors are in fact the same variable – and the decision whether it is a risk or protective factor for an adolescent depends on the severity of the exposure.

For example, many parents would attempt to deny any family conflicts for the benefit of their children's development. They don't realize that conflicts are an unavoidable part of life's experiences. Too few family conflicts may not provide their children with opportunities and may not prepare youth to cope with or solve interpersonal conflicts outside the home. Yet, too many family conflicts may be debilitating and lead youth to feel hopeless and distressed, and considered a risk factor. A moderate amount of family conflict may provide youth with enough exposure to learn from the development and resolution of the conflict. They essentially learn through modeling or vicarious experience. The challenge model of resilience can be considered inoculation (Masten, 1999; Rutter, 1987), if a developmental (i.e., longitudinal) consideration will be included. This model suggests that continued or repeated exposure to moderate levels of a risk factor helps inoculate children and adolescents, so they are prepared to overcome more significant risks in the future. Children learn to mobilize assets and resources as they are exposed to adversity. As youth successfully overcome low levels of risk, they become more prepared to face increasing risk. As people age and mature and continue to be exposed to adversity, their capacity to thrive despite risks may increase or decrease, reflecting the complex relations between factors revealing individual differences (Fergus & Zimmerman, 2005).

In conclusion, the deficit perspective is generally based on the assumption that different types of relationships serve differentiated unique functions that are not interchangeable and each relationship type directly affects loneliness in a specific way. Loneliness is thus considered as an expression of social deficits. Empowering models do not deny deficiencies and difficulties; however, they propose to adopt a more comprehensive approach that recognizes not only the multiple factors but their dynamic and varied interactions and relations, and to examine feelings and behavior within a wider multidimensional and dynamic perspective. This approach that is detailed in the following chapters, exploring a wide range of personal, familial, and educational factors, can provide meaningful guidance to parents and educators in identifying the multiple ways in which children negotiate varied social risk factors and cope with many stressors, across domains, developmental stages, and contexts. The understanding of the interactions between personal and environmental variables will modify children's responses to adversity and may affect their adaptation through developmental paths, and may also propose supportive directions to mental health professionals. Within these empowering models, the salutogenic paradigm and the hope theory are presented as two examples for promoting in-depth theoretical understanding that have practical implications. The salutogenic paradigm is based on the developmental outcomes of past experiences and current activities, while the hope theory is aspiring to bridge the current way of life with the impact of future goals and expectations.

The Salutogenic Paradigm

Antonovsky (1987) coined the term "salutogenesis" from salus, the Latin word for health and wellbeing, to emphasize the focus of his model on health rather than on disease (i.e., pathogenesis) (Kirsten, 2008). The salutogenic model (Antonovsky, 1987) searched for answers to the question: "why some people, regardless of major stressful situations, risk factors and severe hardships, stay healthy and content, while others do not." His proposed explanations to account for the unexpected fact that some people stay relatively well, despite major risk factors and main challenges in their lives, initiated the development of the salutogenic model that explores the origin of health and wellbeing, rather than explaining the varied causes of disease. It should be noted especially that this conceptualization rejects the dichotomous classification of people as either healthy or diseased and proposes that everybody can find his location along the continuum between health and illness. Considering the dynamic approach to understanding wellbeing and the quality of life, the salutogenic paradigm focuses on the identification and examinations of factors that may contribute to a dynamic movement of individuals along the experiencing of the ease/dis-ease emotional and physical continuum. This approach has a special value for loneliness research, directing the conceptualization from the dichotomy (lonely or not lonely) to a continuum conceptualization that examined individuals' experiences between satisfying feelings of strong connectedness, closeness, or relatedness to the hurting experiences of isolation/alienation/loneliness distress, assuming that nobody is completely lonely or fully connected, but dynamically moving along this continuum. This line of thinking is especially valuable for exploring empowering and coping approaches – not striving to "repair" the loneliness but to help the individual to move along this continuum.

   The salutogenic approach has a central position in future public health and health promotion research and practice (Lindstrom & Eriksson, 2005). Tomorrow's society will most probably focus more effort on research that aims at strengthening health, namely the salutogenic (health causing) factors. The shaping of health-promoting settings at work, in hospitals, in schools, and in local communities, has therefore already been significantly supported by the World Health Organization (WHO) (Tellnes, 2009). Within this paradigm, the ability to identify and use internal (personal) and external (contextual) resources for effective coping with challenges such as loneliness was conceptualized as the Sense of Coherence construct (Antonovsky, 1987). The Sense of Coherence has been defined as a global orientation that expresses the extent to which individuals have confidence that their internal and external environments can be viewed and treated as structured and predictable; that resources are available to meet increased demands; and that these demands can be considered challenges worthy of energy investment and engagement. The Sense of Coherence consists of three interrelated components: comprehensibility, manageability, and meaningfulness:

   Comprehensibility refers to the extent to which individuals understand and perceive environmental information as ordered, consistent, and structured, rather than as unpredictable, disordered, and accidental. Individuals with a high sense of comprehensibility are able to understand what is happening to them and why.

   Manageability defines the extent to which individuals consider their available resources as appropriate to meet demands. The individual may control these resources, or they may be available from others, such as support and help provided by friends or professionals.

   Meaningfulness represents the affective-motivational aspect of personal coherence. Individuals view many events and activities in their life as challenging and as worthy of emotional investment and commitment. For example, a mother or a father with a high Sense of Coherence who want to help their child who is struggling in a developmental challenge such as loneliness will explore and examine the challenge until he or she will have appropriate understanding of the difficulty – what is loneliness, and its circumstances – where and why the child is lonely and when he/she is not (Comprehensibility); he or she will consider what they can do to help, or get advice and assistance (manageability) and how important it is for the parent and the child (meaningfulness).

   The Sense of Coherence scale was also known as the "Orientation to life" scale, and has been widely used (in 33 languages) in different cultures. It was related to overall health and adjustment measures, such as stress, depressive affect and anxiety (Flensborg-Madsen, Ventegodt, & Merrick, 2005). Risk factors such as negative emotionality (both anxiety and depression), anger-suppression coping style and cynical hostility were absent among people with high Sense of Coherence (Hart, Wilson, & Hittner, 2006). In another study that explored the self-perceptions during critical illness, patients with a strong Sense of Coherence were found more likely to take an active role in shaping their own health outcomes (Fok, Chair, & Lopez, 2005). A longitudinal study of personality and social development was started when the participants were 8- or 9-year-old children (in 1968). Data gathered again at ages

14, 27, 36, and 42 were used in this study (Feldt, Kokko, Kinnunen, & Pulkkinen, 2005). The results indicated that child-centered parenting in adolescence and a stable career line in adulthood were directly associated with a high Sense of Coherence at age 42. In addition, child-centered parenting, high parental socioeconomic status, and school success at age 14 were associated with Sense of Coherence during adults' age stage (Feldt, Metsäpelto, Kinnunen, & Pulkkinen, 2007). Individuals with high Sense of Coherence also had lower levels of Neuroticism. Thus, Sense of Coherence describes the individual's dispositional orientation to life which has been developed through maturation processes and life experiences.

Family background (child-centered parenting, parental socioeconomic status), school success during childhood and adolescence, and career orientation (education, stability of career line) in adulthood were related to adults' Sense of Coherence. From early childhood, generalized resistant resources (e.g., family and social support, ego strength, intelligence) shape everyday encounters in life to become positive experiences, which gradually build up a high Sense of Coherence, whereas lack of various generalized resistant resources are conducive to a low Sense of Coherence. Longitudinal studies revealed that overall Sense of Coherence was a relatively stable measure when followed over 40 years, but a lower stability value was found for individuals with low Sense of Coherence. In addition, when people faced a major threat to their wellbeing, such as severe illness or the diagnosis of a disabled child in the family; it may have affected stability, focusing attention on the accumulated impact of risk factors. Persons with a high Sense of Coherence were assumed to have a greater variety of generalized resistant resources at their disposal, and therefore they were able to cope better with challenges and negative experiences in life. In addition, Antonovsky suggested that when people with a high Sense of Coherence have viewed a stimulus as a stressor in the first stage of appraisal, they are likely to treat the stressor as a challenge in the second stage of appraisal. They were capable of assessing the nature of the problems they were facing and considered them challenges they were willing to face. They were open to feedback and corrective action (reappraisal). Consequently, high Sense of Coherence individuals coping with life stressors are likely to be more successful than those with lower Sense of Coherence, and therefore life may become even more meaningful, comprehensible, and manageable.

On the other hand, for persons with low Sense of Coherence, life may become a downward spiral, in which negative life events are more often encountered, risk factors are more often viewed as overpowering stressors, and when these stressors are combined with decreased generalized resistant resources, the person is less likely to initiate active coping, and therefore the stability of Sense of Coherence is still threatened even in adulthood. The examination of the protective factors during adolescence revealed and highlighted the value of home environment (Hakanen, Feldt, & Leskinen, 2007).

In a research survey, examining the relations between quality of life and Sense of Coherence, it was reported that Sense of Coherence had an impact on the quality of life; the stronger the Sense of Coherence, the better the quality of life that was reported (Eriksson & Lindstrom, 2007). Sense of Coherence is assumed to promote an individual's health through its central role in generating a more resilient choice of strategies for coping with life stressors. Thus, people with a high Sense of Coherence are assumed to occupy a more favorable position on the health ease/disease continuum than those scoring low in Sense of Coherence. These results are not surprising, since Sense of Coherence helps individuals to understand, manage and find meaning in their world. The salutogenic perspectives emphasizing Sense of Coherence within developmental research on loneliness will be presented in the next chapters, incorporating the protective role of Sense of Coherence in children through different developmental stages, the impact of their personal and interpersonal experiences, and their future expectations including the contributions of the hope theory (Snyder, 2002). A short summary of the hope theory will be presented to exemplify the importance of future perspectives in understanding the impact of past and present experiences.

Hope Theory

The concept of hope has been studied in different environments, such as schools, working places, mental health centers and hospitals, considering it as positive expectations for future goal attainment. Only in the last decade has it been explored more methodologically within the positive psychology trends. Although intuitively one would describe hope in terms of emotion, research used a cognitive approach to understanding and explaining the construct of hope (Parveen & James, 2007). Lynch's early definition of hope was "the fundamental knowledge and feeling that there is a way out of difficulty, that things can work out... that there are 'solutions'... hope is a sense of the possible" (Lynch, 1965, p. 32). Hopes extend the current reality, reflecting cognitive and emotional processes. Snyder focused attention on the cognitive processes and defined hope as "a cognitive set of beliefs based on a reciprocally derived sense of successful (a) agency thinking (goal-directed determination) and (b) pathways thinking (planning of ways to meet goals)" (Snyder, 2002). Snyder's model is based on the assumption that human actions are inherently goal directed. Agency thinking refers to a sense of efficacy (or "will") in working toward one's goals and can be considered the perceived capacity of individuals to initiate and sustain movement along a pathway until the goal is reached. It is the motivational component of hope and often it is manifested in positive self-statements such as "I can do this" (Snyder, 2000). A pathways thinking refers to the ability to develop plans (or "ways") in order to achieve desired goals. It involves not only the production of routes and strategies to a goal, but also the inner confidence in the ability to find these routes (Snyder, 2002).

High-hope people are more convinced in their ability to produce multiple routes to a goal compared to low-hope people. This ability is advantageous when a pathway becomes blocked because it enables the individual to continue pursuing the goal along alternative pathways. As a result, a greater repertoire of pathways thinking will contribute to a higher probability of accomplishing the desired goals.

The emotional aspects in this approach are expressed through the motivational optimistic beliefs, positive self-statements and acquiring personal energy to move efforts toward achieving the desired goals. Hope was related to wellbeing, life satisfaction and psychological adjustment across several life domains (Bailey, Eng, Frisch, & Snyder, 2007; Chang, 2003). It was employed in different environments such as work and schools. It was also related to students' grade expectancies and academic performance (Rand, 2009). A longitudinal study demonstrated the relations between hope components and later academic goal-attainment. It also provided evidence, consistent with the hope-theory assertion, that students adjust their hopes as they experience success or failure in pursuing goals. Thus, the dynamic developmental understanding of the hope construct was demonstrated (Feldman, Rand, & Kahle-Wrobleski, 2009). Another longitudinal study revealed that hope may be considered as a resiliency or protective factor with an effect of reducing the severity of depression symptoms and anxiety measured 1 month later. It is interesting, and perhaps encouraging, that severity of depression symptoms did not have any effect on future levels of hopefulness (Arnau, Rosen, Finch, Rhudy, & Fortunato, 2007).

The value of hope was demonstrated for different populations, different cultures, through different age groups including distressful and challenging realities, such as chronically sick people. In addition, its value to predict effective professional care-taking was also demonstrated (Chang & Banks, 2007; Feudtner et al., 2007; Tennen, Cloutier, Wakefield, Hall, & Brazil, 2009). For example, high-hopes' nurses that provided various aspects of palliative care were more competent in providing care and support to dying children and their families. Similarly, pediatric clinicians with higher hope were able to provide more effective care, to generate varied strategies and tactics to reach their goals when they encountered barriers, and they had the motivation to implement those strategies and tactics. They did not tend to ignore or diminish the severity of the obstacles they faced, but showed a continued persistence in their effort. Likewise, in our studies we found that teachers with high hopes were more ready to invest effort to help children with special needs in inclusive classes, such as children with learning disabilities, than teachers with lower hopes. They did not underestimate the difficulties, but considered them as worthy challenges. High-hopes' teachers recognized the importance of knowledge about disabilities and appropriate training and they expressed personal commitment and wishes to learn better didactic approaches to support effective teaching in heterogenic classes.

Hope theory also provides an in-depth understanding of feelings of regret. Regret has been described as a "comparison-based emotion of self-blame, experienced when people realize or imagine that their present situation would have been better had they decided differently in the past" (Beike, Markman, & Karadogan, 2009). Most people regret their decisions when they wish that they had done something differently in their lives. They may regret actions, but sometimes they may regret inactions (when they did not perform an important action). Individuals experience regrets when they make mistakes as well as when they miss opportunities to act. The experience of regret may lead to ruminations about other paths that could have been taken. Although such ruminations can be painful, they keep incomplete goals in mind so as to maximize the likelihood of acting on future opportunities to fulfill goals. Thus, experiencing regret and its associated ruminations can motivate people to act upon opportunities to remedy the regretted outcome (Beike, Markman, & Karadogan, 2009). Potentially, repeatable outcomes may elicit less regret than non-repeatable outcomes because they offer greater hope. Thus, hope inducing may promote the abilities of individuals to visualize alternative paths, to attempt achieving desired goals and reduce regrets.

In conclusion, the hope construct is related to important indices of behavior, psychological functioning and wellbeing in adults and in children. It may buffer the destructive impact of loneliness and may provide practical guidance to prevention and intervention planning. The developmental conceptualization of hope and its interrelations with childhood loneliness is detailed in Chapter 2.

Conclusions and Implications

The goals of this chapter were to provide an overview of loneliness research as a basis for the developmental discussions that will be presented in the following chapters. In the first stage it was clarified that loneliness is a subjective complex set of painful experiences and feelings, reflecting a gap between existed and expected social relations and connections, and unfulfilled social needs. The paradox between limitless connectivity due to Internet and cell communication, the blurring boundaries between private and public environments, and the distress of social isolation and alienation were pointed out, requesting a more in-depth clarification of these processes. The complexity of the loneliness construct as a multivariable construct was considered by scholars that proposed different interrelated subtypes with different origins and characteristics. The emotional loneliness captured the distress related to the lack of close satisfying interpersonal relations, while social loneliness focused interest on the frustrations emerging from unsatisfactory network connectedness and belonging. The focus of the third type – the existential loneliness – was the personal painful feelings of isolation and worthless, while the fourth type – the representational loneliness – was unique in providing a focus on the conflictual awareness to personal alienation and distance from others whose connectedness enhanced the personal feelings of separation and remoteness.

Loneliness is different from solitude, and staying alone can be enjoyable and a source of satisfaction. Yet, it is connected to loneliness, since people who have difficulties in staying alone may experience increased loneliness. For most adults and children, loneliness is just a temporary unpleasant condition, but special attention has to be offered to those who experience chronic loneliness, and seriously consider it as a threat to their adjustment and wellbeing. Special awareness is needed to children's loneliness that may risk their developmental path. Since loneliness reflects personal characteristics that interact with different contextual conditions, there is a need for comprehensive loneliness models in order to examine the interactions between risk factors and protective factors in predicting resiliency. In this chapter we presented the salutogenic paradigm and the hope theory that will be further discussed in the following chapter within the developmental framework. In the beginning of the chapter we started with loneliness definitions and clarifications and ended with the hope conceptualization, since the value of hope and its applicability for buffering childhood loneliness will be supported by the thorough understanding of development and outcomes.

References

Ackerman, B. P., Izard, C. E., Schoff, K. M., Youngstrom, E. A., & Kogos, J. L. (1999). Contextual risk, caregiver emotionality, and the problem behaviors of 6- and 7-year-old children from economically disadvantaged families. *Child Development, 70*(6), 1415–1427.

Antonovsky, A. (1987). *Unraveling the mystery of health*. San Francisco: Jossey-Bass.

Appleyard, K., Egeland, B., Van Dulmen, M. H. M., & Sroufe, L. A. (2005). When more is not better: The role of cumulative risk in child behavior outcomes. *Journal of Child Psychology and Psychiatry, 46*(3), 235–245.

Arnau, R. C., Rosen, D. H., Finch, J. F., Rhudy, J. L., & Fortunato, V. J. (2007). Longitudinal effects of hope on depression and anxiety: A latent variable analysis. *Journal of Personality, 75*(1), 43–64.

Asher, S. R., & Paquette, J. A. (2003). Loneliness and peer relations in childhood. *Current Directions in Psychological Sciences, 12*(3), 75–78.

Asher, S. R., Parkhurst, J. T., Hymel, S., & Williams, G. A. (1990). Peer rejection and loneliness in childhood. In S. R. Asher & J. D. Coie (Eds.), *Peer rejection in childhood* (pp. 253–273). Cambridge: University Press.

Bailey, T. C., Eng, W., Frisch, M. B., & Snyder, C. R. (2007). Hope and optimism as related to life satisfaction. *The Journal of Positive Psychology, 2*(3), 168–175.

Beasley, M., Thompson, T., & Davidson, J. (2003). Resilience in response to life stress: The effects of coping style and cognitive hardiness. *Personality and Individual Differences, 34*(1), 77–95.

Beike, D. R., Markman, K. D., & Karadogan, F. (2009). What we regret most are lost opportunities: A theory of regret intensity. *Personality and Social Psychology Bulletin, 35*(3), 385–397.

Belsky, J., & Pluess, M. (2009). The nature (and nurture?) of plasticity in early human development. *Perspectives on Psychological Science, 4*(4), 345–351.

Bering, J. M. (2008). Why hell is other people: Distinctively human psychological suffering. *Review of General Psychology, 12*(1), 1–8.

Bottrell, D. (2009). Dealing with disadvantage: Resilience and the social capital of young people's networks. *Youth Society, 40*(4), 476–501.

Cacioppo, J. T., Hawkley, L. C., & Berntson, G. G. (2003). The anatomy of loneliness. *Current Direction in Psychological Science, 12*(3), 71–74.

Cacioppo, J. T., Hawkley, L. C., Ernst, J. M., Burleson, M., Berntson, G. G., Nouriani, B., et al. (2006). Loneliness within a nomological net: An evolutionary perspective. *Journal of Research in Personality, 40*(6), 1054–1085.

Cacioppo, J. T., Hughes, M. E., Waite, L. J., Hawkley, L. C., & Thisted, R. A. (2006). Loneliness as a specific risk factor for depressive symptoms: Cross-sectional and longitudinal analyses. *Psychology & Aging, 21*(1), 140–151.

Cacioppo, J. T., & Patrick, W. (2008). *Loneliness: Human nature and the need for social connection*. New York: W. W. Norton.

Cassidy, J., & Asher, S. R. (1992). Loneliness and peer relations in young children. *Child Development, 63*(2), 350.

Chang, E. C. (2003). A critical appraisal and extension of hope theory in middle-ages men and women: Is it important to distinguish agency and pathways components. *Journal of Social and Clinical Psychology, 22*(2), 121–143.

Chang, E. C., & Banks, K. H. (2007). The color and texture of hope: Some preliminary findings and implications for hope theory and counseling among diverse racial/ethnic groups. *Cultural Diversity & Ethnic Minority Psychology, 13*(2), 94–103.

Chen, X., & French, D. C. (2008). Children's social competence in cultural context. *Annual Review of Psychology, 59*, 591–616.

Chua, S. N., & Koestner, R. (2008). A Self-Determination Theory perspective on the role of autonomy in solitary behavior. *Journal of Social Psychology, 148*(5), 645–648.

Cicchetti, D., & Rogosch, F. A. (2009). Adaptive coping under conditions of extreme stress: Multilevel influences on the determinants of resilience in maltreated children. *New Directions for Child and Adolescent Development, 124*, 47–59.

Cicchetti, D., & Toth, S. L. (2009). The past achievements and future promises of developmental psychopathology: The coming of age of a discipline. *Journal of Child Psychology and Psychiatry, 50*(1–2), 16–25.

Csikszentmihalyi, M. (1996). *Creativity: Flow and the psychology of discovery and invention*. New York: Harper-Collins.

Davidson, R. J., Pizzagalli, D., Nitschke, J. B., & Putnam, K. (2002). Depression: Perspectives from affective neuroscience. *Annual Review of Psychology, 53*(1), 545–574.

Dykstra, P. A., & Fokkema, T. (2007). Social and emotional loneliness among divorced and married men and women: Comparing the deficit and cognitive perspectives. *Basic and Applied Social Psychology, 29*(1), 1–12.

Eriksson, M., & Lindstrom, B. (2007). Antonovsky's sense of coherence scale and its relation with quality of life: A systematic review. *Journal of Epidemiol Community Health, 61*(11), 938–944.

Feldman, D. B., Rand, K. L., & Kahle-Wrobleski, K. (2009). Hope and goal attainment: Testing a basic prediction of hope theory. *Journal of Social & Clinical Psychology, 28*(4), 479–497.

Feldt, T., Kokko, K., Kinnunen, U., & Pulkkinen, L. (2005). The role of family background, school success, and career orientation in the development of Sense of Coherence. *European Psychologist, 10*(4), 298–308.

Feldt, T., Metsäpelto, R., Kinnunen, U., & Pulkkinen, L. (2007). Sense of coherence and five-factor approach to personality: Conceptual relationships. *European Psychologist, 12*(3), 165–172.

Fergus, S., & Zimmerman, M. A. (2005). Adolescent resilience: A framework for understanding healthy development in the face of risk. *Annual Review of Public Health, 26*, 399–419.

Feudtner, C., Santucci, G., Feinstein, J. A., Snyder, C. R., Rourke, M. T., & Kang, T. I. (2007). Hopeful thinking and level of comfort regarding providing pediatric palliative care: A survey of hospital nurses. *Pediatrics, 119*(1), e186–e192.

Flensborg-Madsen, T., Ventegodt, S., & Merrick, J. (2005). Sense of coherence and physical health. A review of previous findings. *The Scientific World Journal, 5*, 665–673.

Fok, S. K., Chair, S. Y., & Lopez, V. (2005). Sense of coherence, coping and quality of life following a critical illness. *Journal of Advanced Nursing, 49*(2), 173–181.

Galanaki, E. P. (2004). Are children able to distinguish among the concepts of aloneness, loneliness, and solitude? *International Journal of Behavioral Development, 28*(5), 435–443.

Galanaki, E. P. (2005). Solitude in the school: A neglected facet of children's development and education. *Childhood Education, 81*(3), 128–133.

Garmezy, N., Masten, A., & Tellegen, A. (1984). The study of stress and competence in children: A building block for developmental psychopathology. *Child Development, 55*(1), 97–111.

Gierveld, J. D. J., & Tilburg, T. V. (2006). A 6-Item scale for overall, emotional, and social loneliness: Confirmatory tests on survey data. *Research on Aging, 28*(5), 582–598.

Haagaa, D. A. F., Dyckb, M. J., & Ernstc, D. (1991). Empirical status of cognitive theory of depression. *Psychological Bulletin, 110*(2), 215–236.

Hakanen, J. J., Feldt, T., & Leskinen, E. (2007). Change and stability of sense of coherence in adulthood: Longitudinal evidence from the healthy child study. *Journal of Research in Personality, 41*(3), 602–617.

Hankin, B. L. (2008). Cognitive vulnerability–stress model of depression during adolescence: Investigating depressive symptom specificity in a multi-wave prospective study. *Journal of Abnormal Child Psychology, 36*(7), 999–1014.

Hart, K. E., Wilson, T. L., & Hittner, J. B. (2006). A psychosocial resilience model to account for medical well-being in relation to Sense of Coherence. *Journal of Health Psychology, 11*(6), 857–862.

Hojat, M. (1982). Loneliness as a function of parent–child and peer relations. *Journal of Psychology, 112*(1), 129–133.

Humphrey, N. (2007). The society of selves. *Philosophical Transactions of the Royal Society B: Biological Sciences, 362*(1480), 745–754.

Izard, C., & Ackerman, B. (2000). Motivational, organizational, and regulatory functions of discrete emotions. In M. Lewis & J. M. Haviland-Jones (Eds.), *Handbook of emotions* (2nd ed., pp. 253–264). New York: Guilford.

Junttila, N., & Vauras, M. (2009). Loneliness among school-aged children and their parents. *Scandinavian Journal of Psychology, 50*(3), 211–219.

Killeen, C. (1998). Loneliness: An epidemic in modern society. *Journal of Advanced Nursing, 28*(4), 762–770.

Kirsten, W. (2008). Health and productivity management in Europe. *International Journal of Workplace Health Management, 1*(2), 136–144.

Kraemer, H. C., Stice, E., Kazdin, A., Offord, D., & Kupfer, D. (2001). How do risk factors work together? Mediators, moderators, and independent, overlapping, and proxy risk factors. *American Journal of Psychiatry, 158*, 848–856.

Larson, R., Csikszentmihalyi, M., & Graef, R. (1982). Time alone in daily experience: Loneliness or renewal? In L. A. Peplau & D. Perlman (Eds.), *Loneliness: A sourcebook of current theory, research, and therapy* (pp. 40–53). New York: Wiley.

Larson, R. W. (1997). The emergence of solitude as a constructive domain of experience in early adolescence. *Child Development, 68*(1), 80–94.

Lavallee, K., & Parker, J. (2009). The role of inflexible friendship beliefs, rumination, and low self-worth in early adolescents' friendship jealousy and adjustment. *Journal of Abnormal Child Psychology, 37*(6), 873–885.

Leary, M. R., Herbst, K. C., & McCrary, F. (2003). Finding pleasure in solitary activities: Desire for aloneness or disinterest in social contact? *Personality and Individual Differences, 35*(1), 59–68.

Lindstrom, B., & Eriksson, M. (2005). Salutogenesis. *Journal of Epidemiology and Community Health, 59*(6), 440–442.

Loewenstein, G. F., Weber, E. U., Hsee, C. K., & Welch, N. (2001). Risk as feelings. *Psychological Bulletin, 127*(2), 267–286.

Long, C. R., & Averill, J. R. (2003). Solitude: An exploration of benefits of being alone. *Journal for the Theory of Social Behaviour, 33*(1), 21–44.

Luthar, S. S., Cicchetti, D., & Becker, B. (2000). The construct of resilience: A critical evaluation and guidelines for future work. *Child Development, 71*(3), 543–562.

Luthar, S. S., & Zelazo, L. B. (2003). Research on resilience: An integrative review. In S. S. Luthar (Ed.), *Resilience and vulnerability: Adaptation in the context of childhood adversities* (pp. 510–550). New York: Cambridge University Press.

Lynch, W. F. (1965). *Images of hope: Imagination as healer of the hopeless*. Baltimore: Helicon Press.

Marcoen, A., & Goossens, L. (1990, April). *Loneliness and aloneness in adolescence: Introducing a multidimensional measure and some developmental perspectives*. Paper presented at the Annual American Educational Research Association, Boston, MA.

Margalit, M. (2004). Second-generation research on resilience: Social-emotional aspects of children with Learning Disabilities. *Learning Disabilities Research & Practice, 19*(1), 45–48.

Masten, A. S. (1999). Resilience comes of age: Reflections on the past and outlook for the next generation. In M. D. Glantz & J. L. Johnson (Eds.), *Resilience and development: Positive life adaptations* (pp. 281–296). New York: Kluwer.

Masten, A. S., Herbers, J. E., Cutuli, J. J., & Lafavor, T. L. (2008). Promoting competence and resilience in the school context. *Professional School Counseling, 12*(2), 76–84.

Mayers, A. M., Khoo, S. T., & Svartberg, M. (2002). The existential loneliness questionnaire: Background, development and primary findings. *Journal of Clinical Psychology, 58*(9), 1183–1193.

Mikulincer, M., & Florian, V. (1998). The relationship between adult attachment styles and emotional and cognitive reactions to stressful events. In J. A. Simpson & W. S. Rholes (Eds.), *Attachment theory and close relationships* (pp. 143–165). New York: Guilford.

Moody, E. J. (2001). Internet use and its relationship to loneliness. *Cyber Psychology & Behavior, 4*(3), 393–401.

Moustakis, C. E. (1961). *Loneliness*. Englewood Cliffs, NJ: Prentice-Hall.

Nilsson, B., Lindstrom, U. A., & Naden, D. (2006). Is loneliness a psychological dysfunction? A literary study of the phenomenon of loneliness. *Scandinavian Journal of Caring Sciences, 20*(1), 93–101.

Page, R. M. (1991). Loneliness as a risk factor in adolescent hopelessness. *Journal of Research in Personality, 25*(2), 189–195.

Parveen, K. G., & James, E. P. (2007). Hope theory: A framework for understanding suicidal action. *Death Studies, 31*(2), 131–154.

Patrick, H., Knee, C. R., Canevello, A., & Lonsbary, C. (2007). The role of need fulfillment in relationship functioning and well-being: A self-determination theory perspective. *Journal of Personality and Social Psychology, 92*(3), 434–457.

Peplau, L. A., & Perlman, D. (1982). Perspectives on loneliness. In L. A. Peplau & D. Perlman (Eds.), *Loneliness: A sourcebook of current theory, research and therapy* (pp. 1–18). New York: Wiley.

Rand, K. L. (2009). Hope and optimism: Latent structures and influences on grade expectancy and academic performance. *Journal of Personality, 77*(1), 231–260.

Rauer, A. J., Karney, B. R., Garvan, C. W., & Hou, W. (2008). Relationship risks in context: A cumulative risk approach to understanding relationship satisfaction. *Journal of Marriage and Family, 70*(5), 1122–1135.

Rokach, A. (2008). Coping with loneliness in North America and Spain. *Psychology Journal, 5*(1), 51–70.

Russell, D., Cutrona, C. E., Rose, J., & Yurko, K. (1984). Social and emotional loneliness: An examination of Weiss' typology of loneliness. *Journal of Personality and Social Psychology, 46*(6), 1313–1321.

Rutter, M. (1979). Protective factors in children's responses to stress and disadvantage. In M. W. Kent & J. E. Rolf (Eds.), *Primary prevention in psychopathology: Vol. 8. Social competence in children* (pp. 49–74). Hanover, NH: University Press of New England.

Rutter, M. (1987). Psychosocial resilience and protective mechanisms. *American Journal of Orthopsychiatry, 57*(3), 316–331.

Rutter, M. (1999). Resilience concept and findings: Implementation for family therapy. *Journal of Family Therapy, 21*(2), 119–144.

Seepersad, S., Choi, M. K., & Shin, N. (2008). How does culture influence the degree of romantic loneliness and closeness? *Journal of Psychology, 142*(2), 209–220.

Snyder, C. R. (2000). *Handbook of hope: Theory, measures, and applications*. San Diego, CA: Academic Press.

Snyder, C. R. (2002). Hope theory: Rainbows in the mind. *Psychological Inquiry, 13*(4), 249–275.

Storr, A. (1988). *Solitude*. New York: Ballantine.

Swami, V., Chamorro-Premuzic, T., Sinniah, D., Maniam, T., Kannan, K., Stanistreet, D., et al. (2007). General health mediates the relationship between loneliness, life satisfaction and depression. *Social Psychiatry and Psychiatric Epidemiology, 42*(2), 161–166.

Tellnes, G. (2009). How can nature and culture promote health? *Scandinavian Journal of Public Health, 37*(6), 559–561.

Tennen, H., Cloutier, M. M., Wakefield, D. B., Hall, C. B., & Brazil, K. (2009). The buffering effect of hope on clinicians' behavior: A test in pediatric primary care. *Journal of Social & Clinical Psychology, 28*(5), 554–576.

Trentacosta, C. J., Hyde, L. W., Shaw, D. S., Dishion, T. J., Gardner, F., & Wilson, M. (2008). The relations among cumulative risk, parenting, and behavior problems during early childhood. *Journal of Child Psychology and Psychiatry, 49*(11), 1211–1219.

Weiss, R. S. (1973). *Loneliness: The experience of emotional and social isolation.* Cambridge, MA: MIT Press.

Werner, E. E., & Smith, R. S. (1982). *Vulnerable but invincible: A longitudinal study of resilient children and youth.* New York: McGraw-Hill.

Woodward, H. (1988). *The solitude of loneliness.* Lexington, MA: Lexington Books.

Zahn-Waxler, C., Shirtcliff, E. A., & Marceau, K. (2008). Disorders of childhood and adolescence: Gender and psychopathology. *Annual Review of Clinical Psychology, 4*, 275–303.

Chapter 2
Abilities, Difficulties, and Developmental Perspectives

Loneliness is a normative experience among children and adults as a part of their day-to-day occurrences. However, there is an urgent need for focused awareness, concerns, and interventions to help those children and adolescents who are often, and chronically, lonely and to reduce the risks for their becoming lonely adults. The goals of this chapter are not only to clarify personal characteristics that may predispose children to loneliness, but also to identify their distinctive assets that may empower them in challenging times, or even prevent their social pains. Loneliness reflects the mismatch between children's social needs and interpersonal desires, and their perceived social environments. Loneliness, rather than peer rejection per se, appears to coincide with emotional distress – as reported by Qualter and Munn's study (2002), which differentiated between three groups of children: children, who were rejected by their peers, yet did not feel lonely; children who felt lonely but were not rejected by their group; and rejected children who also reported experiencing loneliness. This differentiation focused attention on the need for an in-depth understanding of differentiated risk factors that predict social agonies.

Loneliness is not an uncommon experience for many children, and about 10–15% of children reported this distress (Iverson & Eichler, 1992). Luftig (1988) found that 22% of second graders, 20% of fourth graders, and 12% of sixth graders indicated strong agreement with statements such as "I feel alone," "I'm lonely," and "I don't have anyone to play with." The decreased proportions don't necessarily indicate that fewer children experience loneliness, but the fact that many adolescents are reluctant to admit this distress. In a lecture to adolescents, I asked the kids who were often lonely and very few raised their hands. Afterward I said that I knew that many children felt uneasy to share this distress, but I would be grateful if lonely children would hand me a short anonymous message at the end of my talk writing if they were often lonely. I received many notes. The roots of loneliness are varied and its appreciation requests a comprehensive understanding. Although primary factors may predispose children to the loneliness experience, secondary self-related variables are also important, and may maintain, mediate, reinforce, or reduce its impacts. The study of these factors will clarify the extent to which the children are at risk of experiencing relations' difficulties and need to cope with negative feelings of being alienated and different from others in their immediate social

M. Margalit, *Lonely Children and Adolescents*, DOI 10.1007/978-1-4419-6284-3_2,
© Springer Science+Business Media, LLC 2010

environment. They may struggle unsuccessfully to bridge social or interpersonal spaces with accompanying emotional distress.

In order to extend the understanding of lonely children and to illustrate the diverse and interacting characteristics of children who are at risk for experiencing chronic alienation, their abilities and difficulties will be explored. However, unlike most studies on children's loneliness, the focus of this chapter is not at children's difficulties. Comprehensive profiles of their personality are presented, including their abilities and vulnerabilities within the risk and protective paradigm, considering the developmental paths of loneliness, genetic roots, and challenging the outcomes. Most studies focused attention on the children's interpersonal and social networks (as is detailed in Chapter 5), neglecting the study of their personal attributes. This neglect is surprising since research on adults' loneliness focused attention mostly on their personal characteristics. In this chapter children's development of their self-conceptualization will be clarified in line with the dynamic models of changes.

Models of Changes and Development

Lonely children are not lonely all the time. Every child is lonely from time to time, but lonely children are at a higher risk of experiencing loneliness more often and for longer periods than the non-lonely ones. Thus, mental-health professionals attempted to identify the roots of risks for loneliness and processes that promote feelings of social isolation.

One of the most fundamental challenges in children's study is to identify the mechanisms that create developmental changes: day-to-day changes as well as continuous periodical and long-term changes. Researchers often suggested conceptualizing developmental changes through adopting the linear stage model. The key assumption in this stage approach hypothesizes that development proceeds along stepwise, with individuals moving from lower levels to higher ones, leaving earlier steps or stages behind while adopting the new ones. The new stage will appear only after the successful termination of the earlier stage. In addition, the stage model assumes that earlier stages are a necessary condition for reaching more advanced stages. Accordingly, a retreat to an earlier stage has been considered an expression of regression and sometimes even a sign of pathology. Parents often expressed their worries and frustrations when their children, who reached relative independent and friendly social relations with peers, returned to play alone and expressed a reluctance to initiate friendship connections. They searched for causes of this "regression," not realizing that it may, in fact, express the natural day-to-day variations, or a retreat needed during maturation processes to enable a further developmental progress.

A nonlinear dynamic systems theory has proposed a different approach, revealing important principles of pattern formation and changes. Changes are often not gradual and linear, but rather may be characterized by a sudden intrusion and increased variability in the systemic behavior before reorganization is stabilized. During this period of fluctuation, the system is open to new information and to the exploration of potentially more adaptive and mature associations and configurations (Hayes, Laurenceau, Feldman, Strauss, & Cardaciotto, 2007). The proposed dynamic view considered the system as a set of elements that interact and continually evolve over time. Observations of the day-to-day changes in children's emotional experiences and social behavior supported this alternative nonlinear approach. Siegler proposed the wave model (Siegler, 1996, 1997) that considered the conceptualization of developmental changes as dynamic and nonlinear.

The wave model proposed that development moves as successive, overlapping waves, each cresting at a somewhat different time of development. In addition, several modes of thoughts and emotions may appear together within the same time frame, showing that a child's behavior may change from a more mature social behavior to childish expressions, and back. The child's behavior can be friendly and socially interacting on 1 day, but on the next day he or she may be socially shy and isolated, expressing profound distress. By rejecting a linear deterministic stage-related conceptualization, the wave approach to development provides a multidimensional understanding of children's connectedness and loneliness, accepting day-to-day changes, and at the same time also recognizing the more generalized comprehensive tendencies. Thus, retreats from close relations may be accordingly considered as expressions of varied affective fluctuations along a continuation between the urge to be connected and the wishes or needs for solitude periods, and not necessarily as signs of developmental regression or pathology. This clarification of nonlinear developmental processes provides a dynamic approach that can help in understanding the interactions among risks, personal strengths, and contextual conditions. These processes will be further clarified not only for enhancing in-depth consideration for a variety of coping strategies with loneliness trends, but especially for planning effective intervention approaches and directing parental guidance and consideration of their children's individual differences.

In this chapter, in order to answer the question how children understand and conceptualize their loneliness, the results of several studies are provided. The primary genetic and personal characteristics that may predispose children to loneliness development are described, including gender differences, followed by the identification of protective factors.

Young Children Experience and Understand Loneliness

Major scientific debates were raised in the past, if young children could experience loneliness. A pre-requisite to this dilemma was that they could understand the concept. When we asked young children if sometime ago they were lonely, they described their loneliness providing detailed situations when they had been left alone and nobody had cared for them. When we shared these results with parents, appreciating the children's insight, they were not surprised and supported our impressions with their stories. Research has showed that children have fundamental needs for inclusion in their group (i.e., playgroups, neighborhood playgrounds), striving to achieve close relationships and feelings of relatedness (Baumeister &

Leary, 1995). Children described different group activities (play, party, sport, and study or sport groups), when they were not invited or welcomed. Often they described their accompanying negative mood and withdrawn behavior. Researchers that explored the phenomenon of children's loneliness (e.g., Coplan, Findlay, & Nelson, 2004; Youngblade, Berlin, & Beslky, 1999) also reported that children understood the meaning of loneliness even before entering school. Their explanations at the preschool level may be partial and incomplete. However, interviews of 5-year-old children clarified that they generally understand the meaning of this social distress.

Indeed children develop friendship relations at early developmental stages. They reported social dissatisfaction when peers rejected them in playgroups. Research indicates clearly that young children have at least a basic understanding of the concept (Asher & Paquette, 2003). During interviews, they explained that loneliness involved "having no one to play with." They described loneliness as "feeling sad and staying alone." This explanation corresponds fairly well to typical definitions of loneliness in the literature. Their awareness and distress expressions related to social isolation appeared at quite an early age. Their cognitive abilities to share and communicate social distress in a coherent way and to explain what loneliness was, was documented for preschoolers (5–6 years old) in different countries including USA, Israel, Greece, and Canada, showing consistently that young children had experienced loneliness before entering school, and they were able to identify situations in which they had felt lonely. Some children (especially girls) were able to differentiate between loneliness and solitude (between voluntary and involuntary aloneness) (Galanaki, 2004; Kirova, 2003; Margalit, 1998).

Young children were aware not only of their own distress, but also of others' social isolation. They made surprisingly sophisticated distinctions between children's shyness and unsociability in their playgroups, demonstrating differences in terms of attributions of behavioral intent, liking, and sympathetic responses. They were able to differentiate between two groups of solitude behavior: the first group consisted of shy and anxious children who play alone and the second group consisted of withdrawn unsociable children, indicating that the second group was less interested in playing with other children and developing friendship relations (Coplan, Girardi, Findlay, & Frohlick, 2007). In terms of social preferences, young children clearly liked the socially competent children more than the unsociable ones and especially they disliked the aggressive lonely peers. In addition, children differentiated between the two groups of withdrawn children, and between these groups they expressed a greater liking and desire to play with the shy children compared to the unsociable peers. Interviews of children about the conceptualization of aloneness revealed their understanding. They were able to respond negatively to the question "Does someone who is alone necessarily feel lonely?" (Hymel, Tarulli, Hayden Thomson, & Terrell-Deutsch, 1999), distinguishing between solitude and loneliness.

Loneliness is not an uncommon experience at the preschool-age stage. Over 10% of children in preschool samples expressed substantial loneliness and dissatisfaction with their social relationships, a proportion similar to that which has been reported among elementary school-age children (Coplan, Closson, & Arbeau, 2007). The young children's descriptions of their loneliness were found relatively stable, revealing their interpersonal style. Children's descriptions detailed that it was often associated with peer exclusion, poorer friendship quality, and school avoidance (Burgess, Ladd, Kochenderfer, Lambert, & Birch, 1999). Parents are often annoyed when their children refuse to go to school, providing several minor health problems (i.e., tummy ache or sore throat) as excuses for preferring to stay at home. However, when parents persist asking and suggesting, the children share their social agony.

A strong relation was found between loneliness and the attitudes toward the preschool. Children, who felt lonely, did not like school, and adults reported their greater school avoidance even at this young age (a problem that many working parents have to struggle with during many mornings and are not aware of the children's message of social distress). It seems that satisfying social relationships and positive self-perceptions are critical components of school adjustment already at this stage of early childhood. Studies emphasized the need for parents' awareness of children's attempts to avoid school in early childhood, since not only may it reflect concurrent distress, but it would predict continued social, emotional, and academic difficulties in later childhood as well (Coplan, Closson et al., 2007). Children, who experienced higher levels of loneliness, often reported lower perceived peer acceptance and overall decreased self-competence.

Loneliness was also related, in research, to additional developmental difficulties, such as anxiety, shyness, aggression, cognitive difficulties, and may reflect a risk for developmental difficulties such as learning disabilities (Margalit, 1998; Vaughn, Zaragoza, Hogan, & Walker, 1993). The comparisons between groups of preschool children revealed that children who were at risk for developing learning disabilities (when compared to children with typical development), expressed higher levels of loneliness, lower self-perceptions, and had fewer friends even before their cognitive difficulties were formally diagnosed. The awareness of social distress expressed by children with special educational needs has a special importance, since most educational effort and programs are directed at remediation of their cognitive and academic difficulties and the social domain has been often neglected. Repeated examination of the children's loneliness (at the beginning, middle, and the end of the school year) revealed the consistency of the social distress. However, when teachers were trained to target children's loneliness within a comprehensive intervention planning (see Chapter 8), a significant change was noted.

Solitude and Loneliness: Developmental Aspects

Many parents observe worriedly the preference of their children to play alone. However, solitary play by itself is not a sign of developmental problems. A more important question that parents have to explore is related to children's activities when they stay alone. This inquiry is critical for understanding the children's wellbeing and for identifying future risk for social difficulties and loneliness. Rubin and Mills (1988) differentiated between two types of behavioral solitude: passive isolation and active isolation.

Passive isolation has usually been involved with a quite constructive or exploratory behavior. During preschool, this behavior may reflect an interest in mastering nonsocial tasks through exploration and constructive play. Only during elementary-school years, when children spend most of their time in constructive activities (i.e., schoolwork), the child who continues to play alone may be reflecting social anxiety, peer rejection, and an increased risk for developing internalizing disorders, such as anxiety, loneliness, and depression.

The second form of social withdrawal – active isolation – is characterized by cognitively immature behavior and may predict the development of loneliness. Uncommunicative and reticent behavior (i.e., on-looking, staying unoccupied and bored) was related to loneliness especially for boys and less for girls (Coplan et al., 2004). This gender differentiation was found to be consistent across the lifespan and shyness-withdrawal trends in children predicted socio-emotional difficulties, more for boys and less for girls. Socially withdrawn boys described themselves as more lonely, as having poorer social skills, and as having lower self-esteem than their typical peers (Rubin, Coplan, & Bowker, 2009).

Shyness was often related in research to loneliness and social anxiety (Findlay, Coplan, & Bowker, 2009). Shyness is conceptualized as social anxiety accompanied by behavioral responses such as inhibition and withdrawal in response to social and novel situations. Shy children have been considered at risk for a wide range of socio-emotional difficulties including low self-worth, loneliness, and difficulties with peers. However, withdrawn and shy boys were at a greater risk than shy girls. It seems that the roots of the relations between gender identity formation and loneliness in young adults (Blazina, Eddins, Burridge, & Settle, 2007) were established in those early developmental stages of young boys.

It can be concluded that many preschool children understand that loneliness involves a combination of staying alone and a distressed feeling. A lot of children were able to distinguish between solitude and loneliness. Loneliness at this age was related to difficulties with peers (revealing shyness or withdrawn behavior), negative attitudes toward the school, and lower self-perceptions.

As the children grew up – during elementary school – they were able to share and provide more complex and elaborated conceptualizations of loneliness. Children in grades 3–8 were interviewed about their understanding of the meaning of loneliness and were asked (Hymel et al., 1999) open-ended questions such as "What does loneliness mean?" "What kinds of things make a person feel lonely?" "What kinds of things have made you feel lonely?" and "Tell me about a time when you felt lonely." Children's responses suggested that they understood what loneliness was. They perceived and experienced loneliness in terms of three distinct features:

(a) An affective dimension,
(b) A cognitive dimension, and
(c) A set of interpersonal situations or contexts.

Children shared a wide range of distressful experiences, revealing diversity and individual differences. They used emotional terms (e.g., sadness, unhappiness, sorrow, and boredom), and the cognitive component was reflected through their appraisal of relationships (e.g., "I have no friends").

In another study, children from kindergarten to sixth grade in a school in western Canada were interviewed (Kirova, 2003). Using a game format, children's conceptualizations were provided and related to three dimensions – spaces, affect, and cognitions. Children referred to space by describing the distance between them and others due to loneliness. Children portrayed the importance of being loved, the meaning of being not only with others but for others. They realized their need to be of worth to several specific others. They were able to describe painful experiences when they felt separated, excluded, or cut off from the shared world of others. The desire to belong to others' shared world – the world outside the children on the one hand, and the impossibility of reaching this desire on the other hand – created a vacuum not only between children and others, but most of all within the children's selves. This vacuum was described by them as loneliness and inner emptiness. In general, children viewed loneliness as a powerful, overwhelming experience that may expand their awareness and sensitivity toward the world, toward others, and especially toward themselves. They experienced loneliness as pain from not being able to share themselves – their thoughts, truths, feelings, and desires – with those whom they love. Thus, they longed for closeness and communion. In addition, their sense of time was also connected to loneliness. While feeling lonely, they experienced time as being stretched out and very long.

The study of solitude at different age groups furthers the developmental understanding of the complexity of the loneliness construct. Winnicott (1965) proposed that the roots of loneliness and solitude could be found in the interrelations between infants and their parents. In order to develop the capacity to stay alone during adolescence, the infant already had to acquire the ability to stay alone in the presence of a caregiver. Individual differences in the preference for, and capacity to benefit from solitude states, were noted at a very young age. However, solitude has been experienced differently at different developmental stages of the human life span. On average, from birth through old age, individuals will experience more and more time alone, and gradually they will develop abilities to handle the psychological demands of solitude (Larson, 1990; Long & Averill, 2003). As Larson (1997) noted, adolescents may experience solitude more positively than preadolescents because (1) they have developed advanced reasoning skills that allow them to make more constructive use of solitude, (2) their social environment is characterized by increased self-consciousness and conformity pressure, and (3) solitude provides a special opportunity to struggle with pressing issues of identity formation. In order to benefit from solitude, the individual must be able to draw on inner resources to find meaning in a situation when external supports are absent. This perhaps explains why many people, when alone, engage in distracting rather than productive activities (Long & Averill, 2003).

Regardless of the positive benefits of solitude, its dangers should be recognized. Solitude can become addictive and a consistent decrease in social interaction may lead to disengagement from the concerns of others. Spending much time alone could foster ever-increasing disengagement and eventual chronic social withdrawal

(Long & Averill, 2003). However, the individual who evidences a stable preference for occasional solitude, and who is open to new emotional experiences, is poised to enjoy the benefits of solitude. Still, several studies considered the solitude preferences during childhood as vulnerability and a risk factor. Children who prefer to stay alone were considered at risk for developing maladjustment, and lower social competence. In contrast, other studies pointed attention to the heterogenic nature of solitude behavior, demonstrating that some anxious solitude children were well adjusted while others revealed maladjustment and difficulties (Gazelle, 2008). Especially during adolescence, solitude was sometimes linked with wellbeing. It did not mean that solitude was considered a happy period, but several adolescents learned to use it more constructively and expressed wishes for privacy and independence (Larson, 1997). At this age, the solitude has a unique importance, facilitating the growth in the self-consciousness and individual identity. It also provides a rest from struggles with peer pressures to conformity and enabling independence. Adolescents, who spent about 25–45% of their leisure time alone, were viewed by their teachers and parents as better adjusted, reporting positive mood.

It seems that a moderate amount of solitude promoted teens' adjustment, providing time for renewal, enabling self-development and the identification of effective coping strategies. Yet, too much or too little solitude was related to lower indices of adjustment. Overall, most adolescents reported that they were happier while staying with other people, and those individuals who preferred to stay alone most of their time, often had adjustment difficulties (Larson, 1997). Usually children spend solitude periods at home and this may reflect the children's attempts toward separation/individuation from the family pressures.

In conclusion, from early age, children experience and can understand loneliness. They were able to share their distress within age-appropriate interview format. The majority of elementary school children were able to provide a complete explanation, referring to both social deficits and distressing negative emotions. Self-explanations and attributions were often provided spontaneously. Children expressed their worries regarding their competence ("I am failing at school," "am I stupid?") and relatedness ("Who will want me as a friend?"). In addition, children's reports of their loneliness reflected their cognitive ability to conceptualize and describe it (Chipuer, 2004). Children were able to elaborate and provide more detailed multifaceted descriptions of their distress and considered it different from solitude. The ability to stay alone was related to decreased loneliness. Yet, children had to experiment solitude opportunities in order to enhance their ability to stay alone and feel satisfied and engaged.

Loneliness Risk: Developmental Considerations

Parents and educators have a difficulty in deciding which age is at a higher risk for experiencing loneliness, and who goes through deeper and more distressful loneliness – young children or adolescents? It has been commonly accepted that adolescents are at a higher loneliness risk. They tend to experience higher levels of personal distress during their active search for identity, separation from parental dependence, and increased need for peer relations and appreciation. However, only few studies validated the expected developmental increase in loneliness during adolescence. Several others pinpointed attention to the higher incidence of loneliness reported among younger children, whereas many additional studies failed to reveal significant age differences (Margalit, 1994).

The fact that some studies revealed higher levels of loneliness in younger groups of children may be explained in two ways: It may be that, in reality, adolescents do experience higher levels of loneliness as expected, yet the younger children are more open in sharing and disclosing their inner feelings than are their older counterparts and express it more fully. Alternatively, it may be assumed that younger children experience less freedom and decreased mobility to enable them to form friendships outside of school. Thus, in-class rejection from peers may directly affect their feelings of loneliness as measured in the school setting. The inconsistent results of these developmental studies may also reflect sample differences, restricting our ability to make generalized conclusions as to the existence of significant developmental trends.

Short-term longitudinal studies that explored the loneliness experience at different times during the school year revealed individual patterns and also periodical changes. The loneliness experience was more pronounced in the beginning of the school year than toward the end of the year. When children return from their summer vacations, their anxiety may be increased toward meeting new teachers and in considering the probabilities of increased academic demands adaptable to a higher class. Children's self-questioning regarding who will be with them in challenging hours, with whom they are going to sit, and who will provide them with meaningful help if needed, affect their experience of isolation. Many times children asked "will my new teacher in the 5th grade be as helpful and as understanding as my teacher in the 4th grade?" Toward the end of the year, most children felt less anxious and less lonely. However, an examination of these results clearly showed that the study of the averages provided only a partial picture – and there is a need to differentiate between children whose loneliness decreased during the academic year and those children who became lonelier. Generally, it seemed that most children, who were not lonely in the beginning of the year, beyond small insignificant changes, remained sociable and well-adjusted. There was a certain amount of stability in their social experiences. However, among those children who were very lonely in the beginning of the year, several children indeed decreased their loneliness, but many others remained lonely and several even reported increased loneliness and accompanying academic and social challenges, emphasizing the need for early focused intervention on the social distress (Margalit, Mioduser, Al-Yagon, & Neuberger, 1997).

Gender Perspectives

No consistent gender differences in the expressions of loneliness were noted, but the link between loneliness and behavioral withdrawal in early childhood appears to be moderated by child gender and activity during solitary play (Qualter & Munn, 2002).

In this study, socially withdrawn boys were at a greater risk for experiencing loneliness in early childhood, since shyness and social withdrawal appear to be viewed as less socially acceptable for boys than for girls (Rubin & Coplan, 2004). Withdrawn boys were also more likely to be excluded by peers. Young boys who were shy and socially withdrawn may also faced more negative interactions with parents and teachers. This may lead them to feel less positive about themselves and their other social relationships, and less satisfied with their peer experiences at school (Rubin et al., 2009). Shy young girls were socially more accepted and viewed as gentle, delicate, and polite, and thus at a lower risk for developing maladjustment.

Another gender-related difference has been documented: the connections between aggression and loneliness. Overt aggression may be a greater risk factor in terms of negative adjustment outcomes especially for girls more than for boys because it is seen as a less acceptable behavior for girls. Similar to the process previously described for socially withdrawn boys, aggressive girls experienced negative interactions with parents, teachers, and peers (aside from peer exclusion) and expressed more loneliness (Coplan, Closson et al., 2007). Overall, boys and girls did not report different levels of loneliness experiences in various samples of children in different cultures and environments (Bagner, Storch, & Roberti, 2004; Booth-Laforce et al., 2006; Margalit & Al-Yagon, 2002; Margalit & Ben-Dov, 1995), but their social distress was related to different developmental challenges. Since, several children were found at a higher risk than others of experiencing loneliness from very early developmental stages, the survey of recent genetic research may clarify the roots of this risk, and why some children are at a higher risk for developing this challenge.

Genetic Factors and Temperament

Many times people treat the genetic characteristics as deterministic factors that would shape developmental outcomes. Within this context, I would like to present Mary's words that expressed her acceptance of this sad belief:

During a meeting at school, Mary said sadly to the school counselor: "I think that nothing can be done to change this sad situation. My son is behaving exactly like my husband – who has been a loner throughout his life. I think that it runs in their family. He also has two brothers – and they share exactly the same social difficulties..."

Mary pinpointed attention to an important dilemma with developmental and therapeutic critical implications. Indeed, if she was confident that nothing and nobody could provide meaningful help to her child, since he behaved similarly to her husband, there was a good chance that the beliefs would become a self-fulfilling prophecy. However, we have to clarify first – what is the scientific basis for these beliefs? Can we identify genetic roots of loneliness, and even more important – should it be treated as a deterministic factor?

Recently, a growing effort has been made in the examination of this question, aiming to identify the genetic predictors of individual differences of loneliness. The solution to this query is a true challenge, since often it is difficult to separate genetic impacts from family and environmental influences. When we observe children that behave similarly to their parents, it may reflect their similar genetic roots, but it also may reveal their shared family environment. Their behavior may reflect the impact of their relations with their parents and the remaining family members.

In an attempt to separate genetic influences from environmental influences, researchers examined twin and adoption studies (twin children who share the same genetic structures, but were adopted at a very early age and grew up in separate families). These studies provided important information for clarifying this imperative dilemma. The heritability of children's loneliness has been examined within the Colorado Adoption Project and the San Diego Sibling Study (McGuire & Clifford, 2000). The results of these studies revealed a significant genetic impact (of about 55–48%), but also pinpointed attention to the impact of the non-shared environmental contributions to individual differences in loneliness. A similarity was identified among siblings and twins in their levels of loneliness, but the similarity was greater for identical twins than for either fraternal twins or siblings. The studies confirmed that the genetic factors predicted a risk for developing loneliness. However, they also focused attention on the role of environmental influences, such as family climate, parental behavior, and educational settings.

Additional studies explored the genetic and environmental determinants of loneliness in adults (Boomsma, Cacioppo, Slagboom, & Posthuma, 2006; Boomsma, Willemsen, Dolan, Hawkley, & Cacioppo, 2005), based on a large data base of 8,387 adult Dutch twins. The genetic contribution to the loneliness variation was similar (48%) to the hereditary estimates found in the children's study. A unique additional perspective (Bartels, Cacioppo, Hudziak, & Boomsma, 2008) was provided by a longitudinal approach that examined the consistency of the children's loneliness every 3 years. Individual differences in children's loneliness were found in the different age groups (7, 10, and 12 years old). A drop in genetic influences and a rise in environmental influences were observed surprisingly at the age group of 12 years old. Maybe during this transition to adolescence, the children were introduced to new interpersonal relationships, situational factors, and social contextual challenges that decreased the genetic impact. However, as these children continued to grow and demonstrated adaptation to the "new" biological/situational challenges of adolescence, their heritable dispositions began to re-emerge as major influences in their loneliness experiences. This study further confirmed the significance of genetic factors in explaining individual differences in loneliness. However, it also demonstrated the impact of developmental processes and contextual conditions. It can be concluded that heritability estimates of complex traits such as loneliness may reflect changes across the lifespan, as the frequency, duration, and range of exposure to environmental characteristics interact with the genetic influences (Cacioppo et al., 2006), explaining individual and situational differences.

So, can we agree with Mary's words? Can we accept the proposed deterministic belief?

Indeed these studies provided important evidence for the significance of genetic factors in predicting the stability of loneliness and explaining individual differences

(Boomsma et al., 2006). However, in addition to the evidence that development of all human characteristics is genetically influenced, we have to be aware that these characteristics interact with varied environmental conditions to yield individual differences in adjustment and psychopathology. Indeed children, who were identified as feeling lonely at a young age, are considered to be at a higher risk of experiencing chronic feelings of loneliness throughout childhood and adulthood. However, the increasing recognition for the importance of shared environmental influences has suggested that active family-based intervention plans can help in preventing and decreasing children's distress. There is also an opportunity for teaching children effective strategies for coping with loneliness. Thus, an active strategy to help children who show early signs of loneliness is not only important to moderate the possibility that these individuals will develop these feelings chronically, but it may also help in avoiding the long-term effects of loneliness. The examination of developmental characteristics of lonely children will not only further clarify the dynamic interactions between various risks, such as difficult temperament and protective aspects of the self, but also suggest directions for parental guidance and educational implications.

Temperament

Children's temperament has been recognized from their earliest developmental stages. Observations of very young infants have revealed their different reactions to noise, pain, and satisfaction of basic needs. Temperament has been defined as individual differences in reactivity and responding to different stimuli, and the self-regulation abilities. It is assumed to have a genetic and constitutional basis, i.e. the relatively enduring biological makeup of the organism (Rothbart, Ahadi, & Ahadi, 2000). Reactivity refers to levels of excitability or the arousing ability of the behavioral and physiological systems of the organism, whereas self-regulation refers to neural and behavioral processes that modulate this reactivity. The individuals' emotional disposition, including their susceptibility to emotional stimulation, their customary intensity and speed of responses that affect the initiation, inhibition or modification of behavior, including those related to effortful control, and the quality of their prevailing mood are dependent upon constitutional make-up (Denham, Wyatt, Bassett, Echeverria, & Knox, 2009).

Children differ in their vulnerability and susceptibility to environmental relations. A general psychobiological reactivity makes some children more vulnerable to environmental influences than others (Belsky, Bakermans-Kranenburg, & van IJzendoorn, 2007). Although temperament is considered generally to be "constitutional" in origin, it can be altered by environmental processes such as parenting approaches, illustrating the importance of models that examined the joint impacts of genetic endowment and environment interactions for predicting developmental outcomes (Denham et al., 2009). Recent research has clearly challenged deterministic approaches and proposed that aspects of these biologically based temperamental characteristics can change at varying time points from infancy through the adolescent period. Learning processes, environmental elicitation and construal, social comparison processes, contextual selection and manipulation are the processes that produce these changes. During these processes, various aspects of the temperament emerge into individual difference characteristics, including sociability, dominance, negative emotionality, aggressiveness, etc. Thus, differential susceptibility to environmental influences indeed differentiates between children, but children who are especially reactive and vulnerable to adversity may also respond positively and benefit disproportionately from positive experiences. Thus some children may be more affected by developmental experiences due to their genetics – for better and for worse – than others. A growing body of theory and evidence raises the prospect that developmental plasticity may be a function of environmental impact and nurture as well as nature, providing an optimistic realization to the importance of parents' guidance, especially for at-risk children (Belsky & Pluess, 2009).

Children who are born with a disposition to react intensively and with negative affect to stress or novelty may go on to show different patterns of behavior, depending on the degree to which they are exposed to different caring behavior. The plasticity conceptualization for Affective Neurocircuitry Model (Fox, Hane, & Pine, 2007) proposed that early children's temperament influences not only the children's behavior, but also the quality of the care-giving environment, and this quality of the environment in turn shapes attention bias to threat and mediates the relations between early temperament and later behavior. Parents often notice that their care-giving style indeed affects their children's behavior but also reacts to it.

A father told us that for his elder daughter he was the perfect parent. She was a charming baby with an easy and pleasant temperament who slept well at night and continuously smiled at everybody who entered her room, and not surprisingly, everybody smiled back at her. His son presented him with new parental challenges. He was a crying baby with a difficult temperament who was restless and annoyed for unknown reasons most of the time. At the same home, with the same parents, this child grew up in a completely different environment. The tired father found himself getting angry easily and he needed all his abilities to regulate his mood in order to control his annoyance.

Children who experienced frequent and intense levels of negative emotionality, related to their temperament, were often more impulsive, easily aroused emotionally, and less accepted by peers (Henwood & Solano, 1994). A series of observations revealed the predicting role of negative emotionality in the quality of interpersonal relations. Observations at different ages exposed a gradual process. For example, after several months at school, children who showed initially frequent and intense levels of negative emotionality became socially isolated and played alone for a longer time. Gradually these children decreased their social interactions and their classmates did not like them. The high levels of negative emotional arousal contributed to social withdrawal, or shortened the social interactions, and thus these children may not have enough opportunities to become socially engaged and involved. They did not have enough opportunities for developing age-appropriate social skills, while socially competent children were higher on emotion regulation and learned to react in ways that helped them avoid experiencing negative emotions.

The intense negative emotional reactions may disrupt interpersonal interactions, increasing the likelihood of aggressive and hostile behavior. However, the reactivity to environmental influences and the plasticity in the behavior style enable positive changes when the environmental influences are planned with clear goals and structured procedures. Gender differences were noted already at the preschool levels (Henwood & Solano, 1994). Boys showed higher proportions of intense negative emotions, externalizing negative emotions, expressing anger, and demonstrating more aggression. Girls exhibited less anger and aggression and were considered more likeable. Emotions are thought to have an important role in social functions, and recently there is a growing interest in the role of emotion regulation in development and adjustment, and individual differences in emotion regulations may be considered within the risk and protective personal factors. A short description of emotions will provide the background necessary for understanding emotion regulation.

Positive and Negative Emotions

Emotions are considered as biologically prepared capabilities that have a remarkable value for survival. Emotions are a kind of radar and rapid response system, constructing and carrying meaning across the flow of experience. They enable us to appraise experience quickly and prepare ourselves to act (Cole, Martin, & Dennis, 2004). The informational effect of emotions on cognitive representations and behaviors has been extensively established in personality research (Forgas, 1991). People have emotions about things that matter to them and their emotions may affect the contents of cognition ("*what* individuals think") (Forgas, 1995), resulting in considering situations and tasks either as challenges or as threats. A challenge will be conceptualized when the individual experiences sufficient or nearly sufficient resources to meet situational demands, resulting in approach reactions. A threat will be conceptualized when the individual experiences insufficient resources to meet situational demands, resulting in avoidance attempts. This differentiation between emotions may have a clear impact on the effort that children and adults are ready to invest in achieving their goals, thus leading to different outcomes (Margalit, 1999). The challenge perception will promote increased effort and engagement, while the threat experience may trigger attempts to create a distance from the sources of threat and to enhance disengagement. However, the differences between emotions are more comprehensive and long lasting.

Researchers have directed attention to the different impacts of positive and negative emotions (Baumeister, 1999; Baumeister, Vohs, DeWall, & Zhang, 2007), establishing the stronger and longer lasting influences of negative emotions than positive emotions, which justifies the investment in preventive planning to minimize such impacts. Negative emotions narrow people's thought–action repertoire (e.g., either fight or flight), while positive emotions typically broaden people's thought–action repertoire in terms of their attention and information processing, encouraging them to explore and discover novel lines of thought or action and enabling flexible and creative thinking. The impact is immediate, yet with a long-lasting developmental influence, creating a spiral toward improved wellbeing and resiliency and building their psychological resources and coping arsenal for handling future adversities (Fredrickson & Joiner, 2002). The differentiation between automatic emotional reactions and conscious emotional states further extends the understanding of the emotions' impacts on behavior.

Automatic and Conscious Emotions

The rapid, automatic emotional responses help in guiding behavior by informing cognition and behavioral choices to individuals. In contrast, conscious emotional states can be treated as an inner feedback system whose influence on behavior is indirect, yet important. These two different types of emotional responses are interrelated and coordinated, even though they serve different functions within the human system. Conscious emotion commands attention and stimulates analysis, learning, and adaptation, often occurring in the aftermath of behavior and its outcomes. In contrast, automatic affective responses provide direct input to the current situation, usually preserving information from previous emotional experiences (Baumeister et al., 2007). As a result, when individuals learn to anticipate feedback, they may alter their behavior to pursue the feedback that they like and prefer. For example, an unpleasant experience of loneliness may motivate children to act in ways that hold the promise of mood repair (i.e., feeling better) and avoiding feeling of social isolation. In contrast, a lower likelihood of success to change the unpleasant situation will evoke negative emotions, which can lead to various coping strategies, such as disengagement and distancing the individuals from the desired goals, but at the same time also from the social pains (Wrosch, Scheier, Miller, Schulz, & Carver, 2003). The emotion regulation may enable children to achieve their goals, and to avoid threat situations. Two examples are provided to illustrate different regulation processes of children.

Emotion Regulation

These short descriptions of two boys, Guy and Danny, will illustrate the importance of emotion regulation for adaptive functioning.

Guy and Danny were 10-year-old boys who faced the same distress. The boys from their class were playing and they were not invited to join the group. They both felt very angry and extremely lonely. However, after an hour, a major difference between them was noticed. Guy was still very angry, his eyes were full of tears and sadly he sat in a corner, observing from a distance the cheerful group of boys. In fact he felt after an hour lonelier than he had felt before. He was prepared to insult them and to behave aggressively, but he was afraid to get into more trouble.

Danny was not there any more. He was able to regulate his negative emotion (sadness) and got involved in a computer game with another boy at the school computer lab. He tried to distract himself by immersing into the competitive game, but to be honest, he could not forget the rejection of his classmates and his unhappiness. However, meanwhile he was able to find an alternative enjoyable activity. He decided not to think about it now, but to think about the challenging situation later – when he would not be so excited. He decided to try to find ways to get into the preferred group. He was not happy – but he was not overwhelmed with the disappointment.

In the descriptions of the two boys, no true solution to the experience of loneliness and rejection was proposed; however, Danny had more positive opportunities to find an acceptable solution. He was able to regulate his anger and hurtful feelings by creating a distraction. He did not act following his automatic emotional reactions, but decided to use conscious emotions for effective problem-solving.

Emotion regulation has been defined as the set of processes used by people to redirect the spontaneous flow of their emotions. It can be promoted by the external environment and parents may play a key role in regulating children's emotional states. In addition, contextual conditions and cultural norms may also discourage the full expression of emotions and promote their regulation. Emotion regulations are expressed through all modalities of the emotional responding, including behavior, physiology, thoughts, and feelings. Active attempts to manage emotional states request using a wide range of strategies, such as attention focused on the source of the initiation of emotion (trying to understand what happens) and distraction – avoiding/ignoring it (deciding not to think about it). The construct of emotion regulation proposes to account for "how and why" emotions organize or facilitate other psychological processes (i.e., focus attention, promote problem solving, search for an alternative, support relationships) and yet why they can have detrimental effects (i.e., disrupt attention, interfere with problem solving, harm relationships, behave aggressively). This concept integrates the understanding of typical and atypical development (Cole et al., 2004). It determines the offset of emotional responding and is distinct from emotional sensitivity, which determines the onset of emotional responding (Koole, 2009). In everyday life, children are continually exposed to potentially emotion-arousing stimuli, ranging from internal sensations like a headache to external events such as peer rejection. However, many times they actively resist being carried away by the immediate emotional impact of the situations. Emotion regulation emerges as one of the most far-ranging and influential processes at the interface of cognition and emotion, affecting social relations.

Emotion regulation has generally been linked to quality of social functioning, such as children who were able to regulate their feelings were also getting along with their peers. Children with regulation difficulties were often rejected by peers (Eisenberg, 2000). Parallel findings with adults confirm the findings that adults who scored high on measures of emotional control were rated by others as more socially sensitive and friendly (Lopes, Salovey, Cote, & Beers, 2005). Thus, the importance of emotion regulation and self-control has been documented in research. However, since emotion regulation has been demanding on personal energy, expending the self's resources, and producing the condition of ego depletion, it still remain to discuss various positive or negative impacts in terms of personal resources and developmental outcomes (Baumeister, Muraven, & Tice, 2000).

Researchers and clinicians were anxious to examine the emotional price that individuals may pay while improving their capacity for emotion regulation. They debated whether it will narrow or enrich the emotional experiences. Initially it has been expected that children, who don't let themselves the full excitation following an emotionally triggering situation, may develop more superficial and restraining emotional experiences with a developmental disadvantage. However, drawing from Chinese poetics and Confucian philosophy, Frijda and Sundararajan (2007) detailed how emotional restraint may contribute to a deeper and more differentiated appreciation of one's emotions. In line with this approach, empirical evidence indicates that individuals with high emotion-regulation competencies are characterized by greater self-reflexivity, mindfulness, and a more profound awareness of their emotions (Brown, Williams, Barker, & Galambos, 2007). People's emotional lives are thus likely to become enriched as people learn new and more powerful strategies of regulating their emotions.

Developmental and individual differences were documented on the abilities for emotion regulation, predicting children's social relations and personal wellbeing. However, the emotion regulation of several children was delayed or ineffective, due to difficult temperament, personal characteristics, developmental delays, disabilities, and/or environmental influences. Different strategies were used by children to regulate their emotions and to compensate their difficulties, such as repressing and avoiding negative emotions, effective coping, and mindfulness training that involve purposefully paying attention to negative emotions, etc. (Koole, 2009).

Emotion Utilization and Emotion Knowledge

Emotion utilization is conceptually different from direct attempts to regulate emotion and involves spontaneous as well as planned constructive actions and creative endeavors. Emotion utilization (Izard, Stark, Trentacosta, & Schultz, 2008) is defined as an adaptive cognition and action, motivated by emotional experience. Efforts directed toward emotion regulation may facilitate emotion utilization, but they are not necessary for harnessing the inherently adaptive functions of emotions in constructive thought and action. For example, the adaptive functions of anger and sadness are self-assertion and social support seeking, respectively. Given adequate emotion knowledge or understanding of emotion, and a supportive social context, a child can learn to utilize the emotional energy and motivation in anger arousal for positive self-assertion rather than for yelling or becoming aggressive. Similarly, an adolescent can learn to utilize the energy and motivation in sadness to reach out for social support from peers or family rather than withdrawing from the situation that is causing the sadness and staying alone.

Developmental research on emotion regulation is currently adopting a systemic view that integrates behavioral and biological constituents of emotional self-control (Thompson, Lewis, & Calkins, 2008). Emotion regulation is thus considered a network of multilevel processes characterized by feedback and interaction between higher and lower systems, and it becomes increasingly apparent that it is a component of a general emotional activation, reflecting the mutual influence of multiple emotion-related systems and not only the maturation of higher control processes (Thompson et al., 2008). Indeed several maturation processes contribute to emotion regulation, such as the growth of executive cognitive control that enables infants the redirection of attention in order to disengage from emotionally arousing stimuli. The developing language abilities are also incorporated into emotion regulation as self-management develops first through the extrinsic talk (which can also be used to solicit assistance from another) and afterward as an internal speech. In early to middle childhood, emotion self-regulation is also enhanced by growth in cognitive processing such as memory, causal reasoning, and advances in self-efficacy. The maturation of executive functioning (the inner control systems) progressively fosters emotion self-management through processes such as self-directed inhibition, self-distraction, reappraisal, and action monitoring, which are also enlisted into broader forms of strategic control development.

Children continually process internal and external emotion cues, including many that are ambiguous or unclear. Emotion information processing, or the acquisition of emotion knowledge, includes appraisal and attribution processes (self-explanations "why this is happening to me") that activate emotions. Over time, as young children continue to process emotional information and use it to confirm and disconfirm predictions of others' behaviors, the emotion knowledge gradually accumulates. Emotion knowledge includes the understanding of the expressive signals, labels, and functions of emotions. Thus, in conclusion, emotion regulation involves two types of processes and strategies, and each one may influence emotion utilization. First, emotionality influences emotion information processing, emotion regulation, and emotion-related behavior. Second, the cumulative emotion knowledge that results from emotion information processing and socio-emotional learning serves as a continuous source of emotion-regulatory strategies. Moreover, maladaptive emotion information processing may distort emotion knowledge and degrade emotion regulation and utilization.

With increasing age, emotion regulation is influenced by growth in self and others' understanding, emotional understanding and empathy, and developing knowledge of socio-cultural rules. Thus, the emotion regulation represents a network of processes from within and outside the children that contribute to emotional self-management. Consequently, the nature of developmental changes in emotion regulation is also multifaceted. Children become more competent in emotion self-control as they acquire greater self and others' understanding and a greater variety of self-initiated strategies of emotion management. These strategies are more flexibly applied to specific contextual demands and gradually incorporate cultural expectations and norms. Consequently, children also enlist emotion regulatory skills to accomplish increasingly complex social and personal goals and interact with environmental influences (Thompson et al., 2008). Early emerging individual differences in emotion regulation are not very stable over time because they are based on changing combinations of behavioral and neurobiological capacities with different maturational timetables and origins and different interactions with contextual influences.

Over the course of development, for most children, emotional processes appear to interact seamlessly with the contingency structure of the social environment. However, underlying these complex behaviors there are myriad skills – such as decoding and conveying emotional signals with caregivers (Goldsmith, Pollak, & Davidson, 2008). Developmental approaches to emotion are enriched by focusing on how individuals learn to respond to signals in their environments – how their unique characteristics interact with environmental signals – perceive, interpret, understand, and react to them. When such an approach is combined with recent insights regarding the plasticity of neural systems, the understanding of risk and resilience in children will be improved, as well as the significance of the early awareness to childhood loneliness. Perceptual and attention systems are relatively plastic and responsive to environmental input early in development. The relative plasticity of these mechanisms may serve an adaptive function: children learn the contingencies in their environments. However, plasticity may also present risks if emotional input or contingencies are aberrant (for example for abused children), leading children to over or under attend to certain emotional signals.

Emotional development is rapid in the first 5 years of life (Cole, Luby, & Sullivan, 2008). By first grade, most children understand and regulate emotion well enough to learn, form, and maintain friendships, and comply with classroom rules (Cole et al., 2008). Their self-perceptions reflect their developmental history and predict their social and academic adjustment. At this age stage socially competent children as well as lonely children are noticed (Kovacs, Joormann, & Gotlib, 2008).

Social Competence

Social competence is a complex developmental construct reflecting the interactions of cognitive and affective processes and cultural expectations at different ages. Most conceptualizations of social competence emphasize active participation or initiative in social interactions and the appropriateness of the behaviors in social settings (Chen & French, 2008). Social initiative refers to the tendency to initiate and maintain social activities, especially in challenging situations. Behavioral control, representing self-regulatory ability to modulate behavioral and emotional reactivity, is closely related to the maintenance of social appropriateness (Eisenberg & Fabes, 1992). A major cause for loneliness during childhood emerged from developmental delays in social competence. The main factors for predicting social difficulties and loneliness among children with typical development as well as children with developmental difficulties (Gresham & Elliott, 1990) are the knowledge and performance deficits.

Children may fail to acquire age-appropriate knowledge needed for developing satisfactory social relations. They may have difficulties in their social cognition and may struggle in tasks that require understanding of social cues within complex social situations. Several children may understand social dynamics in dyads and manage quite well to play in a small group of friends, but have difficulties when they have to join a larger group or participate in class. Their difficulties may focus on understanding the group interactions, but may also reflect their deficient age-appropriate knowledge how to react to these cues, even when they understand them. Children, who have acquired the needed social knowledge, may still have difficulties in transforming their age-appropriate information into effective interpersonal behaviors due to difficulties in selecting the appropriate behavior because of emotion-regulation difficulties and/or limited opportunities to experiment in social interactions. Social skills are those socially accepted, learned behaviors that enable children to interact effectively with peers and avoid socially unacceptable responses (Gresham, 1986). Strategies for entering into groups, initiating and maintaining interactions, sharing, helping, and requesting help, are just some examples of social skills (Gresham & Elliott, 1990). It is not enough to obtain the knowledge and to understand the rules of adjusted social behavior. Children who acquire these behaviors need enough opportunities for exercising and experimenting with them in order to achieve a fluent performance.

Rejected and lonely children have difficulties not only in acquiring social skills, but also in mastering them, since they have fewer occasions to use them until developing skilled social behavior. Thus, children may be able to understand and explain in detail what the desired social responses are during their interactions with peers. They may have high levels of motivation to interact socially. Yet when in real life they face excitement or frustrations, they may prove unable to perform the socially accepted behavior, reflecting their immature emotion regulation. As the chronic loneliness develops, social skills will become less competent since they had fewer opportunities to use them and/or resulting from motivational deficits.

Several children who find staying alone more difficult than their peers, may be at a greater risk for developing loneliness (Margalit, 2006). The roots of this difficulty are in caregiver–infant relations (Winnicott, 1965), and infants who feel confident in their parents' support and availability will explore the environment with the assurance that they can control the proximity of the caregiver. A delay in the development of children's abilities to stay on their own due to attention difficulties, cognitive delays, or deficient emotional maturation may enhance the desperation of lonely children when they are left on their own. Many times the roots of this struggle are in their difficulties to stay engaged and satisfied in solitude activities without the presence of a supportive adult. Mothers and fathers shared with us their confusion and indecision what to do when their child would complain "I am bored," or "I don't have anything to do." Worriedly they questioned themselves where they had failed if their child could not enjoy solitude activities, and whether they should continue to provide activities. They were worried that by helping their child they would encourage dependency on adults for planning leisure activities. Children, who have difficulties staying alone, and at the same time imagine that their classmates are having an enjoyable time, feel more desperate, frustrated, and lonely.

Lonely children often behave in specific ways – disclosing a typical style to lonely individuals. They relate to other children in ways that convey their expectations to be rejected or ignored. They accept the reputation of isolated individuals (Margalit, 1994). Their interpersonal approach, communication style, and nonverbal cues reveal their alienated self-concept as well as their beliefs in their inability to change this distressing situation and to develop satisfying social relations. Behavior of lonely children often reveals their negative self-perceptions.

Children who have difficulties in acquiring age-appropriate social competence are at risk for developing higher levels of loneliness. However, reciprocal relations exist between social skills and loneliness. Children who do not develop age-appropriate interpersonal skills are less able to initiate, establish, and maintain satisfying relations with peers and will feel lonely. But the experience of loneliness may in turn further affect the children's self-perceptions of their various aspects of competence.

Self-Perceptions

Successful self-regulation is defined as the willingness to exert effort toward one's most important goals, while taking setbacks and accepting failures as opportunities to learn, identify weaknesses and address them, and develop new strategies toward achieving those goals (Crocker, Brook, Niiya, & Villacorta, 2006). Contingencies of self-worth and self-concept can facilitate self-regulation because people are highly motivated to succeed and avoid failure in domains of contingency. The relations between loneliness and low self-perceptions are considered reciprocal and negative patterns of self-perceptions were found to be associated with increased loneliness among children and adults (Hymel et al., 1999).

Even when children behave, talk, and dress similarly (revealing youth culture), they may feel differently about themselves and choose different courses of action, depending on how they construe themselves – what attributes (abilities as well as difficulties) they think they possess, what roles they presume they are expected to play, what they believe they are capable of, how they view they fare in comparison with others, and how they judge they are viewed by others. These are beliefs and perceptions about self that are heavily rooted in one's past achievement and reinforcement history. Yet it is these subjective convictions which play a determining role in individuals' further growth and development. The Sense of Coherence, self-concept, attribution style, and self-efficacy are such self-constructs that have received a lot of research attention related to children's social competence and academic achievements (Bandura, 1997; Bong & Skaalvik, 2003).

Sense of Coherence

The Sense of Coherence construct has been considered a protective factor for children and adults. It has been linked to greater stress-resistance and better health, and a source of support to wider effective coping strategies (Antonovsky, 1993). This is a personal disposition toward seeing the world as comprehensible, manageable, and meaningful (conceptual presentation of the Sense of Coherence construct is presented in the first chapter). We have performed comprehensive studies with children at different ages from preschool to adolescents and young adults (Efrati-Virtzer & Margalit, 2009; Margalit, 1994, 2006). In our studies we included children with typical development and children with developmental disabilities, learning disabilities, and various additional adjustment challenges. Consistent negative relations were found between children's loneliness and their Sense of Coherence. Most children, who reported higher levels of loneliness, experienced a low Sense of Coherence. In several studies, the low Sense of Coherence was related to children's current distress, to early expressions of adjustment difficulties, and to perceived health and somatic complaints (Honkinen et al., 2009; Honkinen, Suominen, Välimaa, Helenius, & Rautava, 2005; Jellesma, Rieffe, Terwogt, & Kneepkens, 2006). Studies also revealed the impact of early adjustment difficulties and developmental difficulties, such as reading difficulties and behavior problems on current lower Sense of Coherence levels (Margalit, 2006). However, many of our studies identified a group of children with developmental or contextual challenges, and yet had levels of Sense of Coherence and loneliness compatible with their typical developing peers.

Within the risk and protective paradigm, research identified factors that contributed to children and adolescents strong Sense of Coherence. This resilience model within an ecological framework promoted the understanding of the role of the Sense of Coherence construct (Marsh, Clinkinbeard, Thomas, & Evans, 2007), revealing its relations with positive and negative emotional expressions. It was also related to family support and to the quality of relations with parents. Children who experienced more support and cohesive family relations during their development, tended to have more self-confidence in themselves and in their world. Thus it is not surprising that Sense of Coherence has been considered a predictor to children's resilience and is related consistently to lower levels of loneliness. In addition to this global and relatively stable measure of self-perception, the self-concept construct extends understanding of protective factors and represents a flexible and differentiated construct.

Self-Concept

Self-concept has been defined as a composite view of oneself, consisting of several domains such as academic self-concept and social self-concept. Children possess a psychologically relevant self-concept from early developmental stages (Goodvin, Meyer, Thompson, & Hayes, 2008). Preschoolers (ages 4–5) have internally coherent views of their psychological distinctiveness, and considerable variability in the characteristics they attribute to themselves. They are able to differentiate between positive and negative attributes and emotions. Preschool children with less positive self-perceptions showed more internalizing problems, reporting loneliness and social-withdrawal (Coplan et al., 2004). They were often excluded by peers and had mothers with less positive parenting styles. These findings indicated that preschool years have to be treated as a formative period for the development of self-concept. This is a period when mental working models of the self are growing quickly and consolidating into coherent perceptions together with their predicted relations to external environmental conditions (Goodvin et al., 2008).

Skaalvik (1997) identified key antecedents to the understanding of the development of the self-concept construct:

(1) *Frames of reference.* The social comparison often serves as the most powerful source of information for self-concept. For example, children judge themselves to be successful in sports or mathematics in comparison to children's achievements in their classes. Individuals' self-concept is influenced by standards against which they judge their traits and accomplishments.
(2) *Causal explanations (attributions).* Individuals explain to themselves and attribute their successes to varied factors. The choice of these factors affects their specific and generalized self-perceptions. For example, children who explained to themselves that they were not invited to participate in a game, because their classmates considered them to be stupid and lazy, would not expect in the future to be invited to a study group by the same children. This attribution affects their self-perceptions and their affective reactions. Self-concept and attributions are related in a reciprocal manner and the types of causal attributions made for previous social failures influence subsequent self-concepts. Thus current self-concept affects later attributions that further contribute to lower self-concept.
(3) *Reflected appraisals from significant others.* Several self-concept approaches suggested that people gradually internalize and view themselves the way they believe that others view them. The socially rejected child may feel that his rejection is justified and understandable. One of the children shared with us "I would not like to be my friend or a friend with a child like me." Another child told his mother sadly about his loneliness at school: "At first in the new school I had many friends. But after they knew me, they did not want to continue hanging out with me. I cannot blame them."
(4) *Mastery experiences.* Self-competence perceptions were developed as outcomes of past experiences in a particular domain. Children, who continuously failed to join the peer group, would develop a lower social self-concept and reduced expectations.

In conclusion, three principal reference points seem to be pertinent for the development of self-concept: first, the image of the self (self-perceptions); second, the internalization of the society's views that in fact is determined by the individual's internal beliefs how others view and evaluate him/her; and third, the individual's belief regarding what he/she wishes to be (the ideal self) (Ittyerah & Kumar, 2007).

Lonely children had, for example, lower self-perceptions and also believed that others didn't appreciate them (Tsai & Reis, 2009). Lonely children perceived themselves more negatively and, in addition, they also believed that others saw them in a negative light. They had doubts about their own competence and, at the same time, they developed relatively negative views about their close friends. Indeed the friends of lonely individuals had negative expectations about interacting with lonely individuals, which may have lead them to respond to a social behavior in a less open, more reluctant manner, thereby triggering interaction sequences that failed to provide desired levels of acceptance and intimacy related to high quality friendship relations (Tsai & Reis, 2009). Attribution style (or explanatory style) extended understanding to sources of individual differences and illustrated the ways that children explained to themselves why they behaved in a certain manner, why events were happening to them, and why other children were treating them in a certain manner.

Attribution Beliefs

Self-concept affects children's interpretations of behavior toward them. Those children, who devaluate themselves, have difficulties believing that their peers may see them positively. Thus it is not surprising that lonely children often feel unloved and incompetent. They explain to themselves the behavior of their peer perceptions, thoughts, and emotional reactions in line with their self-perceptions and their attribution style. Children are constantly trying to understand themselves and their environment, and they start acting on the basis of this knowledge and understanding (Weiner, 2000).

Maladaptive attribution styles contributed to the development and maintenance of loneliness (Anderson, 1999). Children's social responses are in part determined by their interpretations of interpersonal situations. They provide meanings to events that they observe and experience. The meaning that they provide to their objective realities emerges from their self-perceptions and general beliefs and influences their affective, motivational, and cognitive responses to various life events. The attribution theory links internal attributions for success and failure (Weiner, 1986, 2008). Some children attribute their occasional achievement or failures to their poor strategies and improper behavior, whereas others attribute such social failures to lack of ability and to their difficulties that made them unpopular. Results of a recent study (Newall et al., 2009) showed that more strongly endorsing internal/controllable causal beliefs (i.e., believing that making friends depends on personal effort) resulted in greater social participation and lower levels of loneliness. In contrast, external and uncontrollable causal beliefs predicted higher levels of loneliness.

Weiner (2004) suggested that in order to understand the attribution processes, three underlying causal properties have to be recognized and they have cross-situational generality: locus, stability, and controllability.

- Locus refers to the location of a cause, either within or outside the person. For example, ability and effort are considered internal causes of success, whereas chance and help from others are considered external causes.
- Stability refers to the duration of the causes. Some characteristics and talents are considered constant, whereas causes such as luck are considered unstable.
- Controllability refers to the ability of the individual to control the process. A cause such as effort is subject to volitional alteration, and thus it is personally controlled, whereas luck and special talents can be viewed as uncontrollable.

In general, a maladaptive attribution style consists of attributions of bad outcomes to internal, stable, global, and uncontrollable causes (i.e., self-blame such as – "I can understand why they don't want to be my friends – I am failing in everything."). Good outcomes are attributed to external, unstable, specific, and uncontrollable causes such as luck (i.e., "I was just lucky – since they could not find anybody else to participate in their game, so I was included. Tomorrow it will probably be different.").

Most individuals possess a self-protective bias which leads them to attribute positive outcomes to themselves and negative ones to external unstable causes. On the contrary, distressed individuals exhibit a non-self-serving bias (Asher, Parkhurst, Hymel, & Williams, 1990) and they tend to blame themselves for failures and to reject taking credit for social successes. This kind of attribution belief is likely to decrease self-esteem and to heighten feelings of distress (Crick & Dodge, 1994). Adolescents who attribute their social failures in a non-self-protective way feel lonelier than those who have a more positive attribution style (Han & Choi, 2006). The findings of this study emphasized the importance of the relations between loneliness and non-self-serving attributions in interpersonal relations.

Youngsters who were more inclined to attribute peer-related events to stable and/or global factors were more likely to report higher levels of depression and loneliness 2 years later (Toner & Heaven, 2005). Thus, it is more adaptive to perceive causal factors for social situations as relatively transient and specific to this domain, especially during early adolescence. In this age of social exploration and identity formation, the social world of early adolescence is expected to be relatively unpredictable and flexible. Thus, a tendency to attribute social events to stable and/or global attributions at this age stage might be detrimental for two related reasons.

First, a major function of attributions is to provide accurate information to guide goal-directed behavior. Because of the unstable and specific nature of the peer-social domain in early adolescence, stable and global attributions are often inaccurate and maladaptive. Second, the higher outcome expectancies arising from stable and/or global attributions for positive events make an individual less prepared for adversity when it occurs. Thus, negative outcomes are seen as a result of one's own shortcomings rather than being because of external factors over which one has no control. Likewise, positive feedback may be more important to those that attribute their performance to internally controlled factors, as positive outcomes are seen as coming from the individual's proficiency, and enhancing positive self-perception.

The attribution to success and failure shape the personal goals and beliefs in the individuals' abilities to reach them. While attributions, or the ways in which individuals explain events, have long been seen to play a central part in determining behavior, they also reflect individual differences in a consistent manner across a variety of situations (Tiggemann, Winefield, Winefield, & Goldney, 1991). They demonstrated in their studies the stability of attribution style. For example, those individuals with depressed affect and feelings of hopelessness attributed positive experiences as more externally rooted and as less stable, whereas negative experiences were viewed by them as stable and global. In addition, individuals do not use a single attribution to explain a positive or negative outcome, but rather utilize complex sets of related attributions and their true significance can be understood only through the awareness to their networks of dynamic connections. The self-questioning related to loneliness "why I am lonely" (Lunt, 1991; Toner & Heaven, 2005) provided various attributions: children consider the current situation as a stable one (i.e., "I am lonely because nobody will ever agree to hang out with me. I know, it has always been like this, and it will always be the same."). They appraise their inability to control the occurrences or to initiate changes (i.e., "Nobody likes me at school, and I cannot change it, and the teacher cannot truly help".) The causes of the distressful situation are attributed to internal characteristics of the child (i.e., "I am a loner. This is who I am. It is only natural that nobody wants to be my friend.").

Thus, lonely children who believe that what is happening to them at school or during the afternoon are beyond their personal control, who appraised themselves as loners, who have difficulties in "making friends," might believe that loneliness cannot be solved nor avoided. In contrast, when children believe that they have some control over their social situation and can change their realities; children who do not consider their loneliness as stable – but as related to external changes (new school, separation from good friends) – the experience of loneliness may trigger their motivation for intense attempts to change their distress – resulting in initiating interrelations and establishing meaningful social connections. Children, who believe that they may have personal control over events, might believe that they can end their loneliness, reflecting greater hopes and optimism. Children who attribute their social exclusion to their personal unattractiveness or a lack of appropriate social skills may gradually convince themselves of the totality of their difficulties, further reducing their motivation to initiate interactions and their beliefs in the possibility of changes.

In summary, the attributed causes of loneliness, especially in terms of their stability, perceived controllability, or personal responsibility (locus of control) seem to guide loneliness-related negative emotions and withdrawal behaviors. The interrelations among the various beliefs and expectations about self and others' reactions may present personal trends and clarify the impact of individual differences. People continuously engage in attributional activity in their attempts to uncover the meaning and broader implications of the actions of others, developing expectations regarding future behavior and seeking explanations in terms of underlying dispositions (Rusbult & Van Lange, 2003). Their attributed beliefs interact with their self-efficacy beliefs about their abilities to perform challenging tasks.

Self-Efficacy

Similar to self-concept, self-efficacy provides an explanation and prediction of the children's thoughts, emotions, and actions. However, efficacy judgment is less concerned with the children's skills and abilities and more involved with the individuals' believes in what they can do with these skills and abilities that they may possess. While self-concept represents one's general perceptions of the self in given domains of functioning, self-efficacy represents children's dynamic and specific expectations and convictions of what they can accomplish in given situations. Their beliefs in their capabilities to mobilize their cognitive resources affect their actions to exercise control over given events (Ozer & Bandura, 1990). Self-efficacy beliefs (Bandura, 1997) are the beliefs in one's capabilities to organize and execute the courses of action required to produce personal goals. These beliefs influence the actions that individuals choose to pursue and their effort investment. The concept of self-efficacy within the social cognitive theory (Bandura, 1982) provides an explicit account of why children may feel lonely and fail to relate socially. Those who judge themselves as less efficacious in many important age-related tasks are more inclined to visualize themselves as experiencing failure scenarios and to dwell on how things will go wrong. Beliefs about self-efficacy affect the self-regulation of cognitive processes, increasing the feelings of hopelessness related to social alienation and decreasing motivation to stay involved in social relations.

Sources of Self-Efficacy

Self-efficacy beliefs are shaped by four major sources (Bandura & Bussey, 2004; Bandura, 1986):

(1) *Mastery experience*. The children's prior experiences with the relevant tasks provide a reliable basis for the development of efficacy beliefs. Successful performance reinforces the development of self-efficacy, whereas repeated failures undermine it. Nobody can promise the children that they will succeed in every pursuit. Yet, a firm sense of efficacy that will be built on the basis of past successes will be able to withstand temporary and occasional failures.

(2) *Modeling experience*. Children may establish their self-efficacy beliefs not only on the basis of their own activities, but also through observing others' performance on the tasks. Thus, modeling may serve as another effective source of efficacy information.

(3) *Verbal persuasion*. The efficacy beliefs are not always the outcomes of personal experiences. Persuasive communication and evaluative feedback from significant others such as parents, teachers, and good friends may also influence one's judgment of self-efficacy. However, not everyone can convince the children. Verbal persuasion is most effective when provided by people who are considered knowledgeable and credible and when the information is viewed realistic.

(4) *Physiological reactions*. Heightened physiological arousals such as sweating, heartbeats, fatigue, aches, pain, and mood changes also send a feedback signal to children that may affect their self-efficacy appraisal.

In conclusion, self-concept and self-efficacy share many of the presumed antecedents such as past experience, social comparison, and reinforcements from significant people. They also share many of the presumed outcomes related to cognitive, affective, and behavioral functioning. However, there are also differences in how they are conceptualized (Bong & Skaalvik, 2003). The central element of social self-concept is the perceived competence in the social relation domain, while the central element in social self-efficacy is related to the perceived confidence in the ability to develop the desired social relations. The social self-concept is a stable trait, based on past experience, while social self-efficacy is considered more flexible and changeable, based on past experience, but includes future oriented beliefs. An additional personal characteristic that was widely examined as a protective and immunization factor when confronted with the risk of loneliness, was the hope related to future expectations.

Developmental Challenges

Children with developmental challenges are aware of their day-to-day struggles and often report lower self-concepts and decreased self-efficacy. Studies examined children with different difficulties, such as children with high incidence disabilities, (i.e., learning disabilities (LD), emotional and behavioral disorders (EBD), and mild mental retardation (MR)). Overall, research reported that many children with difficulties and disabilities, compared with peers without disabilities, experienced higher levels of depression and lower self-concepts. Many were lonelier and at greater risks for poor adult outcomes. Children with attention deficit and hyperactivity described their symptomatic behaviors, detailing their ambivalence and confusion as they tried to reconcile the internal experiences of their bodies with the impact of their behaviors in the world. They described their internal "jumpiness" or "craziness" saying, "It's crazy, like there are lots of people inside me". . . . Children expressed fear, sadness and social exclusion in relation to all these worries: "I'm always in trouble because of how I behave and it makes me sad."

Many of these children failed at school due to their learning or behavior disabilities, and questioned their overall self-worth (Bakker, Denessen, Bosman, Krijger, &

Bouts, 2007; Bear, Minke, Griffin, & Deemer, 1998; Margalit, 2006; Singh, 2007). Primary factors may predispose these children to the loneliness experience, and secondary self-related or situational variables may maintain or reinforce it. These factors may include in addition to academic challenges, the extent to which the child fails to develop meaningful social relations, to bridge interpersonal space, and to cope with feelings of being excluded and different from others in their educational and social environments. The personal characteristics and difficulties among children with developmental challenges not only may predispose them to loneliness, but also may render it more difficult for them to cope with feelings of loneliness.

For example, in a meta-analysis of 15 studies on depression and students with learning disabilities, results indicated that these students had significantly higher depression scores and displayed lower self-concepts than did students without disabilities (Maag & Reid, 2006; Montague, Enders, Dietz, Dixon, & Cavendish, 2008). Similarly, children with emotional difficulties also experienced more loneliness, hopelessness, low self-esteem, and anxiety (Ammerman, Kazdin, & Hasselt, 1993). Indeed children with developmental challenges are at risk for developing loneliness. However, many youngsters did not report lower self-perceptions than their typically developing peers. Personal strengths, supportive homes, and school environments, as well as positive future expectations may contribute to their resilience. In every chapter of this book, a special section will be devoted to this heterogeneous group of children.

Future Expectations and Hope

Expectancies can be defined as beliefs that we hold about our future. Our deliberate actions depend not only on our past experiences, but also on our future expectations and on our assumptions about how the environment will react in response to our actions. Effort investment and persistence of behavior are assumed to depend significantly on the individual's expectation to do well in a given task (Dickhauser & Reinhard, 2008). Hope is an internal process linked to the experience of meaning and awareness of possibilities. This awareness releases energy and activates thoughts and feelings, enabling the person to make meaningful choices and to set goals promoting expectations of positive outcomes (Benzein, Saveman, & Norberg, 2000).

Indeed past experiences structure our current activities in many ways. Children and adolescents carry with them a mental map of the preschool and school settings drawn according to both: outside – what it was like in these social settings, and inside – how the child handled and experienced them. Home and school impacts are intertwined in these influential inner images. The tremendous importance that children attributed to being with other children affected their experiences and behavior (Torstenson-Ed, 2007). The amount of effort that adolescents invested in their studies at school was predicted by their specific and global self-evaluation, by their social distress (loneliness), and by their hope for achieving future goals. These relations were similar for children with typical achievements as well as for children with developmental difficulties. Considering the importance of the hope conceptualization, especially for understanding coping efforts and planning effective intervention, a survey of research will be provided to emphasize the hope's significance in socialization development.

Snyder, Cheavens, and Sympson (1997) suggested that humans build pathway and agentic thoughts almost from the time of their birth. He proposed that pathway thoughts are related to

(a) The sensing and perceiving of external stimuli,
(b) The learning of temporal linkages between events, and
(c) The forming of goals.

In his writings he specified that in pathways thinking, infants form perceptions of "what is out there," and they learn that certain events co-occur temporally. The infants begin to recognize their needs and to focus on the particular goals that satisfy these needs. Gradually they acquire the basic processes necessary for pathway thinking through learning linkages to goals.

Snyder considered the agentic thinking, as composed of

(a) Self-recognition,
(b) The perception of one's self as the originator of actions, and
(c) The forming of goals.

Barriers play a particularly important role in the development of differences in hope. Barriers produce negative emotions, especially when a child encounters profound blockages. However, the successful pursuit of goals tends to produce positive emotions, especially when barriers are overcome. Through the encouragement of role models (e.g., parents, teachers, or friends), high-hope children learn to find and maintain pathway and agentic thoughts for their goals in the face of barriers. They develop resiliency as a mental health immunization and high-hope thinking often results from successfully overcoming impediments. Thus, high-hope children may actually be protected when they encounter subsequent difficulties.

As children grow up, their life experiences multiply as well, requiring a more complex understanding of their place in the world. They may develop new schemas that reflect their new roles in different life areas with a more context-related sense of hope that differentiates their approach to different circumstances and challenges. Although all people have an overall generalized sense of hope, their specific hopes varies in different situations and environment. An interesting illustration to the differences between high hope's and low hope's students was provided by Snyder. Even good students get low grades from time to time. However, high hope's students treat them differently than low hope's students. The students in the first group, when receiving low grades, often view them as a challenge to work harder and get better ones. In the same situation, low hope's students are often ready to give up. High hope's students enjoy competition because it enables them to test their skills and their ability to invest efforts. Thus, high-hope individuals are effective in goal achievement, but in addition, they also gain pleasure from the process of getting there. They are able to break long-range goals into sub-goals and to enjoy each step (Snyder et al., 1997). High-hope students realize that nobody can avoid mistakes in the pursuit of their goals, but they remain mentally energized (i.e., agentic thinking) and view mistakes as potential clues to find what will work for them (i.e., pathway thinking). Snyder, Cheavens and Sympson concluded (1997) that to embrace the goal pursuit process entails an enjoyment of the sense of personal mastery that comes with the various sub-steps on the way to some larger goal pursuit activity. This pleasure is reinforced by supporting parents and teachers who value the achievements.

Similar processes were conceptualized with regard to the relations of hope development with socialization processes. As children develop, they learn that their desires must operate in the context of a larger group. Children start expressing their hopes by saying "I want. . ." but they soon find out that what they desire may involve other people. As an example, children gradually learn that one can get help toward achieving personal goals if they are ready to reciprocate by helping other children or adults. Additionally, children learn to convince others to help them in achieving their goals. Furthermore, children learn to accept goals that reflect compromises between others and themselves. High-hope children enjoy their interactions with others, they are able to take the perspectives of others, and this probably enables them to interact more easily and to perceive available social support. Furthermore, high hopers are not anxious about their social interactions. For example, high-hope young adults reported that, as children, they formed attachments to their parents and had effective role models for successful social interactions (Snyder et al., 1997). Learning in school cannot be separated from the social interpersonal life. They are intertwined in the children's life world and show the critical role of the current perceptions for future expectations (Torstenson-Ed, 2007).

Why do high-hope students do better than their low-hope counterparts? Part of the answer lies in the benefits derived by finding multiple pathways to desired educational goals, as well as being able to motivate oneself to invest effort in those goals. Another part of the answer to this question probably relates to high-hope students staying on task and attending to the appropriate cues in particular learning environments (Onwurgbuzie & Snyder, 2000). Children, who are raised in an environment that lacks boundaries, consistency, and support, are at risk for failing to learn hopeful thinking. The boundaries and consistency represent a rule structure for determining when it is or is not appropriate to engage in goal-directed behaviors. !!!Children's hopes were related to depression and loneliness (inverse relations with hope) and perceived competency and control (positive correlations with hope) (Snyder et al., 1997). An additional example to the impact of developmental challenges on hope was provided by research on learning disabilities.

Children and adolescents with academic difficulties revealed lower levels of hope and decreased effort (Kotzer & Margalit, 2007; Lackaye & Margalit, 2006). Figure 2.1 presents the comparisons between adolescents with learning disabilities and a comparison group of adolescents with typical development (based on data from Lackaye, Margalit, Ziv, & Ziman, 2006), demonstrating that adolescents with

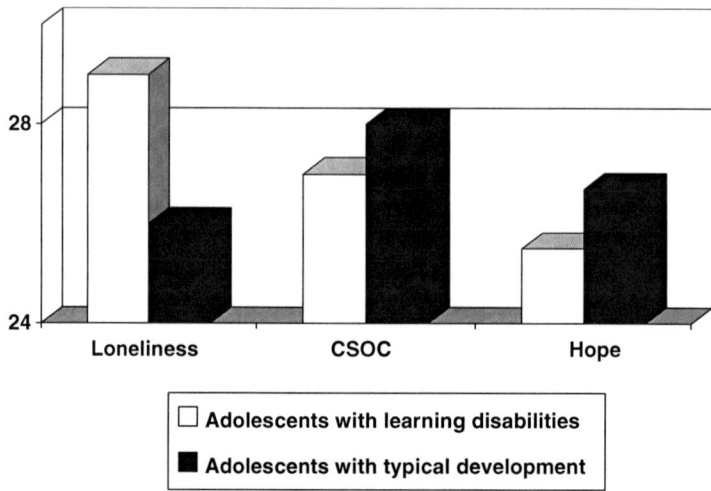

Fig. 2.1 Comparisons between two groups of adolescents

learning disabilities reported lower levels of hope as well as a decreased sense of coherence and increased loneliness.

Future perceptions are, in fact, the extension of the current activities. Thus interventions that will target planned and structured training to articulate goals may enhance children's hope. The goals' pursuits often interact with positive and negative emotions, affecting the readiness to invest effort in academic and social challenges (Aarts, Custers, & Holland, 2007). More detailed intervention approaches will be presented in Chapter 8. In conclusion, the comparisons of the self-perceptions among children and adolescents and their relations to loneliness revealed that all these different variables not only captured different aspects of self-valuation, but they also predicted different outcomes. Self-concept reflects evaluations of self-worth and competence, hope reflects individuals' evaluations of the extent they can achieve their goals (Snyder et al., 2002), and attribution style reflects their beliefs regarding the causes for positive and negative events in their life. Hope theory emphasizes future expectancies (e.g., setting goals), whereas attribution style focuses on explanations of the past (Snyder et al., 2002).

Several longitudinal studies revealed the predictive power of hope. High school students in Australia were followed for 2 years. Children with high hope tended to achieve social acceptance, in addition to their scholastic competence (Ciarrochi, Heaven, & Davies, 2007). Hope was the best predictor for academic achievements, lower ratings of behavioral problems, and increases in positive affect. Similar results were reported in an additional longitudinal study (Arnau, Rosen, Finch, Rhudy, & Fortunato, 2007). Similarly, research that rated 135 Mexican youth (Edwards, Ong, & Lopez, 2007) found that the hope scores were positively correlated with measures of positive affect, life satisfaction, support from family and friends, and optimism. In summary, important determinants for social performance and loneliness distress are the individuals' global and specific self-perceptions of abilities and difficulties as well as their hopes for the future. If individuals believe that they can perform the task, they will have higher expectancies compared to individuals with low self-perceptions of ability.

Conclusions and Implications

This chapter explored the personal characteristics of lonely children. Before starting the discussion it was important to clarify that children's reports of their loneliness are valid and reflect their comprehension from early developmental stages. Their needs for relatedness and social networking can be identified even before entering the first grade. They understand what loneliness is, and gradually learn to define it and differentiate it from solitude. In this chapter the genetic roots of loneliness were presented within a dynamic model that considered the genetic vulnerability as an increased risk within a wide range of interacting risk and protective factors. Children's temperament, emotional style, and emotion regulation continuously interact with personal strengths and difficulties. Since loneliness is a subjective experience, special importance was provided to different self-perceptions and their predictive power. The differentiation between global self-perceptions, such as Sense of Coherence, social self-concept, social self-efficacy beliefs, hope expectations, and attribution styles, were consistently related to loneliness, yet were interlocked within an interrelated network of traits that were also linked to gender and age.

Special attention was devoted to children with special needs, since a simplistic approach may accentuate the expectation that children whose development is marked with a personal history of failures in highly valued tasks are at an increased risk for lower self-competence, decreased social skills, and a different attribution style to their social difficulties, and experience higher levels of loneliness. However, this approach ignores the complexity of the children's network of personality variables, their strengths, their future hopes, and resilience trends.

Loneliness and companionship can be treated as both personal and interpersonal experiences. Individual traits and contextual components jointly and dynamically contribute to human's connections and relations. In addition to research on the personal characteristics related to loneliness, the impact of ecological factors has received major research attention. The study of children's loneliness requires the consideration of environmental conditions that promote or limit the child's abilities and the likelihood of experiencing satisfying human relations. The next chapter will focus on the family context.

References

Aarts, H., Custers, R., & Holland, R. W. (2007). The nonconscious cessation of goal pursuit: When goals and negative affect are coactivated. *Journal of Personality and Social Psychology, 92*(2), 165–178.

Ammerman, R. T., Kazdin, A. E., & Hasselt, V. B. V. (1993). Correlates of loneliness in non-referred and psychiatrically hospitalized children. *Journal of Child and Family Studies, 2*(3), 187–202.

Anderson, C. A. (1999). Attributional style, depression, and loneliness: A cross-cultural comparison of American and Chinese students. *Personality Social Psychology Bulletin, 25*(4), 482–499.

Antonovsky, A. (1993). The implications of Salutogenesis: An outsider's view. In A. P. Turnbull, J. M. Patterson, S. K. Behr, D. L. Murphy, J. G. Marquis, & M. J. Blue-Banning (Eds.), *Cognitive coping, families and disabilities* (pp. 111–122). Baltimore: Paul Brooks.

Arnau, R. C., Rosen, D. H., Finch, J. F., Rhudy, J. L., & Fortunato, V. J. (2007). Longitudinal effects of hope on depression and anxiety: A latent variable analysis. *Journal of Personality, 75*(1), 43–64.

Asher, S. R., & Paquette, J. A. (2003). Loneliness and peer relations in childhood. *Current Directions in Psychological Sciences, 12*(3), 75–78.

Asher, S. R., Parkhurst, J. T., Hymel, S., & Williams, G. A. (1990). Peer rejection and loneliness in childhood. In S. R. Asher & J. D. Coie (Eds.), *Peer rejection in childhood* (pp. 253–273). Cambridge: University Press.

Bagner, D. M., Storch, E. A., & Roberti, J. W. (2004). A factor analytic study of the loneliness and social dissatisfaction scale in a sample of African-American and Hispanic-American Children. *Child Psychiatry and Human Development, 34*(3), 237–250.

Bakker, J. T. A., Denessen, E., Bosman, A. M. T., Krijger, E. M., & Bouts, L. (2007). Sociometric status and self-image of children with specific and general learning disabilities in Dutch general and special education classes. *Learning Disability Quarterly, 30*(1), 47–63.

Bandura, A. (1982). Self-efficacy mechanism in human agency. *American Psychologist, 37*(2), 122–147.

Bandura, A. (1986). *Social foundations of thought and action: A social cognitive theory.* Englewood Cliffs, NJ: Prentice-Hall.

Bandura, A. (1997). *Self-efficacy: The exercise of control.* New York: Freeman.

Bandura, A., & Bussey, K. (2004). On broadening the cognitive, motivational, and sociostructural scope of theorizing about gender development and functioning: Comment on Martin, Ruble, and Szkrybalo. *Psychological Bulletin, 130*(5), 691–701.

Bartels, M., Cacioppo, J. T., Hudziak, J. J., & Boomsma, D. I. (2008). Genetic and environmental contributions to stability in loneliness throughout childhood. *American Journal of Medical Genetics Part B: Neuropsychiatric Genetics, 147B*(3), 385–391.

Baumeister, R., & Leary, M. R. (1995). The need to belong: Desire for interpersonal attachments as a fundamental human motivation. *Psychological Bulletin, 117*(3), 497–529.

Baumeister, R. F. (1999, August). *Bad is stronger than good.* Paper presented at the Annual convention of the American Psychological Association, Boston.

Baumeister, R. F., Muraven, M., & Tice, D. M. (2000). Ego depletion: A resource model of volition, self-regulation and controlled processing. *Social Cognition, 18*(2), 130–150.

Baumeister, R. F., Vohs, K. D., DeWall, C. N., & Zhang, L. Q. (2007). How emotion shapes behavior: Feedback, anticipation, and reflection, rather than direct causation. *Personality and Social Psychology Review, 11*(2), 167–203.

Bear, G. G., Minke, K. M., Griffin, S. M., & Deemer, S. A. (1998). Achievement-related perceptions of children with learning disabilities and normal achievement: Group and developmental differences. *Journal of Learning Disabilities, 31*(1), 91–104.

Belsky, J., Bakermans-Kranenburg, M. J., & van IJzendoorn, M. H. (2007). For better and for worse: Differential susceptibility to environmental influences. *Current Directions in Psychological Science, 16*(6), 300–304.

Belsky, J., & Pluess, M. (2009). The nature (and nurture?) of plasticity in early human development. *Perspectives on Psychological Science, 4*(4), 345–351.

Benzein, E. G., Saveman, B. I., & Norberg, A. (2000). The meaning of hope in healthy, nonreligious Swedes. *Western Journal of Nursing Research, 22*(3), 303–319.

Blazina, C., Eddins, R., Burridge, A., & Settle, A. G. (2007). The relationship between masculinity ideology, loneliness, and separation-individuation difficulties. *Journal of Men's Studies, 15*(1), 101–109.

Bong, M., & Skaalvik, E. M. (2003). Academic self-concept and self-efficacy: How different are they really. *Educational Psychology Review, 15*(1), 1–40.

Boomsma, D., Cacioppo, J., Slagboom, P., & Posthuma, D. (2006). Genetic linkage and association analysis for loneliness in Dutch twin and sibling pairs points to a region on chromosome 12q23-24. *Behavior Genetics, 36*(1), 137–146.

Boomsma, D., Willemsen, G., Dolan, C., Hawkley, L., & Cacioppo, J. (2005). Genetic and environmental contributions to loneliness in adults: The Netherlands twin register study. *Behavior Genetics, 35*(6), 745–752.

Booth-Laforce, C., Oh, W., Kim, A., Rubin, K., Rose-Krasnor, L., & Burgess, K. (2006). Attachment, self-worth, and peer-group functioning in middle childhood. *Attachment & Human Development, 8*(4), 309–325.

Brown, N. R., Williams, R. L., Barker, E. T., & Galambos, N. L. (2007). Estimating frequencies of emotions and actions: A web-based diary study. *Applied Cognitive Psychology, 21*(2), 259–276.

Burgess, K. B., Ladd, G. W., Kochenderfer, B. J., Lambert, S. F., & Birch, S. H. (1999). Loneliness during early childhood: The role of interpersonal behaviors and relationships. In K. J. Rotenberg & S. Hymel (Eds.), *Loneliness in childhood and adolescence* (pp. 109–134). New York: Cambridge University Press.

Cacioppo, J. T., Hawkley, L. C., Ernst, J. M., Burleson, M., Berntson, G. G., Nouriani, B., et al. (2006). Loneliness within a nomological net: An evolutionary perspective. *Journal of Research in Personality, 40*(6), 1054–1085.

Chen, X., & French, D. C. (2008). Children's social competence in cultural context. *Annual Review of Psychology, 59*, 591–616.

Chipuer, H. (2004). Australian children's understanding of loneliness. *Australian Journal of Psychology, 56*(3), 147–153.

Ciarrochi, J., Heaven, P. C. L., & Davies, F. (2007). The impact of Hope, self-esteem, and attributional style on adolescents' school grades and emotional well-being: A longitudinal study. *Journal of Research in Personality, 41*(6), 1161–1178.

Cole, P. M., Luby, J., & Sullivan, M. W. (2008). Emotions and the development of childhood depression: Bridging the gap. *Child Development Perspectives, 2*(3), 141–148.

Cole, P. M., Martin, S. E., & Dennis, T. A. (2004). Emotion regulation as a scientific construct: Methodological challenges and directions for child development research. *Child Development, 75*(2), 317–333.

Coplan, R. J., Closson, L. M., & Arbeau, K. A. (2007). Gender differences in the behavioral associates of loneliness and social dissatisfaction in kindergarten. *Journal of Child Psychology and Psychiatry, 48*(10), 988–995.

Coplan, R. J., Findlay, L. C., & Nelson, L. J. (2004). Characteristics of preschoolers with lower perceived competence. *Journal of Abnormal Child Psychology, 32*(4), 399–408.

Coplan, R. J., Girardi, A., Findlay, L. C., & Frohlick, S. L. (2007). Understanding solitude: Young children's attitudes and responses toward hypothetical socially withdrawn peers. *Social Development, 16*(3), 390–409.

Crick, N., & Dodge, K. A. (1994). A review and reformulation of information-processing mechanisms in children's social adjustment. *Psychological Bulletin, 115*(1), 74–101.

Crocker, J., Brook, A. T., Niiya, Y., & Villacorta, M. (2006). The pursuit of self-esteem: Contingencies of self-worth and self-regulation. *Journal of Personality, 74*(6), 1749–1772.

Denham, S. A., Wyatt, T. M., Bassett, H. H., Echeverria, D., & Knox, S. S. (2009). Assessing social-emotional development in children from a longitudinal perspective. *Journal of Epidemiology and Community Health, 63*, 137–152.

Dickhauser, O., & Reinhard, M. A. (2008). The effects of affective states on the formation of performance expectancies. *Cognition & Emotion, 22*(8), 1542–1554.

Edwards, L. M., Ong, A. D., & Lopez, S. J. (2007). Hope measurement in Mexican American youth. *Hispanic Journal of Behavioral Sciences, 29*(2), 225–242.

Efrati-Virtzer, M., & Margalit, M. (2009). Students' behaviour difficulties, sense of coherence and adjustment at school: Risk and protective factors. *European Journal of Special Needs Education*, 24(1), 59–73.

Eisenberg, N. (2000). Emotion, regulation, and moral development. *Annual Review of Psychology*, 51(1), 665–697.

Eisenberg, N., & Fabes, R. A. (1992). Emotion, regulation, and the development of social competence. In M. S. Clark (Ed.), *Review of personality and social psychology* (Vol. 14, pp. 119–150). Newbury Park, CA: Sage.

Findlay, L. C., Coplan, R. J., & Bowker, A. (2009). Keeping it all inside: Shyness, internalizing coping strategies and socio-emotional adjustment in middle childhood. *International Journal of Behavioral Development*, 33(1), 47–54.

Forgas, J. P. (1991). *Emotion and social judgment*. Oxford: Pergamon.

Forgas, J. P. (1995). Mood and judgment: The affect infusion model (AIM). *Psychological Bulletin*, 116(1), 39–66.

Fox, N. A., Hane, A. A., & Pine, D. S. (2007). Plasticity for affective neurocircuitry: How the environment affects gene expression. *Current Directions in Psychological Science*, 16(1), 1–5.

Fredrickson, B. L., & Joiner, T. (2002). Positive emotions trigger upward spirals toward emotional well-being. *Psychological Science*, 13(2), 172–175.

Frijda, N., & Sundararajan, L. (2007). Emotion refinement: A theory inspired by Chinese poetics. *Perspectives on Psychological Science*, 2(3), 227–241.

Galanaki, E. P. (2004). Are children able to distinguish among the concepts of aloneness, loneliness, and solitude? *International Journal of Behavioral Development*, 28(5), 435–443.

Gazelle, H. (2008). Behavioral profiles of anxious solitary children and heterogeneity in peer relations. *Developmental Psychology*, 44(6), 1604–1624.

Goldsmith, H. H., Pollak, S. D., & Davidson, R. J. (2008). Developmental neuroscience perspectives on emotion regulation. *Child Development Perspectives*, 2(3), 132–140.

Goodvin, R., Meyer, S., Thompson, R. A., & Hayes, R. (2008). Self-understanding in early childhood: Associations with child attachment security and maternal negative affect. *Attachment & Human Development*, 10(4), 433–450.

Gresham, F. M. (1986). Conceptual and definitional issues in the assessment of children's social skills: Implications for classification and training. *Journal of Clinical Child Psychology*, 15(1), 3–15.

Gresham, F. M., & Elliott, S. N. (1990). *Social skills rating system manual*. Circle Pines, MN: American Guidance Services.

Han, E., & Choi, N. (2006). Korean institutionalized adolescents' attributions of success and failure in interpersonal relations and perceived loneliness. *Children and Youth Services Review*, 28(5), 535–547.

Hayes, A. M., Laurenceau, J. P., Feldman, G., Strauss, J. L., & Cardaciotto, L. (2007). Change is not always linear: The study of nonlinear and discontinuous patterns of change in psychotherapy. *Clinical Psychology Review*, 27(6), 715–723.

Henwood, P. G., & Solano, C. H. (1994). Loneliness in young children and their parents. *Journal of Genetic Psychology*, 155(1), 35–46.

Honkinen, P. L., Aromaa, M., Suominen, S., Rautava, P., Sourander, A., Helenius, H., et al. (2009). Early childhood psychological problems predict a poor Sense of Coherence in adolescents: A 15-year follow-up study. *Journal of Health Psychology*, 14(4), 587–600.

Honkinen, P. L., Suominen, S. B., Välimaa, R. S., Helenius, H. Y., & Rautava, P. T. (2005). Factors associated with perceived health among 12-year-old school children. Relevance of physical exercise and sense of coherence. *Scandinavian Journal of Public Health*, 33(1), 35–41.

Hymel, S., Tarulli, D., Hayden Thomson, L., & Terrell-Deutsch, B. (1999). Loneliness through the eyes of children. In K. J. Rotenberg & S. Hymel (Eds.), *Loneliness in childhood and adolescence* (pp. 80–106). New York: Cambridge University Press.

Ittyerah, M., & Kumar, N. (2007). The actual and ideal self-concept in disabled children, adolescents and adults. *Psychology Developing Societies*, 19(1), 81–112.

Iverson, A. M., & Eichler, J. B. (1992, August). *Predicting children's loneliness: Quantity and quality of friendships*. Paper presented at the Annual convention of the American Psychological Association, Washington, DC.

Izard, C., Stark, K., Trentacosta, C., & Schultz, D. (2008). Beyond emotion regulation: Emotion utilization and adaptive functioning. *Child Development Perspectives, 2*(3), 156–163.

Jellesma, F. C., Rieffe, C., Terwogt, M. M., & Kneepkens, C. M. F. (2006). Somatic complaints and health care use in children: Mood, emotion awareness and sense of coherence. *Social Science & Medicine, 63*(10), 2640–2648.

Kirova, A. (2003). Accessing children's experiences of loneliness through conversations. *Field Methods, 15*(1), 3–24.

Koole, S. L. (2009). The psychology of emotion regulation: An integrative review. *Cognition & Emotion, 23*(1), 4–41.

Kotzer, E., & Margalit, M. (2007). Perception of competence: Risk and protective predictors following an e-self-advocacy intervention for adolescents with learning disabilities. *European Journal of Special Needs Education, 22*(4), 443–457.

Kovacs, M., Joormann, J., & Gotlib, I. H. (2008). Emotion (dys)regulation and links to depressive disorders. *Child Development Perspectives, 2*(3), 149–155.

Lackaye, T., & Margalit, M. (2006). Comparisons of achievement, effort and self-perceptions among students with learning disabilities and their peers from different achievement groups. *Journal of Learning Disabilities, 39*(5), 432–446.

Lackaye, T., Margalit, M., Ziv, O., & Ziman, T. (2006). Comparisons of self-efficacy, mood, effort, and hope between students with learning disabilities and their non-LD-matched peers. *Learning Disabilities Research & Practice, 21*(2), 111–121.

Larson, R. W. (1990). The solitary side of life: An examination of the time people spend alone from childhood to old age. *Developmental Review, 10*(2), 155–183.

Larson, R. W. (1997). The emergence of solitude as a constructive domain of experience in early adolescence. *Child Development, 68*(1), 80–94.

Long, C. R., & Averill, J. R. (2003). Solitude: An exploration of benefits of being alone. *Journal for the Theory of Social Behaviour, 33*(1), 21–44.

Lopes, P. N., Salovey, P., Cote, S., & Beers, M. (2005). Emotion regulation abilities and the quality of social interaction. *Emotion, 5*(1), 113–118.

Luftig, R. L. (1988). Assessment of perceived school loneliness and isolation of mentally retarded and nonretarded students. *American Journal of Mental Retardation, 92*(5), 472–475.

Lunt, P. K. (1991). The perceived causal structure of loneliness. *Journal of Personality and Social Psychology, 61*(1), 26–34.

Maag, J. W., & Reid, R. (2006). Depression among students with learning disabilities: Assessing the risk. *Journal of Learning Disabilities, 39*(1), 3–11.

Margalit, M. (1994). *Loneliness among children with special needs: Theory, research, coping and intervention*. New York: Springer.

Margalit, M. (1998). Loneliness and coherence among preschool children with learning disabilities. *Journal of Learning Disabilities, 31*(2), 173–180.

Margalit, M. (1999). Resiliente kinder mit lernstorungen (Resilient children with learning disabilities). In G. Opp, M. Fingerle, & A. Freytag (Eds.), *Was kinder starkt – erziehung zwischen risiko und resilienz* (pp. 204–220). Munchen: Reinhardt Verlag.

Margalit, M. (2006). Loneliness, the Salutogenic paradigm and LD: Current research, future directions and interventional implications. *Thalamus, 24*(1), 38–48.

Margalit, M., & Al-Yagon, M. (2002). The loneliness experience of children with learning disabilities. In B. Y. L. Wong & M. Donahue (Eds.), *The social dimensions of learning disabilities* (pp. 53–75). Mahwah, NJ: Lawrence Erlbaum.

Margalit, M., & Ben-Dov, I. (1995). Learning disabilities and social environments: Kibbutz versus city comparisons of loneliness and social competence. *International Journal of Behavioral Development, 18*(3), 519–536.

Margalit, M., Mioduser, D., Al-Yagon, M., & Neuberger, S. (1997). Teachers' and peers' perceptions of children with learning disorders: Consistency and change. *European Journal of Special
Needs Education, 12*(3), 225–238.
Marsh, S. C., Clinkinbeard, S. S., Thomas, R. M., & Evans, W. P. (2007). Risk and protective
factors predictive of sense of coherence during adolescence. *Journal of Health Psychology,
12*(2), 281–284.
McGuire, S., & Clifford, J. (2000). Genetic and environmental contributions to loneliness in
children. *Psychological Science, 11*(6), 487–491.
Montague, M., Enders, C., Dietz, S., Dixon, J., & Cavendish, W. M. (2008). A longitudinal study
of depressive symptomology and self-concept in adolescents. *Journal of Special Education,
42*(2), 67–78.
Newall, N. E., Chipperfield, J. G., Clifton, R. A., Perry, R. P., Swift, A. U., & Ruthig, J. C. (2009).
Causal beliefs, social participation, and loneliness among older adults: A longitudinal study.
Journal of Social and Personal Relationships, 26(2–3), 273–290.
Onwurgbuzie, A. J., & Snyder, C. R. (2000). Relations between Hope and graduate students'
coping strategies for studying and examination-taking. *Psychological Reports, 86*(3), 803–806.
Ozer, E. M., & Bandura, A. (1990). Mechanisms governing empowerment effects: A self-efficacy
analysis. *Journal of Personality and Social Psychology, 58*(3), 472–486.
Qualter, P., & Munn, P. (2002). The separateness of social and emotional loneliness in childhood.
Journal of Child Psychology and Psychiatry and Allied Disciplines, 43(2), 233–244.
Rothbart, M. K., Ahadi, S. A., & Ahadi, S. A. (2000). Temperament and personality: Origins and
outcomes. *Journal of Personality and Social Psychology, 78*(1), 122–135.
Rubin, K. H., & Coplan, R. J. (2004). Paying attention to and not neglecting social withdrawal and
social isolation. *Merrill-Palmer Quarterly, 50*, 506–534.
Rubin, K. H., Coplan, R. J., & Bowker, J. C. (2009). Social withdrawal in childhood. *Annual
Review of Psychology, 60*, 1–31.
Rubin, K. H., & Mills, R. S. L. (1988). The many faces of social isolation childhood. *Journal of
Consulting and Clinical Psychology, 56*(6), 916–924.
Rusbult, C. E., & Van Lange, P. A. M. (2003). Interdependence, interaction, and relationships.
Annual Review of Psychology, 54(1), 351–375.
Siegler, R. S. (1996). *Emerging minds. The process of change in children's thinking*. New York:
Oxford press.
Siegler, R. S. (1997). Beyond competence – Toward development. *Cognitive Development, 12*,
323–332.
Singh, I. (2007). Clinical implications of ethical concepts: Moral self-understandings in children
taking Methylphenidate for ADHD. *Clinical Child Psychology and Psychiatry, 12*(2), 167–182.
Skaalvik, E. J. E. P. (1997). Self-enhancing and self-defeating ego orientations: Relations with task
and avoidance orientation, achievement, self-perceptions, and anxiety. *Journal of Educational
Psychology, 89*, 71–81.
Snyder, C. R., Cheavens, J., & Sympson, S. C. (1997). Hope: An individual motive for social
commerce. *Group Dynamics: Theory, Research, and Practice, 1*(2), 107–118.
Snyder, C. R., Feldman, D. B., Shorey, H. S., & Rand, K. L. (2002). Hopeful choices: A school
counselor's guide to hope theory. *Professional School Counseling, 5*(5), 298–308.
Thompson, R. A., Lewis, M. D., & Calkins, S. D. (2008). Reassessing emotion regulation. *Child
Development Perspectives, 2*(3), 124–131.
Tiggemann, M., Winefield, A. H., Winefield, H. R., & Goldney, R. D. (1991). The stability of attri-
butional style and its relation to psychological distress. *British Journal of Clinical Psychology,
30*(3), 247–255.
Toner, M. A., & Heaven, P. C. L. (2005). Peer-social attributional predictors of socio-emotional
adjustment in early adolescence: A two-year longitudinal study. *Personality and Individual
Differences, 38*(3), 579–590.
Torstenson-Ed, T. (2007). Children's life paths through preschool and school: Letting youths talk
about their own childhood – Theoretical and methodological conclusions. *Childhood, 14*(1),
47–66.

Tsai, F. F., & Reis, H. T. (2009). Perceptions by and of lonely people in social networks. *Personal Relationships, 16*(2), 221–238.

Vaughn, S., Zaragoza, N., Hogan, A., & Walker, J. (1993). A four-year longitudinal investigation of the social skills and behavior problems of students with learning disabilities. *Journal of Learning Disabilities, 26*(6), 404–412.

Weiner, B. (1986). *An attributional theory of motivation and emotion.* New York: Springer.

Weiner, B. (2000). Intrapersonal and interpersonal theories of motivation from an attributional perspective. *Educational Psychology Review, 12*(1), 1–14.

Weiner, B. (2004). Attribution theory revisited: Transforming cultural plurality into theoretical unity. In D. M. McInerney & S. Van Etten (Eds.), *Big theories revisited* (pp. 13–30). Greenwich, CT: Information Age Publishing.

Weiner, B. (2008). On theoretical co-existence versus theoretical integration. *European Journal of Psychology of Education, 23*(4), 433–438.

Winnicott, D. W. (1965). The capacity to be alone. In D. W. Winnicott (Ed.), *The maturation processes and the facilitating environment* (pp. 29–36). New York: International Universities Press.

Wrosch, C., Scheier, M. F., Miller, G. E., Schulz, R., & Carver, C. S. (2003). Adaptive self-regulation of unattainable goals: Goal disengagement, goal reengagement, and subjective well-being. *Personality and Social Psychology Bulletin, 29*(12), 1494–1508.

Youngblade, L., Berlin, L. J., & Beslky, J. (1999). Connections among loneliness, the ability to be alone, and peer relationships in young children. In K. J. Rotenberg & S. Hymel (Eds.), *Loneliness in childhood and adolescence* (pp. 135–152). New York: Cambridge University Press.

Chapter 3
Loneliness in the Family

Family studies provide important insights to the understanding of children's and adolescents' loneliness, given that the roots of interpersonal relations and loneliness experiences can be identified within this context. Children learn, construct, and experience their first social understanding in their families. They experiment basic interactions and intimate relations with their parents and siblings. They develop relatedness to their close and extended family system and structure their social identity. Within this context, they experience acceptance and rejection. They acquire close relations, and participate in angry conflicts. They struggle for love and develop trust. Indeed children learn about the complexity of relations in their family, and these early interactions provide them not only with the fundamental knowledge about relations, but also with vital experiences that will serve as the basis for their social growth and peer interactions. The infant's development as a separate individual with a coherent self-identity depends in the beginning of life upon his or her interactions with parental figures. Early socialization processes in the family, with parents, as well as with siblings, gradually shape the child's social behaviors and attitudes. Parenting abilities and vulnerabilities, interpersonal relations, the family climate, and other components of this systemic experience jointly contribute to children's social functioning and development.

In this chapter, the impact of the family environment on children's loneliness will be discussed, including research on early relationships with parents and the development of vulnerability to loneliness. A special section will identify the role of children with chronic difficulties on parents and family dynamics. Multidimensional risk and resilience models will be presented to provide a comprehensive dynamic framework for identifying the complex, interacting circumstances that influence and predict diverse children and family outcomes.

Research proposed that parental psychological resources and difficulties, as well as their own developmental histories, influence their parenting qualities and family climate characteristics, and thereby affect their children's development (Belsky & Barends, 2002; Belsky, 1984). Only for the clarity of the discussion, the different family factors related to children's loneliness will be presented separately. Nevertheless, throughout this chapter we have to remember that there is not a single characteristic of persons and environments that affect children's development and

M. Margalit, *Lonely Children and Adolescents*, DOI 10.1007/978-1-4419-6284-3_3,
© Springer Science+Business Media, LLC 2010

adaptation. Loneliness will be considered in this chapter within systemic models, reflecting the ongoing joint impact of three groups of factors:

(1) The parents' characteristics,
(2) The child's characteristics, and
(3) The different contextual conditions.

In the first part of this chapter, the relations between early social experiences and children's later thinking and feeling about themselves in their social world will be presented within the context of (a) the attachment theory and (b) the family systemic models.

Attachment

Numerous studies focused interest in the early dyadic relations between parents and their infants – exploring the attachment paradigm as the basis for learning, self-identity, the development of intimacy, and the roots of loneliness. Before discussing the current research, the attachment construct will be characterized.

What Is Attachment?

Attachment has been defined as an interactive process in which mother (or father) and infant affect one another, thus reflecting the quality of the emotional ties within the mother–child unit (Winnicott, 1965). It refers to the experience of togetherness and emotional linkage – the assurance that, if needed, intimacy and closeness will be available. The conceptualization of the loneliness experience has been consistently related to the attachment conceptualization. According to the attachment paradigm, infants become attached to adults who take care of them (usually parents) and are sensitive and responsive to their needs. The infants have a basic innate need for a secure relationship with adult caregivers. Attachment conceptualization has been considered an active process of getting closer to someone, actually or symbolically, in order to reduce anxiety (Josselson, 1992). This model enhances awareness to the togetherness concept within the family as the roots for later interpersonal intimacy.

Through this connection, the infant gradually develops mental representations of people and relationships, or as named by Bowlby, "internal working models." These representations are interpretive filters for social perceptions, expectations, and memories that cause children to approach social situations and social partners in specific manners, based on the security of their attachment during their infancy (Bowlby, 1969; Raikes & Thompson, 2008).

Basic assumptions have been identified in the formation of these internal working models (Fivush, 2006; Keller, 2008):

1. Internal working models emerge from earlier experiences, based on actual care-giving behaviors.
2. Internal working models are reasonably stable over time. However, they will become gradually more elaborated, flexible, and adaptable to specific contexts (i.e., at first the infant learns that if he cries, his mother will leave everything and come running. Gradually he learns that usually his mother will come. But if she is angry, tired, or very busy, she will not come to alleviate his distress).
3. Internal working models are generalized representations; they provide general models of self, other, and the world.
4. Internal working models may be transmitted across generations. It means that securely attached mothers have a higher probability of having securely attached infants who grow up to be securely attached mothers and fathers with their own infants and so on.

Attachment research has confirmed associations between early attachment and later outcomes of children's self-concept, emotional understanding, and social relations, revealing children's working models of the self in addition to interpersonal relationships. The quality of infant–parent attachment and interactions has been consistently associated with the later development of satisfactory interactions with peers (Sroufe, Egeland, Carlson, & Collins, 2005). Before presenting the attachment research related to children's loneliness, parental anxious self-questioning will be exemplified.

During many of my lectures, after learning the importance of early relations with their children, fathers and mothers often asked worriedly: "Can we change these early experiences?" Some parents further share their distress, providing more details to their anxious reflections: "We were young parents, inexperienced, preoccupied, and/or stressed and probably made many mistakes. Can we change the situation?" The current chapter and the chapters on coping and intervention present insights from family studies in order to point at directions for explaining how children learn to form connectedness, when do they experience loneliness, and most importantly, how can parents change early patterns of social relations, based on the plasticity paradigms. But first, several additional basic concepts have to be explained.

Secure-Base Behavior

The concept of the secure-base behavior has been a central tenet of the attachment theory, calling attention to the interplay of individuality and exploration needs, together with the basic human needs for relatedness and closeness. This terminology – the "Secure base" – was proposed by Bowlby (1988), who considered the role of care giving to a baby in terms used to describe an army officer who provides "a secure base" to his soldiers. The "secure base" is the place ". . . from which an expeditionary force sets out and to which it can retreat, should it meet with a setback. Much of the time, the role of the base is a waiting one, but it is none the less vital for that. For it is only when the officer commanding the expeditionary force is confident his base is secure that he dare press forward and take risks" (p. 11). Similarly, individuals (babies, as well as children and adults) who believe that they have "a secure base" that is there for them, can "make sorties into the outside world" (p. 11), knowing that they can return for comfort, reassurance, and/or supportive assistance if they encounter difficulties along the way.

Winnicott (1965) identified the roots of loneliness in the interplay between attachment relations and the ability to stay alone. The mother (and/or the father) provides "a secure base" for the baby, enabling (and even encouraging) him/her to explore the environment while feeling safe in her presence. Paradoxically, during typical development, infants can develop their separate identity when they have confidence in the existence of the adults' connections and support. Winnicott assumed that in order to move away from the mother (or the father), to develop separateness, and to use this ability for actively exploring the environment, the baby must have already internalized a sense of feeling close to the parent and protected, even when physically he (or she) is not close. The basis of the capacity to stay alone is the experience of being alone in the presence of a reliable individual who provides an ego-support. The development of this capacity to stay alone is also related to children's ability to get in touch with themselves, to discover what they need or want, irrespective of what others expect from them, and to be able to express their inner feelings. Thus, the capacity to be alone may be conceptualized as a sign of inner security, rather than as an expression of a withdrawn state.

Individuals who lack confidence in the availability of their caregivers, anxiously attempt to remain in close proximity to their caregivers in order to ensure that the dependable adults are available when needed (Bowlby, 1973). Separation from the caregivers may be experienced by them as initiating loneliness and may reduce their wishes to explore their environment. Through repeated daily experiences, individuals learn that their attachment figures are accessible, available, and responsive when needed. Bowlby (1969) hypothesized that by 3 years old, children had begun to develop generalized representations of the caregiver as supportive or unsupportive, and of the self as worthy or unworthy, based on repeated experiences with the caregiver across a variety of situations. It can be concluded that individuals, whose caregivers have been emotionally available, especially during periods of stress, construct internal working models of the self as worthy, the others as trusting and relationships as worthwhile, pleasant and important. Conversely, individuals with a history of caregiver insensitivity or emotional unavailability, construct negative working models of the self, others, and relationships.

These attachment models are expected to color the individual's approach to relationships and views of the self throughout the lifespan (Bowlby, 1988). Through the formation of expectations and the filtering of the individuals' cognitive processing, such as their attention and memory, they affect the development of interpersonal interactions (McElwain, Booth-LaForce, Lansford, Wu, & Dyer, 2008). A child who has received repeated rejection and hostility from attachment figures may be at risk of expecting similar treatment from others. Children who do not develop secured attachment, will have lower trust and may provide aggressive and anxious explanations to ambiguous social situations. Patterns of verbal and nonverbal communication between the caregivers and the children, especially about emotions, are important to the development and maintenance of these expectations, which are gradually supported by the children's rapidly growing language and cognitive skills, and by interactions outside home (Thompson, 2000).

Parental Perceptions and Behavior

Studies attempted to find out why parents behave differently toward their infants. What are the roots of their attachment styles? Individual differences in the quality and/or effectiveness of infant–caregiver attachment relationships were considered largely the product of the history of the parents' interactions with their own parents, and the variations in attachment quality were the foundation for future individual differences (Bowlby, 1969). Parents' behavior emerged from their beliefs and expectations that were structured during their development. Many times we hear boys and girls who state that they will not behave toward their children similarly to their parents. At the same time you can hear many fathers and mothers who will recognize unhappily that they are treating their children similarly to their parents, even though they were determined to be different. Parental history is reflected in their parenting attachment, but the concept of attachment is not linear, nor deterministic. Bowlby proposed a nonlinear conceptualization, a transactional model, in which every partner (the parent and the infant) in the interaction affects and is affected by the behavior of the other. The mother–child dyad can be considered as a nonlinear dynamic system, since the developmental outcomes are determined by the mutual relations between partners. Thus, even small changes may sometimes produce complex effects and the outcomes may not be proportional to the experiences, and can lead to different developmental directions (Olthof, Kunnen, & Jan, 2000).

Mothers and fathers approach their newborn baby with certain assumptions and beliefs about the infant's needs and abilities, and also with their own priorities and competencies as parents. Their expectations and convictions are reinforced by signals from the infant, indicating the fathers' and mothers' importance to their baby. If their perceptions of the infant's needs and abilities are incomplete, due to a number of reasons (for example, their own emotional stress related to the infant's development, marital conflicts or stress at work), the child may receive a limited input, such as too little attention, and an incomplete range of shared parent–child activities. Early parental neglect may therefore develop in later years into relational problems. On the other hand, too much attention and emotional closeness may lead to fusion or intrusion and result in a difficulty to form the kind of socio-emotional bond that will enable the development of separate self-identity, and the ability to stay alone may be delayed (Vaughn et al., 2006). Thus, significant relations were found between the level of loneliness in young children and the level of their mothers' loneliness (Henwood & Solano, 1994).

Mary Ainsworth complemented Bowlby's conceptual approach by specifying the relations between attachment qualities and different characteristics of parental behavior. She identified maternal sensitivity and consistent responses toward infant's signals, and considered them as the essence of effective care-giving during the first year of life (Ainsworth, 1990; Keller, 2008). She concluded that infants who receive sensitive and responsive care-giving will view themselves as worthy of care, view others as trustworthy, and the world as a safe place. In contrast, infants who do not receive sensitive care-giving will view themselves as unworthy of care, others as untrustworthy, and the world as unsafe (Fivush, 2006). Yet, a child may be anxiously attached to one caregiver and may develop secure attachment with another, and these relationships will be jointly reflected in the developing perceptions of the child's identity (Sroufe & Sampson, 2000). Research showed that children's self-understanding was jointly influenced by prior different interpersonal relations, and further affected their future social interaction and loneliness vulnerability (Goodvin, Meyer, Thompson, & Hayes, 2008).

Studies explored the development processes not only of infants but also of parenting perceptions. Maternal structuring in the early interactions with their infants predicted maternal representations, including a mothers' capacity to develop realistic positive views about herself as a mother (Shamir-Essakow, Ungerer, Rapee, & Safier, 2004). During interviews, mothers of securely attached children provided realistic and balanced descriptions of their children that reflected their sensitivity to their infants' developmental needs. On the whole, they showed awareness of their children's perspectives. Although they were able to acknowledge both positive and negative characteristics of their children, their overall view was predominantly positive and accepting. Conversely, mothers of insecurely attached children provided a more negative view of their care-giving role and a less-balanced description of their children. They described themselves as less competent in their knowledge of their children's needs and as ineffective in satisfying those needs. Furthermore, their perception of their children was distorted by the defensive exclusion, or misinterpretation, of affect and/or information regarding their children.

Intergeneration relations of attachment were documented, and disclosed complex relations and adaptation to changing contextual conditions (Button, Pianta, & Marvin, 2001; Slade, Belsky, Aber, & Phelps, 1999). Recent studies (Goodvin et al., 2008; Reese, 2008) provided support to two types of links: a connection between children's attachment security and their social and emotional development, and their self-perceptions and the relations between mothers' own attachment and their children's self-concept. Mothers, who viewed themselves as secured individuals, also had children who overall reported a positive self-concept, and a stronger interpersonal sense of self, with higher levels of social closeness, social conscience, and lower levels of alienation and aggression.

However, children of secure and insecure mothers did not differ in aspects of the self-concept that were more individual or intrapersonal (i.e., achievement, stress reactivity, harm avoidance, and overall wellbeing) (Reese, 2008). Attachment security was found consistently related to children's peer-related thoughts and feelings and to their reports of loneliness and social problems (Raikes & Thompson, 2008).

In addition, different parenting characteristics, such as sensitivity and depressive symptoms, were differentially associated with children's peer-related thoughts and feelings. Parental sensitivity predicted children's social problem-solving solutions, and parental depressive symptoms were associated with negative attributional style. In conclusion, both parenting quality and attachment early in life predict the children's social competence, suggesting them as the foundations for the children's later cognitive and emotional processing of social satisfactions, frustrations, and loneliness. Longitudinal studies, such as the Minnesota study of parents and children, may clarify the development complexity of social relations from infancy to adolescence and adulthood.

The Minnesota longitudinal study of parents and children from birth to adulthood (Sroufe, 2005; Suess & Sroufe, 2005) presented the ongoing impact of early relationship with a parent that was embedded in the changing family contexts. In this study, researchers recruited an urban sample of more than 200 mothers during the mid-1970s, who were considered as being at risk for parenting difficulties due to the challenges associated with poverty. The follow-up through childhood and adolescence in this comprehensive longitudinal study revealed the cumulative nature of different experiences and their continual impact during different developmental stages. The results of this study showed that relations were not dependent on one side. All partners, the parents and the children alike, shared the responsibility for structuring family interrelationships and developmental adjustment. The ongoing interplay between experiences, representations, and continuing adaptation during different developmental stages structured the outcomes. Clearly, a nonlinear and probability model was exposed, and variations in infant–caregiver attachment were not directly related to outcomes only within the context of complex developmental systems and processes. These results established the value of early parents–children relations only within a wider developmental model and had practical implications for worried families who were anxious to introduce changes in their parental style to assist their children during different stages of development. This issue will be further detailed in the coping and intervention chapters.

The early relations between parents and their children did not determine development in a rigid conceptualization, but as integrated with later experiences. During the developmental processes it was connected to arousal modulation, emotional regulation, curiosity, and emotional competence, to name just a few additional functions (Sroufe, 2005). For example, children who had emotionally available caregivers during childhood, who fostered open discussions and encouraged sharing of emotions, would have many opportunities for learning about emotions and emotion regulation (Laible, 2007). Secure children were found more emotionally competent and capable of maintaining organized behavior even in times of excitement, conflicts, and emotional arousal. They would be able to develop higher levels of empathy than insecure children, and would be more successful at regulating their emotions. In contrast, insecure individuals were more prone to being either overregulated or under regulated in their emotional expressions (Mikulincer & Florian, 2001). Studies linked parental characteristics with disrupted early attachments that had adverse effects on mental representations of the self and others and increased risk for children's loneliness (de Minzi, 2006; Jackson, 2007; Wiseman, Mayseless, & Sharabany, 2006). These studies focused attention on parental characteristics as well as their parenting styles.

Parental Characteristics

Authentic voices of fathers and mothers online enabled research to probe into parenting distress and happiness as related to their individual characteristics and contextual conditions.

A young and single mother wrote on a discussion board: "Being a mother can at times be very lonely . . . alone all day and then at night, alone again, talking mainly to someone who doesn't understand and then at night, talking to no one, whispering words in front of computer screens . . ." An angry father wrote "I'm not always loving, laughing, kind, generous, and in a good mood. . ." Within the risk and protective paradigm, parental difficulties, such as loneliness, negative affect, and depression; their psychological resources such as their Sense of Coherence, positive mood, and hope may shape their parental skills and behavior. In order to provide optimal child-care, parents need sufficient psychological resources, manifested in their abilities to be sensitive to children's needs (Belsky, 1984). Parental emotions and moods, their values and attitudes regarding social relations on the one hand, and their feelings toward their parenting and children on the other hand, may jointly affect their interactions and reactions to their children's social difficulties and loneliness. In-depth awareness to the impact of parental emotions may extend the understanding of their children's emotional development.

Parental Positive and Negative Affect

Parental emotions were associated with the perceptions of themselves, their children, and their family life. These links were bidirectional, and the perception of familial processes may also have reciprocally influenced the emotions in individual family members. General positive emotions enhanced perceptions of better family functioning. Mothers with positive affect often had children with positive affect as well as with higher emotion regulation abilities. This result was confirmed for children with typical development as well as for children at risk (Feng et al., 2008). Indeed positive affect was related to children's positive mood and to maternal active and enthusiastic involvement in various areas of life. Similarly, negative and depressive maternal affect was also related to children's negative mood. Studies explored the impact of depressive parents on their children's development. However, before reporting research on depressive parents and its impact on the children's adjustment, parental expressions of loneliness will be presented. Parents often felt reluctant to share their social distress – but described it freely online. For example, a distressed mother wrote on a discussion board "I guess you understand how lonely I am as a mother and a woman." Another wrote "This feeling of loneliness and despair is terrible. . ." "Feeling of being all alone and why isn't there anyone to pick me up at the end of a bad day? . . . someone there for me and with me." A desperate father wrote "Why are evenings always my worst enemies?"

The traditional roles of mothers and fathers have been challenged both by ideology (i.e., feminism) and events (i.e., the increased opportunities for economic and social independence of women, increased proportions of single-parent families and divorce). One manifestation of these changes is the growing participation of mothers in all levels of the workforce, with a proportionate decrease in the time they can spend in the caring and upbringing of their children. Another manifestation is expressed in the role changes that fathers experienced (for example, a father wrote on a blog: "I've now given up my job and am looking after my daughter full time as house-husband."). Facing life stresses, day-to-day hassles, and self-questioning regarding their self-perception and life satisfaction initiate many times feelings of loneliness and thoughts that nobody truly understands them and/or provides meaningful and empowering support. The protective and risk impacts of social support will be further discussed in Chapter 7.

Parental depression is another example of negative affect that may impair fathers' and mothers' abilities and may challenge their emotional resources to provide responsive attention and meaningful answers to children's needs. Most studies focused attention on maternal depression, demonstrating its impact on their abilities to interact in an optimally sensitive manner with their children and, therefore, the ability to create an emotional environment that fosters mother–child relationships (Campbell et al., 2004; Cummings & Cicchetti, 1990).

Mothers' Depression

Studies that examined mothers' depression detailed their sadness, anxiety, fatigue, irritability, as well as social and emotional withdrawal. These mothers experienced a general incompetence, helplessness, and ineffectiveness in their role as parents. Generally, a depressed individual is concerned with depressive themes of inadequacy, failure, loss, and worthlessness, as well as biased perceptions, interpretations, and memories of personally relevant experiences that influence their interpretation of past and current events. Maternal depression has a negative impact not only on their life quality, but also on their children's development. The experience of depression after childbirth is quite common and, although the majority of episodes resolve spontaneously within the first few months postpartum, a significant proportion of mothers continue to report persistent depressive symptoms during their children's preschool years. In order to clarify the impact of depression, the thought processes of mothers and their behavior were examined (Trapolini, Ungerer, & McMahon, 2008).

This research reported that depressive symptoms may result in the mothers' psychologically unavailability to their family members and a decrease in their sensitive interactions with their children. In addition, the mothers' insecure state of mind did not start with the birth of their children. In fact, it triggered earlier difficulties that these mothers experienced in their own childhood. Thus, insecure attachment and maternal depression may both be considered as risk factors for effective parenting. For example, children who were insecurely attached at 24 months and their mothers continued to experience depressive symptoms (for an additional $2\frac{1}{2}$ years), had lower social problem-solving skills compared to insecure children whose mothers did not report high levels of depressive symptoms.

Thus, insecurity and maternal depressive symptoms have to be considered as cumulative risks to children's social development (Raikes & Thompson, 2008), and not as separate factors. In addition, reports regarding protective factors, such as the maternal sensitivity and positive affect toward their children, extended the dynamic understanding of their behavior. Mothers' abilities to be responsive to the children's emotional needs have also a unique protective value for depressive mothers, moderating the association between depression and adverse child outcomes. In conclusion, children, who were exposed to their mothers' depression, were at a developmental risk, yet they performed better on various tasks when their mothers were able to stay sensitive to their kids, regardless of their depression (Feng et al., 2008; NICHD Early Child Care Research Network, 1999).

Interestingly, in another study, it was found that a substantial proportion of mothers with depression were able to provide a sensitive and supportive environment to their children in spite of their negative mood (McMahon, Barnett, Kowalenko, & Tennant, 2006). Those mothers, who were able to reflect upon their own childhood attachment experiences, were more likely to demonstrate sensitivity to their children's needs – a capacity to describe and understand the thoughts and feelings underlying their children's behavior (Trapolini et al., 2008). Additionally, children's strengths such as emotional understanding and executive functions (i.e., the ability to plan, concentrate, and solve problems) act as protective processes, demonstrating that any consideration of risk situations needs to include a comprehensive consideration for many factors, thus rejecting a deterministic approach (Hughes & Ensor, 2009).

Most studies examined mothers' depression and only a few studies recognized the impacts of fathers' depressive moods as well as their supportive role in the family dynamics. More studies are needed to examine the impact of fathers' depression on their children. Overall, these results call for sensitizing mothers and fathers to the impact of their emotional availability on their parenting style and children's development, the possible influence of their mood regulation, and the impact of their own attachment relations with their parents. Thus, awareness not only to parental risks, but also to parental protective resources, may expand the understanding to the children's developmental outcomes. Parents' Sense of Coherence is an example of mothers' and fathers' characteristic, that was related to children's adjustment. Parents' individual characteristics, such as their ability to regulate emotions and find ways to meet their own needs, have been related to their Sense of Coherence.

Sense of Coherence

A global personality construct such as Sense of Coherence (Antonovsky, 1987) provides an important index of parental functioning (see Chapter 1 for an extended discussion of the construct). Parental Sense of Coherence has been considered an important resource for establishing relatedness and cohesiveness in the family system. Mothers, who were less anxious and reported higher levels of Sense of Coherence, had children who were less lonely (Al-Yagon, 2008). Individuals with a strong Sense of Coherence often see life as being meaningful and they have a strong sense of purpose in life. Nobody can avoid some degree of life stresses. But parents' Sense of Coherence was considered a protective factor that contributed to effective coping with stressors (Oelofsen & Richardson, 2006). Sense of Coherence enhances wellbeing and emotional regulation (Hart, Wilson, & Hittner, 2006), and thus, it is not surprising that mothers with a strong Sense of Coherence were more effective in their parenting skills. This construct was also related to family adaptation in different contexts and cultures. Lonely school-age children often had mothers who experienced lower levels of Sense of Coherence.

Hope and Future Visions

Not only are past and present circumstances important for predicting the future outcomes of development, but also the individual's expectations for new goals structure the current patterns of adaptation. Hope was considered a relatively stable characteristic and parents' narratives of hope and optimism showed a modest level of consistency, yet with fluctuations related to different situations (Pratt, Norris, Van de Hoef, & Arnold, 2001; Snyder, Sympson, Michael, Cheavens, & Chang, 2001). Strong relations were found between parental hope and adaptive individual (i.e., self-esteem) and familial functioning (i.e., parent–child relationships, social adjustment). Considering the reciprocal nature of family systems, the degree to which high-hope parents report enacting prosocial behaviors, participating in a cohesive and stimulating family environment (i.e., social integration outside the family), and perceiving less stress, may indirectly affect children. Thus the development of children's hope was based on parents' "coaching" behaviors (Shorey, Snyder, Yang, & Lewin, 2003). Hope was associated with active coping approaches (i.e., positive reinterpretations, planning), negatively associated with maladaptive passive behaviors (i.e., avoidance, behavioral disengagement, self-handicapping), and predicted parental effective functioning. Thus, parental hope may be considered an important resource for creating collaborative, productive, and fulfilling relationships among the family members while simultaneously meeting ones own desired needs and outcomes.

Even for parents who have been confronted with challenging behaviors of their children, hope and self-efficacy may be essential to personal and interpersonal performance, and predictive of the family functioning (Kashdan et al., 2002). Parental hope was examined as a resiliency factor for the daily challenges of raising children with disruptive behavior. Among parents of impulsive, noncompliant, oppositional, and defiant children, fathers and mothers who succeeded in setting clear goals, who believed that their goals were obtainable, and persevered despite obstacles, may have been likely to obtain more positive outcomes. The protective role of hope was also documented by studies that examined wellbeing of parents to children with disabilities such as mental retardation (Al-Yagon & Margalit, 2009). In addition, to understanding parental characteristics, family climate studies expand the awareness of the reciprocal interactions of a wide range of risk and protective systemic factors.

Family Characteristics

Family system conceptualization explored factors which may either exacerbate feelings of stress or may serve a stress-resistance role that contribute to empowering families and promote their happiness (North, Holahan, Moos, & Cronkite, 2008). Within the systemic approach, family members affect and are affected by the relations within the family, the behavior of its members, and their beliefs. The cohesion and support styles among family members as well as parental social activities jointly provide a model for their children's developing interpersonal style or experiencing social isolation (Margalit, 2006). Several studies reported that the family structure (Jones, Carpenter, & Quintana, 1985; Uruk & Demir, 2003) and communication styles were predictors in the development of loneliness within the family. The social-ecological model of Family Climate (Moos & Moos, 1994) assessed family environment in terms of three major underlying domains: relationship, personal growth, and system maintenance.

The relationship domain provides information about meaningful interpersonal relations and closeness among the family members. Parents' emotional availability (i.e., parents who express and display warmth, support, and availability during parent–child interactions), indicates to children that parents have the ability to successfully manage stress while maintaining family harmony (Sturge-Apple, Davies, Winter, Cummings, & Schermerhorn, 2008). Lower levels of family cohesion have predicted children's loneliness, while high Cohesion and a strong emotional bonding among the family members were considered protective factors. The relationship domain also deals with expressiveness, the extent to which family members are encouraged to communicate openly and to express their feelings directly. The third aspect of this domain has been related to conflicts in the family, including expressions of anger, participation in quarrels, and disagreement interactions (Holahan et al., 2007). Inter-parental conflicts were often associated with children's insecure representations of the parent–child relationship through its association with diminished parental emotional availability, predicting higher levels of children's loneliness and school avoidance.

The personal growth domain reflects the family's support for the development of its members, encouraging expressions of individuality, achievements, and independence, the ability of the system to accept, and even encourages personal development and progress. This domain refers to the extent to which the family members can feel independent, self-sufficient, and assertive, without a threat to the family cohesiveness. It expresses a competitive and achievement-oriented framework as well as the degree of participation in social, intellectual, and recreational activities, and involvement in the community (Moos, 2002).

The system maintenance domain reflects the family's needs and emphasizes order and control; the clarity of its norms, rules, and habits as well as the expectations from the family members in protecting the wellbeing of the system. It also reflects the levels of responsiveness to changes and rigidity or flexibility.

Social systems tend to maintain or accentuate individual characteristics that are congruent with their dominant aspects. Thus, in families that emphasize Cohesion and intimate relations, children will develop emotional connections, happiness, and there is a smaller risk for feelings of social isolation (North et al., 2008). More supportive and cohesive relationships among family members and a greater emphasis on their personal growth predicted increased wellbeing and fewer complaints of physical or emotional symptoms (Moos, 2002). Youngsters in families that value independence, achievement, and intellectual and recreational pursuits are more likely to develop self-confidence and autonomy, but may be at a higher risk for loneliness. Some emphasis on each of the three domains enhances positive emotional and behavioral development, but too much focus on any one domain may lead to distress and dysfunction. Highly achievement-oriented and rigidity structured families can create anxiety and erode youngsters' self-confidence. Moderate emphasis on system maintenance factors helps to promote ego control among individuals who prefer a well-structured setting. But a strong focus on these factors, especially among independent-minded and internally oriented persons, may restrict individual growth and foster passivity (Moos & Holahan, 2003). Moos (1991) reported that higher levels of self-esteem and sociability were reported by adolescents from cohesive, expressive, and well-organized families.

Parental conflicts were the focus of several studies, since they were considered predictors for children's loneliness and emotional distress. Children who were exposed to high levels of parental conflicts were more vulnerable to a wide range of emotional, behavioral, social, and academic problems (Oppenheim, 2006). Yet, it is not the quality of the conflicts or their intensity that shaped the youngsters' wellbeing. The adolescents' cognitive appraisals of marital conflict, rather than the actual conflicts had a wide-range influence. In addition, peer relations interacted and moderated the effect of marital conflict on adolescents' positive affect (Xin, Chi, & Yu, 2009). Interestingly, marital conflicts had different relations with positive and negative affect. The conflicts in the family predicted increased adolescents' negative affect, even when these youngsters had good peer relationships. But for the positive affect, the situation was different. Though adolescents may have been exposed to frequent parental conflicts, if they were popular among their peers, high levels of positive affect would be predicted. Yet, if these kids were not popular, the conflicts at home would have a stronger negative impact on their affect. In conclusion, if adolescents cannot obtain social provisions from their families, they can alternatively get them from their friends, such as encouragement, closeness, and cooperation. But some special provisions, such as close relations with parents, the sense of family order and harmony, cannot be obtained outside families. In their absence, children and adolescents will be at risk for experiencing more negative affect.

Conditions in one social environment often influence those in other settings (i.e., the family and school) in several ways. Researchers have identified three general patterns of interface between settings: (1) positive carryover, in which one setting enriches the other; (2) negative carryover, in which problems in one setting create tension in the other; and (3) compensation, in which the lack of resources in one setting impels a quest for substitute resources in another. For example, when the family emphasizes social connections, children who grow up developing and appreciating social competence may develop appropriate friendship relations at school. Yet, conflictual family environments may encourage children to look for meaningful social relations outside their homes. It can be concluded that the conceptualization of environments has progressed from a static model in which structural factors are related (i.e., poverty level was expected to be linked to indices of community pathology), to a dynamic model of neighborhood interacting processes and experiences, focusing on characteristics such as social integration, community resources and support (Moos, 2002). Additional sources for individual differences were also noticed. Several children were attuned to the environment and open to the power of contextual factors, whereas others were more apt to shut out external stimulation and resist outside forces. Certain personal factors reflected an individual's receptiveness to environmental influence, such as field dependence, external control orientation, and the need for social approval, whereas others reflected an individual's tendency to resist or overcome the force of the environment with a strong self-identity.

Moos' Family Climate model provided an elaborated profile of family characteristics, emphasizing the dynamic interrelations between a wide range of domains and several contextual conditions. The Circumplex Model of Marital and Family Systems extended the understanding of families through the awareness to the value of balanced dynamic relations (Olson, Gorall, & Tiesel, 2007). It focused the discussion on two central dimensions (Olson, 2000): cohesion and adaptability/flexibility, and explored the consequences of their extreme versus balanced relations. Accordingly, not only low Cohesion or flexibility may predict risks to family members, but also too much Cohesion and flexibility may predict difficulties.

Circumplex Model of Family Systems

The basic hypothesis in this conceptualization is that families who find balance on two family dimensions – cohesion and adaptability/flexibility – will function better than those in the unbalanced range. Extreme scores represent maladaptive systems, and moderate scores lead to adjustment and wellbeing of the family members (DeFrain & Asay, 2007; Larson & Olson, 2004).

Family Cohesion reveals the extent to which family members are close, connected, and involved with one another, including commitment and enjoyable time together. It assesses how much the family members feel good about their own family, trusting that their needs will be met, and the development of relationships flows smoothly (Olson, 2000). Family Cohesion enhances the systemic confidence that problems are comprehensible and manageable (Black & Lobo, 2008; McCubbin, Balling, Possin, Frierdich, & Bryne, 2002). Well-functioning family members tend to interact among themselves on a daily basis, providing nurturance and compliments, and reinforcing each others' efforts. This dimension can range from the extremes of disengaged (very low connections) to enmeshed (very high connections). It may change to meet needs such as in times of crisis, and the members of the families may become closer and turn to each other for support. Their Cohesion scores will be higher and these changes will be considered protective factors for promoting resilience.

Family adaptability or flexibility reflects the flexibility and adaptation capacity of the family system to changes due to internal developmental processes, as well as due to external pressures and challenges. It can range from the extremes of rigid families (very low acceptance for changes) to chaotic families (very high acceptance for changes with very low permanence and regulation). According to Olson (2000), families prefer stable and orderly patterns, yet function best when a balance is achieved between moderate amounts of structure and flexibility. It is common for most families to resist and even try to avoid changes, yet resilient families do not view changes in their life with helplessness; rather, roles are reorganized and changes are viewed optimistically as challenges to build a new equilibrium. Thus, dysfunctional parents, tend to operate at the extremes of being either overly rigid or chaotically unstructured (Black & Lobo, 2008).

Research documented specific associations between family environment and children's personality, adjustment, and behavior. Flexible and cohesive family climate was related to adolescents' higher self-perception and children's feeling of higher control of their life (Vandeleur, Perrez, & Schoebi, 2007; Zdanowicz, Janne, & Reynaert, 2004). Idan, Sade and Margalit (2009) examined the relations between children's personal sense of coherence, family climate, hope expectations, effort investment, and children's loneliness, and identified unique interactions – as presented on Fig. 3.1. Children from cohesive families were more hopeful, felt lower levels of loneliness and were more ready to invest effort in their school work. Similarly, children with high sense of coherence also reported lower levels of loneliness and higher levels of hope, and hopeful children were ready to invest effort. This study presented the connections' complexity. Indeed personal and familial factors predicted children's loneliness, but it did not explain directly lower levels of effort investment. However, the impact of loneliness was mediated by hopeful thinking. Thus, lonely children who were able to remain hopeful were ready to continue learning and investing effort at school regardless their social frustrations.

Comparisons between the family functioning levels reported by parents of lonely and non-lonely adolescents (Efrati, 1993), revealed that the parents of the lonely youngsters viewed their family members as less competent and communicative. In

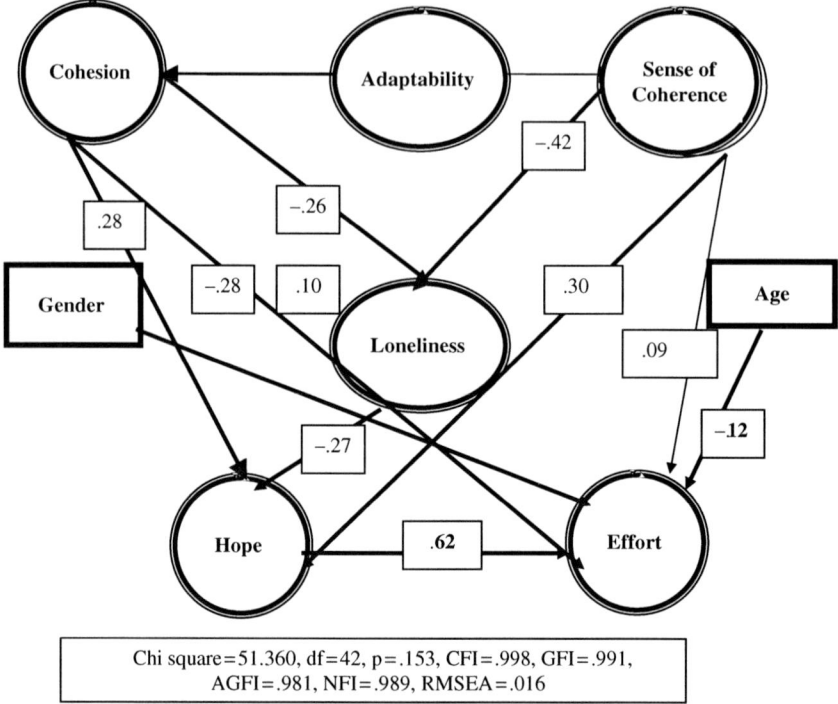

Fig. 3.1 Structural equation model for typically achieving students

addition, their family systems were perceived as less cohesive and committed and as demonstrating lower levels of coping. Olson (2000) also proposed that a higher level of cohesion in family climate was related to youngsters' better social functioning, since, in a closer, more involved family system, children's needs were better addressed.

   All families have strengths that constitute their valuable resources, even though many times the family members are not aware of their powers. Family strengths are the competencies and capabilities of the family unite and its members. These characteristics are used to promote the family's effective functioning in response to crises and stress. Research explored the resilience of struggling families, and identified systemic and parental strengths (Dunst, 2002). Research examined in addition to parents' sources of stress, the family's capacity for successful adjustment even under stressful conditions. This paradigm examined factors which either exacerbated feelings of stress or served a stress-resistance role that contributed to empower families and to promote their happiness (North et al., 2008). The conceptualization of family functioning style implies a unique, systemic (interpersonal and intra-familial) manner of dealing with life events, including crises, and of meeting the needs and promoting the growth and development of individual family members. Every family is characterized by a specific combination of strengths and competencies that systematically define the style in which it affects the growth, socialization, and maturation of its members. Within this family functioning approach, the following qualities of strong family systems were proposed, with the understanding that no one family would be expected to display all of these qualities. Instead, these qualities that follow were considered dynamic, interrelated, and interactive (Dunst, Trivette, & Deal, 1988): commitment to the family system and its members, communication among the family members, Cohesion, competence, and effective coping.

In conclusion, considerations of social contexts expand the understanding of attachment development of children within the family environment. The joint impact of parental distinctiveness and environmental characteristics were presented through several different conceptualizations of family climate, which shared appreciation to family cohesiveness and structure. These different models and approaches treat the family's close and supportive relations as a source of empowering their children. In addition, within the family environment, different parenting styles further affect children's social development, relatedness, and social exclusion (Keller, 2008). Studies of parenting style will illustrate their cumulative effect to the conceptualization of family functioning and children's loneliness.

Parenting Style

The links between parenting styles and children's social competence, development, and loneliness are complex, involving the interplay between parenting beliefs, attitudes, emotional climates (such as acceptance or dominance), and specific behaviors (parenting practices). Research often defines parenting along separate attitudinal and behavioral dimensions, expecting family experiences and processes to shape children's peer competence and the quality of relationships (Ladd & Pettit, 2002). Parents spent many hours with their children, and gender differences were noticed within different age groups. For example, mothers had more responsibility for adolescents' discipline, daily care, and recreational activities (Phares, Fields, & Kamboukos, 2009). They reported spending more time with their adolescents than did fathers. Developmental patterns were found for some aspects of time involvement, with both mothers and fathers reporting higher involvement with the younger groups of children. The actual parenting behaviors differed across distinct ages. For example, the activities of mothers with their preschool children differed from their activities with school-age children, reflecting varied levels of age-appropriate social connections, networking, and close companionship.

Not any single measure of parenting styles predicted children's adjustment. Only the different cumulative aspects of parenting practices determined outcomes. Direct and indirect influences of parental styles were identified. Direct modes of influence included parents' active efforts to socialize or "manage" children's social development. Indirect modes of influences emerged from parental beliefs, attitudes, social behavior, and emotional climate. Parents supervised actively several aspects of their children's social connections in different age stages, fulfilling several different "roles" (Ladd & Pettit, 2002). They may act as designers, mediators, supervisors, and advisors or consultants.

Direct Parenting Style

Parents may act as designers when they seek to control or influence their children's behavior through structuring the settings in which children meet and interact with peers. They can provide them with access to different environments (i.e., their choice of afternoon activities, neighborhood relations, and even the choice of schools), and avoid others. They can arrange their room, structure the play settings at home, and provide games and toys that will initiate certain types of peer interactions.

Parents act also as mediators, especially for young children, providing help and assistance for meeting with peers. Mothers and fathers arrange "play dates," talk with parents of other children, and drive children to their friends. They regulate the frequency their children meet or don't meet particular play partners. Slowly and gradually parents decrease their levels of mediating activities, enabling their children to start negotiating their own social connections. The change can be gradual. For example, sometimes at the end of the school day a 5-year-old shy girl asked hesitantly the mother of another girl if she could come to play at their home after school. Her mother stood by her daughter's side – letting her take over the mediation resourcefulness and perhaps encouraging these early experimentations of independent social initiatives.

Parents' supervision is expressed through parents' efforts to control and regulate children's ongoing interactions and activities, and by monitoring their relations with peers. Children may accept the supervision, or may angrily oppose parental intervening, considering it an insult to their independence and judgment. Angry adolescents may react negatively to parental regulation of their social activities

Parents' roles as advisors may seem less controlling, but they provide children with beliefs, guidance, and suggestions evaluating playmates' choices and activities. Fathers and mothers may start discussions with their children, proposing how to initiate friendships, to manage conflicts, and to maintain preferred relations. Such conversations may be proactive or reactive in nature: they may prepare children for future challenges or may react to their expressed distress regarding upsetting peer experiences. As consultants, parents may be relatively didactic, providing "expert" advice to peer problems, or they may just listen to children's views and experiences, enabling reflections, expressions of emotions and providing empathic listening, understanding, and support. Children differ in their reactions to parents' consultation. Some children request parental insight and appreciate the suggestions while others may angrily reject adults' advice (Ladd & Pettit, 2002).

Indeed parenting is a complex process, involved in multiple levels of organization that change in and through integrated, mutually interdependent relationships with children, within the family contexts. It is complex, since we rear our children, and at the same time they rear us. Studies showed that the impact of children on their families (Beaver & Wright, 2007), and the impact of families on their children cannot be studied in isolation. Thus, parenting processes are rarely the result of a single event or an exclusive characteristic, but reflect multiple interacting factors through time. Transactional models of development suggest that various aspects of parents, children, and family factors (both intra-familial and extra-familial) interact jointly and longitudinally across time in complex ways, and affect dynamically the development of parenting style. Indirect parenting style is expressed in parent–child interactions during different day-to-day activities, reflecting parental beliefs and practices including disciplinary style. All these aspects are related to children's peer competence and social difficulties (Hart, Ladd, & Burleson, 1990; Haskett & Willoughby, 2007; Madden-Derdich, Estrada, Sales, Leonard, & Updegraff, 2002).

Indirect Parenting Style

Indirect influences consist of attitudes, perceptions, and beliefs that underlie parenting behavior and modeling socialization practices. Although they include a wide variety of different processes, research identified two major complex dimensions of parenting style: responsiveness and demandingness (Maccoby & Martin, 1983).

Responsiveness refers to the extent to which parents foster individuality and self-assertion by being attuned and supportive to children's requests; it includes warmth, autonomy support, and reasoning. Parental responsiveness reflects the affective dimension. Responsive mothers have a positive impact on children's adjustment, reducing the impact of risk predictors (Weaver & Prelow, 2005).

Demandingness refers to the monitoring and supervision of the children and to the enforcement of parental guidelines and rules. It refers to claims that parents make on children to become integrated into the family system and into society by behavior regulation, direct confrontation, maturity demands (behavioral control), and supervision of children's activities (monitoring). The interactive dynamics of responsiveness and demandingness, rather than focusing only on a single parenting process, would clarify the variability in children's behavior and adjustment. Different combinations of demanding and responsiveness were related to children's behavior and development (Baumrind, 1991; Heaven & Ciarrochi, 2008). Three parent configurations were identified as a prototype: authoritative, permissive, and authoritarian. They represent a complex exemplifying of the distinctive features of the group, as well as an explicit description of parenting behaviors that characterize each group member.

Authoritative parents are demanding and responsive. They exercise firm, negotiated control within a warm and loving environment. These parents share with their children the reasons for particular rules and expectations, praise competencies, and their children show the highest levels of internalization of parental standards. Children of authoritative parents were more successful at setting achievable goals for themselves, finding the means to achieve these goals, and overcoming barriers to their goals, or as proposed by Snyder (Snyder, 2002), they modeled higher levels of hope. Youth reared by authoritative parents were more skilled at hopeful thinking than youth who reported other parental styles (Heaven & Ciarrochi, 2008). Thus, "high-hope homes" were structured by parents who model hopeful thinking, competent behaviors, and appreciation of effort.

Permissive parents believe that any form of parental control or discipline may inhibit the children's natural tendencies and prospects of self-actualization. These parents don't see themselves as responsible for shaping and altering the child's ongoing and future behavior. Permissive parents do not enforce rules firmly but tend to have a "laissez faire" attitude toward childrearing (Baumrind, 1978, 2005).

The third category – *authoritarian parenting* style – involves parental power assertion without warmth, nurturance, or two-way communication. These parents tend to use punitive discipline styles in order to control the behavior of their children. Perceived authoritarian parenting was related to children's low self-esteem, since often children fail to achieve the exact standards that parents expect from them. Both authoritarian and permissive parenting styles were generally associated with poorer self-perceptions among school aged children and adolescents and increased loneliness.

The most positive development of children was reported when they experienced parenting that was high in both responsiveness and demandingness (authoritative parenting). At the other extreme, children revealed the most problematic development when parents scored low on both of these dimensions (indifferent parenting). Punitive discipline was most likely to be used by indifferent parents and least likely to be used by authoritative parents. Indifferent parents were characterized by a lack of closeness in parent–child relationships and had children with the highest levels of externalizing behavior (Lim & Smith, 2008).

A similar approach of conceptualizing parenting styles explored the impact of autonomy promotion as it was related to parental control. Early attempts to map the domains of parenting, described parental autonomy-support and control as opposite ends on a single continuum. In a large-scale factor analysis, Schaefer (Schaefer, 1965) identified a factor defined by parental behaviors such as "intrusiveness," "possessiveness," and "control through guilt." Additional studies differentiated between these concepts and treated them as two separate constructs (Silk, Morris, Kanaya, & Steinberg, 2003). The relation between perceived parental psychological control and autonomy-support depended on how autonomy-support was conceptualized. Parental promotion of independence would or would not co-occur with psychological control (Silk et al., 2003). Recently research identified two groups of parents' who encouraged children's independence: parents who were considered as non-controlling and those who were considered as controlling (Soenens, Vansteenkiste, & Sierens, 2009). The former group encouraged their children to make decisions independently; moreover, this independent functioning was allowed in a volitional way. Parents had confidence in their children's ability to act independently in a responsible manner and, therefore, would provide their children with opportunities and choices to develop their own point of view and to make their own decisions. However, not all parents encouraged independence in a non-controlling fashion. Another group of parents were high in promoting independence and psychological control. These parents were perceived as encouraging independence in a pressuring way. They would not allow their children to be dependent, even when their children would actively seek parental guidance. Instead, they would induce guilt and blame their children for being immature and childish when children requested parental support.

In consequence, these youngsters experienced their parents' promotion of independence as an obligation rather than as a choice. The lack of independence promotion may also have occurred within a controlling or a non-controlling parenting environment. Parents, who kept their child within close physical and emotional boundaries, were taking an overprotective stance, infantilizing their children, and restricting expression of independent thought and behavior. However, not all promotion of dependence occurs in a pressuring fashion, and parents may enable dependency with or without implementing psychologically controlling tactics. Children who may need parental guidance when making decisions, and may perceive their parents as meeting this need for guidance in an empathic and thoughtful manner, described their parents as promoting dependency without control. Parents allow their child's dependence and refrain from intrusive tactics because the children freely choose to ask for parents' advice and support and, as such, fully stand behind their reliance on their parents.

Children without control fared generally better than those in the two controlling groups. The studies demonstrated the complexity of parenting impact on children's feelings of competence and their developing self-conceptions as able to function independently, or lonely, when forced to avoid dependence. Many times parents were not aware of their children's distress, if they were not used to sharing and being attentive to expressions of emotions. The expressions of children's and parents' emotions have to be considered within age-appropriate cultural conventions. Children learn in their families how to express their positive and negative emotions, to sensitize adults to their loneliness distress and social dissatisfaction. Parental sensitivity to children's initial expressions of emotions and thinking has developmental importance. Children learn emotional expressions, rules (i.e., when and how to express feelings in acceptable and unacceptable manners), and regulations (how to control emotional outbursts and when to let go) in their families. Parental reactions to children's emotions are an example of ways in which parents can directly socialize children's emotion-related reactions.

Parental Styles of Emotional Expressions

In everyday life, children frequently express positive and negative emotions. Parental reactions to displays of emotions are likely to provide varied opportunities for emotional socialization, related to the adaptability of the emotional expression to the contextual conditions, the culture and the beliefs of the parents. Fathers and mothers can react in supportive or unsupportive ways to a child's expressions of emotion. For example, fathers can avoid contact with the child or respond negatively to verbal communication and actions that minimize the legitimacy of the child's emotional experience (i.e., crying when he/she is not expected to cry, or laughing at the misfortune of another child), with attempts to comfort the distressed child, or with efforts to teach the child ways to control the emotion and the stressful context or to adapt the emotion to expected social conventions (Eisenberg, Cumberland, & Spinrad, 1998). Caregivers' meta-emotion philosophy predicted child emotion understanding and emotion regulation, which also predicted children's behavior adjustment and social skills (Cunningham, Kliewer, & Garner, 2009). The emotional communication and expressiveness between parents and children has been used as an index of family cohesiveness and functioning (Cassidy, Parke, Butkovsky, & Braungart, 1992). Parents' support of children's emotional expressions (Yap, Allen, & Ladouceur, 2008) and their own manifestations of positive and negative affect expressed their styles of emotional socialization. Through modeling of feelings, parents provided patterns and timing for appropriate affective messages (Edwards, Shipman, & Brown, 2005). They suggested the children the suitable emotional valence and intensity for specific occasions and regulated the children's social-emotional development (McDowell & Parke, 2005).

Indeed parents can affect their children's emotions, yet their own emotional communication reflects their children's characteristics. Positive parental affect will often be related to successful and adjusted children. Similarly, children with a difficult temperament often trigger unintentional angry reactions from their parents. However, only the joint impact of unique parental characteristics and children's behavior problems predict their stress and even abusive parenting style (McPherson, Lewis, Lynn, Haskett, & Behrend, 2009). It is not clear if the happy child affects the parental positive mood, or maybe the positive mood that parents express contributes to the child's happiness.

It is difficult to be parents. Fathers and mothers face conflicting and demanding roles embedded within the day-to-day stresses. These roles affect the quality of parenting and the functioning of the family system, which in turn influence the quality of the child's developmental functioning across the wide spectrum of social, affective, and cognitive domains. Parents' responses to their children are based upon their ways of thinking about the care-giving relationship, which, in turn, are strongly influenced by their own parenting history and interactions with children's characteristics and contextual conditions. Parents, who feel that they have a low impact on their children's behavior and development, view them as a potential source of threat to their sense of control (Bugental, 2004). This complexity often contributes to feelings of helplessness (i.e., in a meeting a father described that on his way home from work he had often made decisions to be a smiling and encouraging father). However, when he opened the door to their apartment, confronted with his crying baby, complaining wife, or insulting teenage son, he could feel the growing anger inside him like a "frightening monster that he had to control." The mother added that she was afraid to be as dominating as her mother had been, but often felt unable to change her style. They both agreed that they suspected they were incompetent parents to their challenging children.

Intervention research has pointed out that there are several possibilities for empowering families, which are further explained in Chapter 8. Family risks, such as conflicts between parents, and/or co-parenting of divorced parents, may add to the day-to-day stresses such as work demands and personal needs and wishes. For most families, everyday stresses of parenting have important adverse implications on their parental abilities. When parents experience increased stress and fewer available resources, they may face difficulties in their effort to monitor and regulate their children's activities or in setting clear rules and boundaries. Their diminished personal resources may reduce their sensitivity and responsiveness to their children's needs. Children with difficulties often provoke parental unique reactions. Parents often become less proactive in their parenting practice and rely on more reactive and punitive strategies of child management, as a result of decreasing sensitivity and challenges to their personal resources (Ladd & Pettit, 2002). The studies of these risk factors and the search for empowering approaches cannot be explored in isolation. Cultural attitudes and environmental conditions are also reflected in the families' circumstances, adding to the understanding of the dynamic complexity of intervening processes.

Parenting Style in Different Environments and Cultural Contexts

Different contextual conditions and cultural attitudes have been reflected in parenting styles and children's outcomes. Differences in family dynamics and the childrearing styles across social classes and different cultures have long-term consequences. For example, an ethnographic research (Lareau, 2000) showed the effects of social classes on parental styles. They reported that middle-class parents attempted to foster the talents of their 10-year-old children through organized leisure activities and extensive reasoning. In contrast, working-class and poor parents of the same age group of children were engaged in appreciating the accomplishments of natural growth, providing the conditions under which children could grow up, but leaving leisure activities to the children's initiatives. These parents often used directives rather than reasoning communication style in their parent–child dialogues.

As family members moved out of the home and interacted with professionals from formal institutions, such as teachers and pediatricians, middle-class children were able to negotiate more valuable resources, explanations, and outcomes than their working-class and poor counterparts. Thus, parenting styles affected children's coping with different challenges outside their families. However, we should be careful in generalizing these results, since research consistently showed the richness of varied childrearing styles, calling for a dynamic understanding and appreciation. For example, although strong relationship between poverty and child neglect has been widely documented by studies, research has also showed clearly that most poor families did not neglect their children and economic affluence did not predict optimal caring. In order to explore in-depth the predicting factors of behavior and outcomes of neglecting parents, comparisons of neglectful with non-neglectful low-income parents were performed. The results identified the critical impact of parental experience of loneliness and distress, beyond and above the impact of the economical constrains and cultural levels. Neglectful parents reported experiencing more life stresses. They suffered from frequent depressive moods and increased levels of loneliness. They also described weaker social supports. In these families, loneliness was associated with life stresses and decreased availability of network supports (Gaudin, Polansky, Kilpatrick, & Shilton, 1993). Ethnic minority groups are disproportionately exposed to a myriad of contextual stressors, including poverty, poor quality neighborhoods, and cultural stressors. In a study that examined parenting style of at-risk Mexican-American families, parental behavior and negative mood were important determinants of child development and mental health outcomes (White, Roosa, Weaver, & Nair, 2009). It can be concluded that similar parenting processes affect children's social competence within different contextual conditions. International studies further supported these conclusions.

The comparisons of parental practices among different countries revealed cultural differences in attitudes toward children's social competence and loneliness. Chao and Tseng (2002) presented the Japanese metaphor, "river crossing," as an illustration to childrearing beliefs. This metaphor reflects Japanese views on the type of assistance and support that parents have to provide in order to help their children "cross the river." Such a metaphor may imply that the parents will stay on the other side of the bridge, urging and encouraging their children to cross. In Japanese society, adults provide parental assistance by staying on the same side of the bridge together with the children and walking them through to the other side – to the adult world. This assistance suggests a dynamic process of socialization involving the interactive experiences of both parents and children. Japanese parents feel that this assistance necessitates closeness and the physical presence of the parent because of the potential risk and particularly the loneliness that may be entailed in the "bridge crossing" challenge.

Comparisons between Chinese and American cultures documented parenting practices with regard to authoritarian and authoritative parenting style, and revealed similarities regardless of cultural differences (Chen, Dong, & Zhou, 1997). This study of Chinese and American children showed that in both cultures the authoritarian parenting, as represented by parental enforcement, punishment, and negative affect, may lead to confusion, frustration, and feelings of insecurity in children which, in turn, may lead to deviant social behaviors, increased loneliness, and peer rejection at school. Furthermore, given that authoritarian parents provide little explanation, guidance, and emotional support in child rearing in the two cultures, their children may be less likely than others to develop intrinsic achievement motivation and will experience difficulties in academic performance, which may in turn lead to further parental disappointment and rejection. In contrast, authoritative parenting based on warmth, induction, and encouragement of exploration may be associated with confidence and positive orientation toward the world which, in turn, may lead to the child's competent behavior in the peer group and high academic motivation and achievement in both cultures.

Inconsistent results in the comparisons between parental approaches and children's adjustment revealed the variability richness of different practices. In conclusion, research traditions attempted to explain the root of children's loneliness in parental behavior. The results proposed that in order to provide optimal childcare, parents must possess personal resources, such as sensitivity, in responding to children's needs and abilities to regulate impulses, feeling secure in their own lives, and finding ways to meet their own needs. Parents affect their children's wellbeing and, at the same time, children affect their parents' thinking, feeling, and managing of their different roles and challenges. Thus, parenting is not an isolated process. Many factors within and outside the family intervene, mediate, and dynamically affect and are affected by each other. Siblings also affect and are affected by the development and structuring of relatedness experiences within the family, and their role are considered in the next section.

Siblings

Siblings play a significant role in the lives of individuals from infancy throughout the entire lifespan. Overall, relations with brothers and sisters may provide opportunities for experimenting social connections, negotiating conflict, and enjoying meaningful and dependable social support. Studies examining the influence of childhood sibling relationships on children's social skills proposed positive connections between close sibling relations and many adaptive socio-emotional outcomes (Cicirelli, 1995). Individuals, who received sibling support, reported lower levels of loneliness and significantly higher self-esteem and life satisfaction than those who reported low sibling-support conditions. In different families, several mechanisms were identified in order to clarify the varied support paths to adjustment and increasing self-esteem (Milevsky, 2005).

Sibling support even compensated children for low support levels in the family or the community (i.e., low support from fathers, mothers, and friends) (Hymel, Tarulli, Hayden Thomson, & Terrell-Deutsch, 1999; Milevsky, 2005). The quality of the relations with brothers and sisters predicted loneliness, regardless of age related differences between them (Sherman, Lansford, & Volling, 2006). Consistently, research showed that participants, who had harmonious (high warmth, low conflict) relationships with siblings, had the lowest loneliness and highest self-esteem scores, and those who reported intense affect (high warmth, high conflict) in their sibling relations had the highest loneliness and lowest self-esteem scores (Sherman et al., 2006). Close, warm, and supporting siblings' relations may not only support children and adolescents' self-esteem and adjustment (Yeh & Lempers, 2004), but also help them in avoiding loneliness in the family and outside home, even compensating for parental distance.

It is not clear if children who acquired age-appropriate social competence would be able to enjoy satisfactory relations with siblings and peer alike, or whether developing close relations with siblings prepared children for developing satisfactory social relations with peers. In addition, we have to remember that relations within the family are also related to stability and family cohesiveness, and together they can be viewed as protective factors for children at risk for developing loneliness. However, in our times, families often encounter a wide range of diverse instabilities due to many changes in their contextual factors that may shape dramatically the children's feelings of confidence, and in consequence, their experience of loneliness.

Instabilities in Family Life

Before reporting research, the story of Gail may illustrate the emotional impact of parental divorce on their children – regardless of their age. Gail was a 22-year-old successful student in a prestigious college. She could not stop crying when her parents told her that they decided at this point when she and her younger brother had left home, that divorce was their best solution. All she was able to say with tears was "how could you do this to me?" This is an intriguing statement, exemplifying children's reactions to instability in their families. In this circumstance, Gail was already a young adult who had left home and was living in her college. Yet, her first reaction was a strong experience of loneliness and it was very difficult for her to accept that home would not remain the same. She felt betrayed and frustrated. Her parents' words only made her angrier. They explained that they had waited until she left home, had a loving boyfriend, new social networks at college, and exciting learning experiences. She was grieving the loss of her secure base – the family life that she had known. Considering Gail's reactions, we can imagine how difficult the reactions of young children were, when their family faced changes such as relocation, parental separation, and divorce.

Many sources may contribute to children's experience of family instability. Major changes may be initiated by factors outside the family which affect family life (i.e., major economic changes when one of the parents changes the work place and/or working conditions). Transitions to new places may introduce major life changes. When families move to a new neighborhood, children enter new schools, interact with new peers, and lose their old social networks and close companions. Family experience of instability may also emerge from parental separation, divorce, or severe illness. Children who experience a family transition are at a greater risk of experiencing subsequent transitions and their concomitant stresses, although the disruptions in the family context that follow divorce and re-partnering are typically temporary. However, several families that undergo multiple transitions may continue experiencing uncertainty. The association between family instability and children's behavior were sometimes not direct, but they were related to parental levels of stress and emotional availability. When parents' personal resources were challenged or diminished due to their personal stress, they would be less able to respond to their children's difficulties. Parents' roles in these transitions were critical, as documented in research describing the impact of maternal stress and poor mothering on children's behavior (Osborne & McLanahan, 2007). Thus, children who experience multiple transitions faced more developmental risks than those who experienced no transition or only one (Cavanagh & Huston, 2008).

The children's developmental stage when they faced family instabilities was a critical factor in predicting outcomes. Cumulative family instabilities from birth were associated with poorer social adjustment on most indicators at the end of elementary school. Children who underwent more and longer family instabilities reported feeling lonelier and less satisfied with their friendships (Bullock, 1993). They also manifested increases in behavior difficulties and lower peer competency during the elementary school years, in comparison to their classmates. This pattern was especially noted for boys who were more susceptible to the stress and uncertainty associated with family instability (Cavanagh & Huston, 2008).

The effects of early cumulative instabilities in the family (i.e., prior to elementary school) may have a more profound impact than later instabilities, leaving children less able to navigate peer relationships, less popular with peers, and lonelier. One explanation for the importance of early childhood experiences is related to attachment processes. If children's primary relationships with attachment figures are disrupted, then their working models for later relationships can be affected. Complementary explanations focused attention on the parents' diminished emotional availability to their young children due to their emerging needs to cope with new stress and growing difficulties emerging from the separation, and to channel their personal energies toward building a new future. At the time of divorce, fathers and mothers undergo considerable stress combined with anger, feelings of loss, loneliness, decreased self-esteem, and lowered self-confidence.

Since divorce proportions and parental separation are continuously growing in many countries, there is a growing need to empower parents in their effort to support the development of their children in times of family crises. The importance of sensitizing parents to these processes was emphasized by research that demonstrated the developmental impact of family transformations. For example, associations between parental divorce and children's behavior problems were widely documented (Amato & Cheadle, 2008). Parental individual differences as well as gender differences were documented. Many fathers and mothers reported anger, loneliness, and depression (Weinraub, Horvath, & Gringlas, 2002).

The post-divorce world is also a lonely struggle for parents and offspring alike, consisting of risks for chaos for the household emerging from the children's movement between two different households (with different rules and different parenting practices), new lovers, friends coming and going, and parental feelings of depression (Cohler & Paul, 2002). The divorced parent may find it difficult to maintain the authority of two parents. Sometimes adolescents reported enhanced conflicts with their parents regarding typical adolescent issues such as daily routine and use of control and punishment. However, the parents' exhaustion affected their effective managing skills and increased their experience of desperation.

Interestingly, although divorce and remarriage may confront parents and children with stresses and new challenges, in many families it also offers an escape from unsatisfying or conflictual family relationships and an opportunity for developing more fulfilling family relationships and personal growth. Thus, as families negotiate divorce and remarriage, a more comprehensive understanding is requested in order to strive for the dynamic balance between risk and protective factors unique to each family system and to each family member. This new balance may predict adjustment, and enable positive hope for future satisfactory relations (Brodzinsky & Pinderhughes, 2002). In these taxing times, social support is very important such as the support provided by extended family members, particularly grandparents. Grandparents may provide diverse types of support. Not only instrumental support (i.e., child care, financial support), but also substantial emotional support. Indeed this is also a challenging time for the grandparents, who share the pain and anger of their children, wishing to provide meaningful help, yet have also to identify the limits of their new roles. A careful balance has to be developed between providing the needed support, and at the same time respecting the autonomy and independence of their children who are struggling adults and not kids. To this complicated situation, children's individual differences, as well as the distress expressions of their grandchildren, may add to the challenging emotional realities.

Children's Characteristics

Additional risk factors for effective parenting are related to children's individual differences. Parents interact differently with their different children. Dan's story displays the impact of children's characteristics on parents' behavior.

Dan is a famous and highly appreciated psychologist. He wrote several books about successful parenting and in his clinic he consulted many families. He is considered an expert in parental style. In one of his well-attended lectures at an international conference for psychologists he shared the following with the audience: "I was an ideal father for my elder son. I was very proud of my parenting skills, feeling competent and pleased with his development. I used him as an example in my many lectures. Yet, when my Ron, my energetic, hyperactive, and restless son was born, my self-perception as a parent and as a professional was challenged. As a child, he did whatever came to his mind, without considering the consequences. I was often called to school by his teachers who felt lost. During that period I think that I made every possible mistake as his father, every strategy that I had advised parents to avoid. I was a completely different father. Most of the time I was angry and frustrated; I had many conflicts with my wife, shouted angrily at everybody, and felt that nothing worked. I even started questioning my abilities as a professional who could not help himself." Many parents shared similar stories with us to demonstrate that parenting skills were in many ways dependent not only on the parents or the family climate, but also on the interactions with the children's temperament and distinctive personalities.

Research documented these interactions from early infancy. Mothers, who perceived their babies as difficult, appraised themselves negatively when they described their maternal competence and reported more depressive symptoms (Church,

Brechman-Toussaint, & Hine, 2005). Similarly, maternal ratings of child behavior difficulties among school-age children were associated with their feelings of sadness and anger (De Los Reyes, & Kazdin, 2005). Children with social and behavior difficulties need more support and understanding from their parents, yet they often evoke the opposite approaches. Research explored parental relations among several groups of aggressive children who were or were not rejected by peers, identifying different connections with their parents (Verschueren & Marcoen, 2002). For example, the rejected non-aggressive group of children perceived their relationship with their fathers as being less secure than did popular non-aggressive children. They felt that they could not rely on their fathers in times of stress, experiencing them as being less responsive to their unique needs and less available. Thus, they were less open when they communicated with their fathers about their daily distresses. This example demonstrated the impact of individual differences that jointly operate at the level of behavioral, emotional, and representational organization (Sroufe & Sampson, 2000). In conclusion, discussions of parenting styles are not complete without considering the joint impact of children's unique characteristics. Research on children's difficulties and disabilities may further clarify these interacting forces, with particular awareness of the impact of children with disabilities on parental stress.

Families of Children with Special Challenges

Families of children with special needs experienced increased stress than families with typical developing children. Special needs refer to a wide range of children's difficulties from high prevalence difficulties such as learning disabilities, attention disorders, and dyslexia to sensory disabilities such as hearing and vision impairments as well as severe disabilities. Family functioning style is considered the end-product of the interactions between four factors:

(a) The family's subjective definitions of their challenges – the children's disabilities.
(b) The severity of the child's handicapping condition and its consequences (i.e., prolonged dependency, increased needs for adults' monitoring, etc.).
(c) The availability of resources to meet the extended needs.
(d) The quality and efficiency of the coping strategies employed to introduce systemic changes and re-organize the family's functioning (McCubbin & Patterson, 1983).

Many parents of children with special needs reported feeling exhausted, less able to participate in social activities, isolating themselves from friends and relatives and often feeling lonely. Family members reported less-supportive relations within the family system, and fewer opportunities for open expression of feelings

(Margalit & Al-Yagon, 2002). These families often faced increased difficulties in providing satisfactory support to their children's initiating and maintaining companionship relations with peers, or for modeling close interpersonal relations to promote their children's effective coping strategies with loneliness. Indeed being parents to children with disabilities is a demanding role, challenging personal strengths and beliefs in self-competence. Thus it is not surprising that, for instance, mothers of children with learning disabilities often reported a lower sense of personal coherence and lower family cohesion (Al-Yagon, 2003). The children's early interactions with mothers and fathers, who struggle with stress and increased demands for parental resources, resulted in higher levels of loneliness and lower levels of self-confidence. In order to explore the impacts of contextual conditions, the interrelations among family functioning, children's social competence, and loneliness were examined in different cultures. The study of relations between children's loneliness and family climate among children with learning disabilities in China (Yu, Zhang, & Yan, 2005) furthered the understanding of the complex interactions between individual and systemic factors in different cultures. In this study, the social status of the children (rated by peers) was predicted by family functioning. Children's loneliness was related to a lower level of popularity, and indirectly to family functioning.

In order to clarify the impact of different contextual conditions, and to examine whether the limited parental capacity to invest in their own personal growth resulted from their lower personal resources, such as time, energy, and financial resources or from a subjective feeling of distress, parents of disabled children were investigated in the Israeli kibbutz environment (Margalit, Leyser, Ankonina, & Avraham, 1991). The kibbutz society, at the time of the study, provided its members' individualized needs (such as food, lodging, medical care, recreation, and education). Thus the increased needs of parents for resources necessary for raising their disabled children were met by the community. Surprisingly, children with disabilities in the kibbutz and in the city alike affected similarly family climate patterns. These families were less supportive and less cohesive than families of typical developing children in the adaptable environments. In addition, they were less able to provide their members with enough opportunities for personal growth in intellectual and cultural areas. This study substantiated the impact of the subjective distress on families with disabled children, despite differences in objective ecological conditions. Even when all of the increased needs were provided through systemic support, materialistic provisions did not help to relieve the extreme parental stress, focusing attention on parental strengths and their Sense of Coherence.

Fathers' and mothers' Sense of Coherence represents their beliefs in their abilities to cope effectively with challenges within their family and community, and it is expected to be relatively stable in a typical life course. In order to study how unexpected severe stress affects this parental self-confidence within their contextual conditions, a series of studies explored families who had children with mild and severe disabilities. Our research examined families of children with various special needs from mild difficulties, such as reading difficulties, to severe and chronic difficulties, such as moderate intellectual disabilities and behavior difficulties. Consistently, results of our studies and studies of different research groups showed that parents of children with disabilities and difficulties reported lower levels of Sense of Coherence than parents of typical developing children (Al-Yagon, 2008; Mak, Ho, & Law, 2007; Margalit et al., 1991). These results confirmed that having children with disabilities challenged fathers' and mothers' basic confidence in their comprehensibility and understanding why this unexpected challenge had happened, and what it meant in the long run. They also felt lower levels of manageability since their parenting skills were continuously challenged by this new, demanding, and difficult reality. The reduced personal resources of the parents were also expressed in their decreased abilities to form secure attachment with their children as well as with their children's pronounced loneliness (Al-Yagon, 2003). In addition, parental difficulties in identifying meaningful answers to the critical question "Why is this happening to us?" and to visualize how their child would be able to cope with challenges in the future, often lead to a decreased feeling of control in the environment, resulting in lower levels of Sense of Coherence. These worries may also contribute to their social isolation.

Parental Loneliness

Interviews of parents to children with disabilities often revealed that not only did children with special needs often experience increased loneliness, but their parents may have also suffered from social alienation and loneliness. They shared distress related to their feelings of social exclusion. One of the mothers said "I can't rejoice with the other parents when they begin to talk about 'school stuff', and I can't seem to brag about my son's education. I am backing into a corner so no one notices me and we don't have to talk about how my daughter is learning to read. . ." Parents are often reluctant to share their loneliness. In order to present the authentic voices of mothers to children with learning difficulties and disabilities, Raskind and Margalit (2008) presented their research in the 2008 annual meeting of the IARLD. The objectives of this study were to examine the personal meaning of loneliness as described online by mothers of children with learning disabilities and attention deficit disorder. The goals of this study were to identify the different sources of mothers' loneliness. The sample consisted of 398 mothers who were registered on a parental website hosting an online community of parents to children with learning difficulties. These online messages were identified through key word searches using "loneliness," "loner," "lonely," and "alone" by means of the website search engine.

The analysis of the loneliness messages revealed the alienation experienced by these mothers and their feelings of isolation and distress (i.e., they described their life as a "lonely road"). They explained that their distress emerged from the fact that nobody could truly understand the problems that they faced (i.e., "I guess you understand how lonely I am as a mother and a woman". . .), with accompanying emotions of guilt, fear, anger, and shame (i.e., "Parenting these kids can be difficult and lonely."; "This journey of trying to help your kids with their learning issues can be a very desperate and lonely one."; "It's like a huge life-long grieving process – I think you will feel this way over and over again.").

Three major challenges were identified in this study:

(a) Conflicts with schools (viewed by them as "lonely battles," i.e., "For years I would walk out of those IEP meetings feeling so alone, so hopeless.");
(b) Anxious concerns related to children's academic difficulties and/or disruptive or isolated behavior (i.e., "I remember feeling so isolated and lonely in my search for help for her");
(c) Frustrations related to unsatisfied needs for support/understanding in their families, including their spouses.

The loneliness of single mothers and their exhaustion were elaborated in several messages demonstrating the cumulative stress and increased needs for networking (i.e., ". . . the loneliness of being a single mom in which everything feels like it's on your shoulders"). Being alone was conceptualized by most mothers as a threat, but also as a sad reality. Negative mood and distressed behavior (such as crying) were detailed. Mothers were anxious when they considered the present difficulties as well as future options (i.e., "I am . . . very scared about his future and find myself feeling very alone . . .").

Studies reported that these families were less supportive, less connected, and experienced distant family interrelations and a decrease in social and recreational activities, within a more rigid and restrictive household. Parents and adolescents perceived their family relations as more disengaged and less connected than did families of typical developing children, and related to children's psychopathology measures (Prange et al., 1992). Family relations enabled only restricted levels of emotional expressions and limited opportunities for conflict resolution. Fewer opportunities were available in the family to pursue personal activities or to enhance the personal growth of its members (Margalit & Almougy, 1991; Margalit et al., 1991). However, supportive social networks reduced stress by serving as a buffer against threatening situations, decreased parental feelings of being overwhelmed by parenting tasks, contributed to parental coping strategies, and furnished parents with additional community resources such as child-rearing advice and information. High levels of social and emotional support in families were linked to children's better social interactions, higher academic achievements, and overall enhanced social and emotional wellbeing. In contrast, mothers who reported a high level of social isolation (limited social support and few friends) were more likely to perceive their children negatively and to engage in coercive interactions (Margalit, 1994).

In conclusion, family distinctiveness and parental characteristics interact with children's abilities and difficulties and jointly predict their social alienation at school and among their peers. Yet, for some children, home is a lonely place. Family characteristics not only predict children's loneliness outside the home, but also contribute to distress inside the family, expressed in overt conflicts or by children distancing themselves from the remaining family members.

Children's Loneliness Inside Families

Most studies explored children's loneliness at school, examining peer relations. However, the loneliness experiences of many children start early at home. Children rely on the warmth, structure, and consistency of family and marital relationships for their development. Family loneliness may emerge from parental characteristics or parenting styles, such as parental lower emotional availability due to personality uniqueness or stress. Children and adolescents, who felt that their family members were remote and not providing intimacy and support, reported that they were experiencing alienation in their homes. When they sensed that nobody in their home was listening to them or had a true interest in their day-to-day happening, they experienced social isolation in their families, and often reduced their emotional communication. Insensitive parenting and less secure child–mother attachment, when joined with children's temperament, may initiate the loneliness experience at home and later in school (Booth-LaForce & Oxford, 2008).

Indeed, the family environment may be a lonely place for children who feel that their parents don't understand them, and several risk factors were identified for developing this distress, such as parents that were described by their children as distant, uninvolved, busy in their challenges and roles, and not available to them. In addition, conflicts among parents further contributed to children's experiences of emotional isolation (Sturge-Apple et al., 2008), and parental separation or divorce would increase this distress (Bullock, 1993). Children often report higher levels of sadness and loneliness following parents' conflicts. Paradoxically, families who want to protect their children during difficult times, when families are struggling with demanding economic constrains or family illness, may initiate increased family loneliness by being reluctant to communicate and talk openly about the difficulties. Several parents tend to keep struggles as a secret, sometimes in order to "protect the children." The children often feel the family tension and do not have enough information for self-explanation, and will thus react negatively to the isolation and parental distancing intended to protect the children from distress. Parents may also distance themselves temporarily as a reaction to changes outside the family that caused various distresses such as economic hardship, health difficulties, and additional obligations (i.e., a sick grandparent).

Growing up in a comforting home, experiencing warm, stable, and secure relationships with parents and siblings is a valuable base for developing socialization, which extends far beyond the boundaries of family life itself. Family connectedness was considered a protective factor for the adjustment of children and adolescents (McGraw, Moore, Fuller, & Bates, 2008). Often children feel reluctant to share their loneliness inside their family. However, online blogs and forums often provide authentic voices of their inner experiences. For example, a girl wrote about her mother in her blog:

"When I feel alone, I just close my eyes and think about her, she who loves me truly, cares for me in my loneliness." Another adolescent wrote about his family "The worst kind of loneliness is when you discover that no one around you listens to you nor really cares much about you." An additional girl shared openly her unsatisfied need for connectedness inside her family "When we want to talk, really talk with our mother, I never feel like she wants to hear anything we have to say. My sister and I can't really open our mouths because we are told to be quiet." It is not easy for children to share their disappointment from their family and to share their loneliness inside their homes. The anonymity of the Internet enabled this self-disclosure – as will be further discussed in the chapter on the Internet (see Chapter 6). Connectedness has been described a protective factor against emotional distress. Unsupportive family environments take a toll on children and adolescent mental health, whereas the experience of consistently supportive environments is associated with higher levels of emotional wellbeing.

In conclusion, the quality of the family relations and the functioning of the family unity were related to children's experience of closeness and confidence with the family members (Dickstein, Seifer, & Albus, 2009), while conflicts promoted the children's and adolescents' experience of distress and alienation. Thus, it is not surprising that the children's conflict resolution strategies were related to children's loneliness (Çiftçi, Demir, & Bikos, 2008). It seems that lonely adolescents will try to avoid direct confrontations in their families. Different explanations were proposed regarding the nature of the links between children's loneliness and parents' characteristics and family social functioning (Cochran & Brassard, 1979). First, parents may directly model friendship for their children, who may observe and imitate specific behaviors, attitudes, or expectations. In addition, the social support that parents receive from friends may directly affect their parenting abilities and thus indirectly affect their children's peer relationships. Parents' friendship satisfaction negatively predicted child's peer rejection. This finding may be a result of both direct and indirect influences, as Cochran and Brassard (1979) suggest in their theory linking parental friendships and child outcomes. In terms of direct influences, parents who are satisfied with their friendships may believe that friendship is important, model strong friendships for their children, initiate play-dates, or intervene when children are upset about their own friendships. In these ways, parents may facilitate good peer relationships for their children. Parental management of conflicts with their friends were beneficial to their children by providing a model for the children's appropriate ways to negotiate and resolve conflicts, to regulate emotions during conflict, and ultimately, to repair and maintain strong relationships with others (Romano, Hubbard, McAuliffe, & Morrow, 2009).

Summary and Conclusions

In summary, there is not a single factor in the family that can explain or predict children's loneliness. Children's loneliness was presented in this chapter as related to the joint impact of individual and systemic experiences. Different approaches have considered the nature of parent–child interactions to be the roots of social competence, providing children with the confidence, knowledge, and experience that will serve as the basis for later social growth and peer relations. The present paradigm attempted to identify those factors which may either exacerbate parental feelings of distress and children's social difficulties, or may serve a stress-resistance role in buffering stressful realities and in empowering parental active coping and children's social growth. The recognition that parents may feel desperately alone in their parenting roles and responsibilities, yet, sometimes they also wish for time alone to empower themselves, exemplify the dynamic complex interactions between the need to be connected and the necessity for solitude.

From the early stages of development, the need for human intimacy appears and finds its expression in the infant's desire for continuous contact with the parents. Research showed that the conceptualization of attachment as a dynamic process continuing throughout the life cycle predicted social connections and isolation. Children and adolescents are continually renegotiating the balance between being connected to others and being independent and autonomous as they encounter new developmental challenges. The established attachment is considered stable, yet paradoxically it constantly develops, undergoing transformations and reintegration with subsequent personal achievements, such as emerging autonomy and entrance into the peer world. Family climate and parental interpersonal behaviors inside and outside the family, with family members as well as with friends and work mates, provide their children with social role models.

The systemic approach in family studies attempted to identify critical elements and processes that are locked together in promoting the children's growth and affecting their abilities to develop meaningful and satisfying social interrelations. Parent–child interactions were considered the end product of parental characteristics including their reactions to different types of stress, as well as disability-related stress, children's characteristics including their specific needs, and family resources as well as family climate. Parents' Sense of Coherence, the family's strengths and capacity for successful adjustment, and parental beliefs, attitudes, and coping abilities, all join together in presenting children with an environment that may either promote their capacity to form meaningful companionship and intimacy or may be considered as a risk for their development, predicting social isolation and alienation. Children's characteristics, strengths, and disabilities interact with these familial factors, predicting loneliness at home and among peers. The next chapter will present children's relations with peers and social exclusion. The wide range of parental activities has a cumulative impact on the different aspects of peer competence, recognizing its variability within different age-appropriate social activities such as the initiation of positive interactions with peers (i.e., utilizing specific peer-related social skills), the formation of affiliate ties (i.e., acquiring friendships and peer-acceptance) and high-quality relationships with peers (i.e., stability, support, security), the avoidance of debilitating social roles (i.e., victimization, rejection, and social withdrawal), and the interpersonal and emotional consequences of these aspects (i.e., loneliness, anxiety, and wariness).

References

Ainsworth, M. D. (1990). Some considerations regarding theory and assessment relevant to attachments beyond infancy. In M. T. Greenberg, D. Cicchetti, & E. M. Cummings (Eds.), *Attachment in preschool years* (pp. 463–488). Chicago: University of Chicago Press.

Al-Yagon, M. (2003). Children at-risk for developing learning disorders: Multiple perspectives. *Journal of Learning Disabilities, 36*(4), 318–335.

Al-Yagon, M. (2008). Maternal personal resources and children's socioemotional and behavioral adjustment. *Child Psychiatry and Human Development, 39*(3), 283–298.

Al-Yagon, M., & Margalit, M. (2009). Positive and negative affect among mothers of children with intellectual abilities. *British Journal of Developmental Disabilities, 52*(2), 109–127.

Amato, P. R., & Cheadle, J. E. (2008). Parental divorce, marital conflict and children's behavior problems: A comparison of adopted and biological children. *Social Forces, 86*(3), 1139–1161.

Antonovsky, A. (1987). *Unraveling the mystery of health*. San Francisco: Jossey-Bass.

Baumrind, D. (1978). Parental disciplinary patterns and social competence. *Youth, & Society, 9*(3), 239–277.

Baumrind, D. (1991). The influence of parenting style on adolescent competence and substance use. *Journal of Early Adolescence, 11*(1), 56–95.

Baumrind, D. (2005). Patterns of parental authority and adolescent autonomy. *New Directions for Child, & Adolescent Development, 2005*(108), 61–69.

Beaver, K. M., & Wright, J. P. (2007). A child effects explanation for the association between family risk and involvement in an antisocial lifestyle. *Journal of Adolescent Research, 22*(6), 640–664.

Belsky, J. (1984). The determinants of parenting: A process model. *Child Development, 55*, 83–96.

Belsky, J., & Barends, N. (2002). Personality and parenting. In M. H. Bornstein (Ed.), *Handbook of parenting* (Vol. 3, pp. 415–438). Mahwah, NJ: Erlbaum.

Black, K., & Lobo, M. (2008). A conceptual review of family resilience factors. *Journal of Family Nursing, 14*(1), 33–55.

Booth-LaForce, C., & Oxford, M. L. (2008). Trajectories of social withdrawal from grades 1 to 6: Prediction from early parenting, attachment, and temperament. *Developmental Psychology, 44*(5), 1298–1313.

Bowlby, J. (1969). *Attachment and loss: Vol.1. Attachment*. New York: Basic Books.

Bowlby, J. (1973). *Attachment and loss: Vol. 2. Separation: Anxiety and anger*. New York: Basic Books.

Bowlby, J. (1988). *A secure base*. New York: Basic Books.

Brodzinsky, D. M., & Pinderhughes, E. (2002). Parenting and child development in adoptive families. In M. H. Bornstein (Ed.), *Handbook of parenting* (Vol. 3, pp. 279–311). London: Lawrence Erlbaum.

Bugental, D. B. (2004). Thriving in the face of early adversity. *Journal of Social Issues, 60*(1), 219–235.

Bullock, J. R. (1993). Children's loneliness and their relationships with family and peers. *Family Relations, 42*(1), 46–50.

Button, S., Pianta, R. C., & Marvin, R. S. (2001). Partner support and maternal stress in families raising young children with cerebral palsy. *Journal of Developmental and Physical Disabilities, 13*(1), 61–81.

Campbell, S. B., Brownell, C. A., Hungerford, A., Spieker, S. J., Mohan, R., & Blessing, J. S. (2004). The course of maternal depressive symptoms and maternal sensitivity as predictors of attachment security at 36 months. *Development and Psychopathology, 16*(2), 231–252.

Cassidy, J., Parke, R. D., Butkovsky, L., & Braungart, J. M. (1992). Family-peer connections: The roles of emotional expressiveness within the family and children's. *Child Development, 63*(3), 603–619.

Cavanagh, S. E., & Huston, A. C. (2008). The timing of family instability and children's social development. *Journal of Marriage and the Family, 70*(5), 1258–1270.

Chao, R., & Tseng, V. (2002). Parenting of Asians. In M. H. Bornstein (Ed.), *Handbook of parenting* (Vol. 4, pp. 59–93). Mahwah, NJ: Lawrence Erlbaum.

Chen, X., Dong, Q., & Zhou, H. (1997). Authoritative and authoritarian parenting practices and social and school performance in Chinese children. *International Journal of Behavioral Development, 21*(4), 855–874.

Church, N. F., Brechman-Toussaint, M. L., & Hine, D. W. (2005). Do dysfunctional cognitions mediate the relationship between risk factors and postnatal depression symptomatology? *Journal of Affective Disorders, 87*(1), 65–72.

Cicirelli, V. G. (1995). *Sibling relationships across the lifespan.* New York: Plenum Press.

Çiftçi, A., Demir, A., & Bikos, L. H. (2008). Turkish adolescents' conflict resolution strategies towards peers and parents as a function of loneliness. *Adolescence, 43*(172), 911–926.

Cochran, M. M., & Brassard, J. A. (1979). Child development and personal social networks. *Child Development, 50*(3), 601–616.

Cohler, B. J., & Paul, S. (2002). Psychoanalysis and parenthood. In M. H. Bornstein (Ed.), *Handbook of parenting* (Vol. 4, pp. 563–599). Mahwah, NJ: Lawrence Erlbaum.

Cummings, E. M., & Cicchetti, D. (1990). Toward a transactional model of relations between attachment and depression. In M. T. Greenberg, D. Cicchetti, & E. M. Cummings (Eds.), *Attachment in preschool years* (pp. 339–372). Chicago: University of Chicago Press.

Cunningham, J. N., Kliewer, W., & Garner, P. W. (2009). Emotion socialization, child emotion understanding and regulation, and adjustment in urban African American families: Differential associations across child gender. *Development and Psychopathology, 21*(1), 261–283.

De Los Reyes, A., & Kazdin, A. (2005). Informant discrepancies in the assessment of childhood psychopathology: A critical review, theoretical framework and recommendations for future study. *Psychological Bulletin, 131*(4), 483–509.

de Minzi, M. C. R. (2006). Loneliness and depression in middle and late childhood: The relationship to attachment and parental styles. *Journal of Genetic Psychology, 167*(2), 189–210.

DeFrain, J., & Asay, S. M. (2007). Family strengths and challenges in the USA. *Marriage, & Family Review, 42*(3), 281–307.

Dickstein, S., Seifer, R., & Albus, K. E. (2009). Maternal adult attachment representations across relationship domains and infant outcomes: The importance of family and couple functioning. *Attachment, & Human Development, 11*(1), 5–27.

Dunst, C. J. (2002). Family-centered practices: Birth through high school. *Journal of Special Education, 36*(3), 139–148.

Dunst, C. J., Trivette, C. M., & Deal, A. G. (1988). *Enabling and empowering families.* Cambridge, MA: Brookline.

Edwards, A., Shipman, K., & Brown, A. (2005). The socialization of emotional understanding: A comparison of neglectful and nonneglectful mothers and their children. *Child Maltreatment, 10*(3), 293–304.

Efrati, M. W. (1993). *Family functioning and adolescents' social competence.* Unpublished master's thesis, Tel Aviv University.

Eisenberg, N., Cumberland, A., & Spinrad, T. L. (1998). Parental socialization of emotion. *Psychological Inquiry, 9*(4), 241–273.

Feng, X., Shaw, D. S., Kovacs, M., Lane, T., O'Rourke, F. E., & Alarcon, J. H. (2008). Emotion regulation in preschoolers: The roles of behavioral inhibition, maternal affective behavior, and maternal depression. *Journal of Child Psychology and Psychiatry, 49*(2), 132–141.

Fivush, R. (2006). Scripting attachment: Generalized event representations and internal working models. *Attachment, & Human Development, 8*(3), 283–289.

Gaudin, J. M., Polansky, N. A., Kilpatrick, A. C., & Shilton, P. (1993). Loneliness, depression, stress and social supports in neglectful families. *American Journal of Orthopsychiatry, 63*(4), 597–605.

Goodvin, R., Meyer, S., Thompson, R. A., & Hayes, R. (2008). Self-understanding in early childhood: Associations with child attachment security and maternal negative affect. *Attachment, & Human Development, 10*(4), 433–450.

Hart, C. H., Ladd, G. W., & Burleson, B. R. (1990). Children's expectations of the outcomes of social strategies-relations with sociometric status and maternal disciplinary styles. *Child Development, 61*(1), 127–137.

Hart, K. E., Wilson, T. L., & Hittner, J. B. (2006). A psychosocial resilience model to account for medical well-being in relation to sense of Coherence. *Journal of Health Psychology, 11*(6), 857–862.

Haskett, M. E., & Willoughby, M. (2007). Paths to child social adjustment: Parenting quality and children's processing of social information. *Child: Care, Health, & Development, 33*(1), 67–77.

Heaven, P., & Ciarrochi, J. (2008). Parental styles, gender and the development of hope and self-esteem. *European Journal of Personality, 22*(8), 707–724.

Henwood, P. G., & Solano, C. H. (1994). Loneliness in young children and their parents. *Journal of Genetic Psychology, 155*(1), 35–46.

Holahan, C. J., Moos, R. H., Moerkbak, M. L., Cronkite, R. C., Holahan, C. K., & Kenney, B. A. (2007). Spousal similarity in coping and depressive symptoms over 10 years. *Journal of Family Psychology, 21*(4), 551–559.

Hughes, C., & Ensor, R. (2009). Independence and interplay between maternal and child risk factors for preschool problem behaviors? *International Journal of Behavioral Development, 33*(4), 312–322.

Hymel, S., Tarulli, D., Hayden Thomson, L., & Terrell-Deutsch, B. (1999). Loneliness through the eyes of children. In K. J. Rotenberg & S. Hymel (Eds.), *Loneliness in childhood and adolescence* (pp. 80–106). New York: Cambridge University Press.

Idan, O., Sade, S., & Margalit, M. (2009, August). *Loneliness and hope: Risk and protective factors for predicting adolescent students' academic effort.* Paper presented at the XIV European Conference on Developmental Psychology, Vilnius, Lithuania

Jackson, T. (2007). Protective self-presentation, sources of socialization, and loneliness among Australian adolescents and young adults. *Personality and Individual Differences, 43*(6), 1552–1562.

Jones, W. J., Carpenter, B. N., & Quintana, D. (1985). Personality and interpersonal predictors of loneliness in two cultures. *Journal of Personality and Social Psychology, 48*(6), 1503–1511.

Josselson, R. (1992). *The space between us.* San Francisco: Jossey-Bass.

Kashdan, T. B., Pelham, W. E., Lang, A. R., Hoza, B., Jacob, R. G., Jennings, J. R., et al. (2002). Hope and optimism as human strength in parents of children with externalizing disorders: Stress in the eye of the beholder. *Journal of Social and Clinical Psychology, 21*(4), 441–468.

Keller, H. (2008). Attachment – Past and present. But what about the future? *Integrative Psychological and Behavioral Science, 42*(4), 406–415.

Ladd, G. W., & Pettit, G. S. (2002). Parenting and the development of children's peer relationships. In M. H. Bornstein (Ed.), *Handbook of parenting* (pp. 269–309). Mahwah, NJ: Lawrence Erlbaum.

Laible, D. (2007). Attachment with parents and peers in late adolescence: Links with emotional competence and social behavior. *Personality and Individual Differences, 43*(5), 1185–1197.

Lareau, A. (2000, August). *Invisible inequality: Social class and childrearing in black families and white families.* Paper presented at the Annual meeting of the American Sociological Association, Washington, DC.

Larson, P., & Olson, D. (2004). Prepare/enrich: A multifaceted systemic couple assessment tool. *The Family Psychologist, 20*(4), 4–9.

Lim, S., & Smith, J. (2008). The structural relationships of parenting style, creative personality, and loneliness. *Creativity Research Journal, 20*(4), 412–419.

Maccoby, E. E., & Martin, J. (1983). Socialization in the context of the family: Parent–child interactions. In E. M. Hertherington (Ed.), *Handbook of child psychology: Socialization, personality and social development* (Vol. 4, pp. 1–101). New York: Wiley.

Madden-Derdich, D. A., Estrada, A. U., Sales, L. J., Leonard, S. A., & Updegraff, K. A. (2002). Young adolescents' experiences with parents and friends: Exploring the connections. *Family Relations, 51*(1), 72–80.

Mak, W. W. S., Ho, A. H. Y., & Law, R. W. (2007). Sense of coherence, parenting attitudes and stress among mothers of children with autism in Hong Kong. *Journal of Applied Research in Intellectual Disabilities, 20*(2), 157–167.

Margalit, M. (1994). *Loneliness among children with special needs: Theory, research, coping and intervention.* New York: Springer.

Margalit, M. (2006). Loneliness, the Salutogenic paradigm and LD: Current research, future directions and interventional implications. *Thalamus, 24*(1), 38–48.

Margalit, M., & Al-Yagon, M. (2002). The loneliness experience of children with learning disabilities. In B. Y. L. Wong & M. Donahue (Eds.), *The social dimensions of learning disabilities* (pp. 53–75). Mahwah, NJ: Lawrence Erlbaum.

Margalit, M., & Almougy, K. (1991). Classroom behavior and family climate in students with learning disabilities and hyperactive behavior. *Journal of Learning Disabilities, 24*(7), 385–448.

Margalit, M., Leyser, Y., Ankonina, D. B., & Avraham, Y. (1991). Community support in Israeli kibbutz and city families of children with disabilities: Family climate and parental coherence. *Journal of Special Education, 24*(4), 427–440.

McCubbin, M., Balling, K., Possin, P., Frierdich, S., & Bryne, B. (2002). Family resiliency in childhood cancer. *Family Relations, 51*(2), 103–111.

McCubbin, H. I., & Patterson, J. M. (1983). The family stress process: The double ABCX model of adjustment and adaptation. In H. I. McCubbin, M. B. Sussman, & J. M. Patterson (Eds.), *Social stress and the family: Advances and developments in family stress theory and research* (pp. 7–37). New York: Haworth Press.

McDowell, D. J., & Parke, R. D. (2005). Parental control and affect as predictors of children's display rule use and social competence with peers. *Social Development, 14*(3), 440–457.

McElwain, N. L., Booth-LaForce, C., Lansford, J. E., Wu, X., & Dyer, W. J. (2008). A process model of attachment-friend linkages: Hostile attribution biases, language ability, and mother–child affective mutuality as intervening mechanisms. *Child Development, 79*(6), 1891–1906.

McGraw, K., Moore, S., Fuller, A., & Bates, G. (2008). Family, peer and school connectedness in final year secondary school students. *Australian Psychologist, 43*(1), 27–37.

McMahon, C., Barnett, B., Kowalenko, N., & Tennant, C. (2006). Maternal attachment state of mind moderates the impact of postnatal depression. *Journal of Child Psychology and Psychiatry, 47*(7), 660–669.

McPherson, A., Lewis, K., Lynn, A., Haskett, M., & Behrend, T. (2009). Predictors of parenting stress for abusive and nonabusive mothers. *Journal of Child, & Family Studies, 18*(1), 61–69.

Mikulincer, M., & Florian, V. (2001). Attachment style and affect regulation: Implications for coping with stress and mental health. In G. Fletcher & M. S. Clark (Eds.), *Blackwell handbook of social psychology: Interpersonal processes* (pp. 537–557). Oxford: Blackwell.

Milevsky, A. (2005). Compensatory patterns of sibling support in emerging adulthood: Variations in loneliness, self-esteem, depression and life satisfaction. *Journal of Social and Personal Relationships, 22*(6), 743–755.

Moos, R. H. (1991). Connections between school, work and family settings. In B. J. Fraser & H. J. Walberg (Eds.), *Educational environments: Evaluation, antecedents and consequences* (pp. 29–53). Oxford: Pergamon.

Moos, R. H. (2002). The mystery of human context and coping: An unraveling of clues. *American Journal of Community Psychology, 30*(1), 67–88.

Moos, R. H., & Holahan, C. J. (2003). Dispositional and contextual perspectives on coping: Toward an integrative framework. *Journal of Clinical Psychology, 59*(12), 1387–1403.

Moos, R., & Moos, B. (1994). *Family environment scale manual* (2nd ed.). Palo Alto, CA: Consulting Psychologists Press.

NICHD Early Child Care Research Network (1999). Chronicity of maternal depression symptoms, maternal sensitivity, and child functioning at 36 months. *Developmental Psychology, 35,* 1297–1310.

North, R. J., Holahan, C. J., Moos, R. H., & Cronkite, R. C. (2008). Family support, family income, and happiness: A 10-year perspective. *Journal of Family Psychology, 22*(3), 475–483.

Oelofsen, N., & Richardson, P. (2006). Sense of coherence and parenting stress in mothers and fathers of preschool children with developmental disability. *Journal of Intellectual, & Developmental Disability, 31*(1), 1–12.

Olson, D. H. (2000). Circumplex Model of marital and family systems. *Journal of Family Therapy, 22*(2), 144–167.

Olson, D. H., Gorall, D. M., & Tiesel, J. W. (2007). FACES IV, & the circumplex model: Validation study. *Journal of Family Therapy, 29*(2), 144–154.

Olthof, T., Kunnen, E. S., & Jan Boom (2000). Simulating mother–child interaction: Exploring two varieties of a non-linear dynamic systems approach. *Infant and Child Development, 9*(1), 33–60.

Oppenheim, D. (2006). Child, parent, and parent–child emotion narratives: Implications for developmental psychopathology. *Development and Psychopathology, 18*(3), 771–790.

Osborne, C., & McLanahan, S. (2007). Partnership instability and child well-being. *Journal of Marriage and the Family, 69*(4), 1065–1083.

Phares, V., Fields, S., & Kamboukos, D. (2009). Fathers' and mothers' involvement with their adolescents. *Journal of Child and Family Studies, 18*(1), 1–9.

Prange, M. E., Greenbaum, P. E., Silver, S. E., Friedman, R. M., Kutash, K., & Duchnowski, A. J. (1992). Family functioning and psychopathology among adolescents with severe emotional disturbances. *Journal of Abnormal Child Psychology, 20*(1), 83–102.

Pratt, M. W., Norris, J. E., Van de Hoef, S., & Arnold, M. L. (2001). Stories of hope: Parental optimism in narratives about adolescent children. *Journal of Social and Personal Relationships, 18*(5), 603–623.

Raikes, H. A., & Thompson, R. A. (2008). Attachment security and parenting quality predict children's problem-solving, attributions, and loneliness with peers. *Attachment, & Human Development, 10*(3), 319–344.

Raskind, M. H., & Margalit, M. (2008, June). *Between loneliness and aloneness: Mothers to children with LD and ADHD.* Paper presented at the Annual meeting of the IARLD, Toronto, ON, Canada.

Reese, E. (2008). Maternal coherence in the adult attachment interview is linked to maternal reminiscing and to children's self concept. *Attachment, & Human Development, 10*(4), 451–464.

Romano, L. J., Hubbard, J. A., McAuliffe, M. D., & Morrow, M. T. (2009). Connections between parents' friendships and children's peer relationships. *Journal of Social and Personal Relationships, 26*(2–3), 315–325.

Schaefer, E. S. (1965). A configurational analysis of children's reports of parent behavior. *Journal of Consulting Psychology, 29*(6), 552–557.

Shamir-Essakow, G., Ungerer, J. A., Rapee, R. M., & Safier, R. (2004). Caregiving representations of mothers of behaviorally inhibited and uninhibited preschool children. *Developmental Psychology, 40*(6), 899–910.

Sherman, A. M., Lansford, J. E., & Volling, B. L. (2006). Sibling relationships and best friendships in young adulthood: Warmth, conflict, and well-being. *Personal Relationships, 13*(2), 151–165.

Shorey, H. S., Snyder, C. R., Yang, X., & Lewin, M. R. (2003). The role of hope as a mediator in recollected parenting, adult attachment, and mental health. *Journal of Social and Clinical Psychology, 22*(6), 685–715.

Silk, J. S., Morris, A. S., Kanaya, T., & Steinberg, L. (2003). Psychological control and autonomy granting: Opposite ends of a continuum or distinct constructs? *Journal of Research on Adolescence, 13*(1), 113–128.

Slade, A., Belsky, J., Aber, J. L., & Phelps, J. L. (1999). Mothers' representations of their relationships with their toddlers: Links to adult attachment and observed mothering. *Developmental Psychology, 35*(3), 611–619.

Snyder, C. R. (2002). Hope theory: Rainbows in the mind. *Psychological Inquiry, 13*(4), 249–275.

Snyder, C. R., Sympson, S. C., Michael, S. T., Cheavens, J., & Chang, E. C. (2001). Optimism and hope constructs: Variants on a positive expectancy theme. In E. C. Chang (Ed.), *Optimism, & pessimism: Implications for theory, research, and practice* (pp. 101–125). Washington, DC: American Psychological Association.

Soenens, B., Vansteenkiste, M., & Sierens, E. (2009). How are parental psychological control and autonomy-support related? A cluster-analytic approach. *Journal of Marriage and the Family, 71*(1), 187–202.

Sroufe, L. A. (2005). Attachment and development: A prospective, longitudinal study from birth to adulthood. *Attachment, & Human Development, 7*(4), 349–367.

Sroufe, L. A., Egeland, B., Carlson, E. A., & Collins, W. A. (2005). *The developing person: The Minnesota study of risk and adaptation from birth to adulthood.* New York: Guilford.

Sroufe, L. A., & Sampson, M. C. (2000). Attachment theory and systems concept. *Human Development, 43*(6), 321–326.

Sturge-Apple, M. L., Davies, P. T., Winter, M. A., Cummings, E. M., & Schermerhorn, A. (2008). Interparental conflict and children's school adjustment: The explanatory role of children's internal representations of interparental and parent–child relationships. *Developmental Psychology, 44*(6), 1678–1690.

Suess, G. J., & Sroufe, J. (2005). Clinical implications of the development of the person. *Attachment, & Human Development, 7*(4), 381–392.

Thompson, R. A. (2000). The legacy of early attachments. *Child Development, 71*(1), 145–152.

Trapolini, T., Ungerer, J. A., & McMahon, C. A. (2008). Maternal depression: Relations with maternal caregiving representations and emotional availability during the preschool years. *Attachment, & Human Development, 10*(1), 73–90.

Uruk, A. C., & Demir, A. (2003). The role of peers and families in predicting the loneliness level of adolescents. *Journal of Psychology, 137*(2), 179–193.

Vandeleur, C. L., Perrez, M., & Schoebi, D. (2007). Associations between measures of emotion and familial dynamics in normative families with adolescents. *Swiss Journal of Psychology, 66*(1), 5–16.

Vaughn, B. E., Verissimo, M., Coppola, G., Bost, K., Shin, N., McBride, B., et al. (2006). Maternal attachment script representations: Longitudinal stability and associations with stylistic features of maternal narratives. *Attachment, & Human Development, 8*(3), 199–208.

Verschueren, K., & Marcoen, A. (2002). Perceptions of self and relationship with parents in aggressive and nonaggressive rejected children. *Journal of School Psychology, 40*(6), 501–522.

Weaver, S. R., & Prelow, H. M. (2005). A mediated-moderation model of maternal parenting style, association with deviant peers, and problem behaviors in urban African American and European American adolescents. *Journal of Child and Family Studies, 14*(3), 343–356.

Weinraub, M., Horvath, D. L., & Gringlas, M. B. (2002). Single parenthood. In M. H. Bornstein (Ed.), *Handbook of parenting* (Vol. 3, pp. 109–140). Mahwah, NJ: Lawrence Erlbaum.

White, R. M. B., Roosa, M. W., Weaver, S. R., & Nair, R. L. (2009). Cultural and contextual influences on parenting in Mexican American families. *Journal of Marriage and the Family, 71*(1), 61–79.

Winnicott, D. W. (1965). The capacity to be alone. In D. W. Winnicott (Ed.), *The maturation processes and the facilitating environment* (pp. 29–36). New York: International Universities Press.

Wiseman, H., Mayseless, O., & Sharabany, R. (2006). Why are they lonely? Perceived quality of early relationships with parents, attachment, personality predispositions and loneliness in first-year university students. *Personality and Individual Differences, 40*(2), 237–248.

Xin, Z., Chi, L., & Yu, G. (2009). The relationship between interparental conflict and adolescents' affective well-being: Mediation of cognitive appraisals and moderation of peer status. *International Journal of Behavioral Development, 33*(5), 421–429.

Yap, M. B. H., Allen, N. B., & Ladouceur, C. D. (2008). Maternal socialization of positive affect: The impact of invalidation on adolescent emotion regulation and depressive symptomatology. *Child Development, 79*(5), 1415–1431.

Yeh, H. C., & Lempers, J. (2004). Perceived sibling relationships and adolescent development. *Journal of Youth and Adolescence, 33*(2), 133–147.

Yu, G., Zhang, Y., & Yan, R. (2005). Loneliness, peer acceptance and family functioning of Chinese children with learning disabilities: Characteristics and relationships. *Psychology in the Schools, 42*(3), 325–331.

Zdanowicz, N., Janne, P., & Reynaert, C. (2004). Family, health, and adolescence. *Psychosomatics, 45*(6), 500–507.

Chapter 4
School Is a Lonely Place

"School can be a very lonely place" concluded Rick (a 10-year-old boy who had just moved with his parents and sisters to a new apartment). He talked with his father about the new school, summarizing his first week's experiences: "I am so alone there, and not only because I don't know the children in my class, but I feel that my teachers are not there for me. I don't know why they don't like me. Sometimes I feel that they don't see me. I hate school."

Children's and adolescents' loneliness at school is not identical to their social isolation or peer rejection, but may be related to it. Indeed loneliness at schools has reflected children's social status and friendship relations. Children who are rejected by their classmates and those who are not satisfied with their friendship relations often feel lonely, as will be discussed in Chapter 5. However, research has also documented that several children and adolescents experience loneliness at schools, sometimes regardless of their social status, their friendship networks, or their behavioral profile (Galanaki, 2007). Interviews of students, aged between 8 and 10 years (Berguno, Leroux, McAinsh, & Shaikh, 2004), revealed that many children described periods of loneliness at school, and that these experiences were often associated not only with their friendship relations, but also with the quality of their relations with teachers, their level of classroom participation, activities and success experiencing during school, tendencies to withdraw into day dreaming, and a passive attitude toward social interactions during recesses. Moreover, children who invested in very few friendships were more vulnerable to becoming isolated. Similarly, there was a connection between expressions of aggression and bullying and the children's loneliness distress with lonely children being more at risk to be victimized by peers. Children's prolonged loneliness at school was noted, even in preschools, closely related to their unsatisfactory relations with their teachers and to their unhappiness and difficulties at school. Several times the feelings of alienation was also initiated by life transitions such as moving to a new class, or having a new teacher, and supported by challenges and conflicts at school.

Playtime (recess) periods provide children with opportunities to relate to each other with minimal intervention on the part of teachers. This is the time when children have to initiate contacts with others, and to negotiate playing activities within groups of peers, or to feel isolated, challenged, and/or neglected. Children who use this opportunity to establish a wide network of friends or playmates appear to be

M. Margalit, *Lonely Children and Adolescents*, DOI 10.1007/978-1-4419-6284-3_4,   111
© Springer Science+Business Media, LLC 2010

less vulnerable to loneliness and bullying. Children may experience loneliness at school, followed by boredom and withdrawal. In consequence, the lonely children spend most of their free time at school on their own, lost in their own thoughts, slowly developing a passive attitude toward their school environment. It may gradually become more difficult for them to initiate contacts with the playing children. In addition, a child who is perceived by peers to be often alone may become the target of bullying, an experience which is likely to lead to an intensification of their experience of social isolation and distress.

The goals of this chapter are to provide expanded views of children's loneliness, as related to their wellbeing at school, including their success or failure and the outcomes in terms of their self-perception of academic competence. Two theoretical models guided the discussions in this chapter: the Transactional Model of Development (Sameroff & Mackenzie, 2003), and the Ecological and Dynamic Model of Transition (Rimm-Kaufman & Pianta, 2000). The Transactional Model places emphasis on the bi-directional nature of interactions between persons and environments. At the core of this model is the idea that neither individuals nor environments alone account for individual outcomes. Rather, it is the ongoing interplay between individuals and environment – such as the transactions between children and their teachers and schools – that dictates outcomes, with attributes of each one influencing the other. Development is best understood when considering ongoing transactions between children and their contexts, and how they contribute to important children's outcomes, such as teacher–child relationship quality. Thus the development of children is a product of the continuous dynamic interactions of the children and the experience provided by their social contexts such as their classes in addition to their families.

Relations with Teachers

The Ecological and Dynamic Model of Transition (Rimm-Kaufman & Pianta, 2000; Rimm-Kaufman & Sawyer, 2004) explored elements of the Transactional Model at periods of transition to school to clarify the dynamic relations between children and educational environments. The central distinction of this model is its emphasis on the development of relationships over time. This model posits that children's successful transitions to school are multi-determined and emerge from combinations of child and contextual characteristics. In addition, this model asserts that the interactions between child and context are bi-directional and always changing, having implications for relationships that impact development. Specifically, teachers influence children and children influence reactions from teachers. These relationships become more structured and stable over time as participants create perceptions, expectations, and behavior patterns in accordance with those expectations, reifying their beliefs about each other in actual contacts and interactions. Research informed by the Ecological and Dynamic Model of Transition reflects an emphasis not only on the relationships among contexts, but how these connections form patterns that develop to affect transition outcomes. For example, a teacher may turn to help a child with difficulties because she believes from her past experience with children with similar competence that "she can make a difference." Another teacher may distance the child with difficulties since she doesn't feel capable to attend to his or her problems, and is afraid to fail. As children make the transition from preschool to kindergarten, a new ecology associated with formal schooling begins to form. Thus, the development of this ecology itself is a key focus for understanding transition processes and outcomes.

The distinctiveness of students' relations with teachers and the attachment processes will be presented in their connections with loneliness. The intrapersonal experience will also be the focus of interest in order to clarify factors that predict wellbeing and inoculate against loneliness. Teachers' attitudes and perceptions of children's competence will be clarified and reviews of research will be provided in order to demonstrate the impact of teachers' beliefs, classroom climate, competitive or collaborative working style, and values on children's experiences of social isolation. In conclusion, children's characteristics that contribute to their vulnerability to loneliness at school such as giftedness and learning disabilities will be presented to exemplify the complexity of the interacting contextual factors in the educational environments.

A great deal of consensus already exists concerning the perceived importance of early and different patterns of relations for the development of satisfying social competence throughout life, not only inside the family contexts – with family members, but also within the school context, with teachers and peers (Rubin & Mills, 1988). The significant role of teachers in children's social and emotional development has been investigated less systematically than the role of parents and peers. Research demonstrated the important role of teachers' expectations and beliefs and their affective expressions to the children's wellbeing and their varied reactions to children's behavior (Arbeau & Coplan, 2007). Several assumptions were proposed in order to explain the nature of the relationship between teachers' and children's loneliness, accentuating the teachers' importance for children's development. Overall, children's school adjustment was facilitated by obtaining close relationships with the teacher, whereas teacher–child conflicts, and to a lesser extent dependency, predicted the children's poorer adjustment (Ewing & Taylor, 2009). These relations are complex and multidirectional, and for some children they have a tremendous impact on their wellbeing, even when teachers are not aware of their origin and manifestations. Age and gender differences were identified in the relations' formation and levels of closeness. For example, girls benefited more from the close relations than boys, but both genders valued teachers' closeness, especially at the preschool and first grades stages.

Teacher–Child Relations at the Preschool

Relationships are key resources for young children, and the quality of their relationships with teachers predicts social and academic performance in school. Without these social resources, children are more likely to attempt avoiding school, report experiencing loneliness, and display low levels of academic and social competence (Birch & Ladd, 1997). Adam's story exemplifies young children's reports of their unsatisfactory relations with teachers.

Adam (a 5-year-old boy) returned home after a few days with a new teacher and told his mother that tomorrow he was not going back to school. "My teacher does not like me, I am alone in class all day" he said. "Many times she just ignores me. When I answer her questions, she says 'very good' but I am almost sure that she does not listen to me. When I talk, she seems distracted and quickly asks other children for another answer. She rarely talks to me if I don't talk to her first, or sits with me." The mother suggested that maybe this was the teacher's style in her new class and that she treated all the kids the same way. But Adam insisted "She likes many children, she sits with them, helps them and laughs with them. She rarely smiles at me." The mother was surprised at her child's detailed observations and his abilities to express his agony. Usually he was an easy-going boy, and expressed his happy mood and feelings quite openly with short and simple answers. This time it seemed that he thought a lot about the situation and tried to find the right words to explain the complicated and most distressful situation. To his mother's worried inquiry if the teacher was expressing her anger due to his misbehavior or a conflict, he declared, "Nothing has happened! The teacher did not shout at me or punish me." Then he started to cry and said that maybe the teacher liked those naughty children that she shouted at them more. This was a worrying remark, especially when it was expressed by a child who was usually cheerful and well-behaved. The mother immediately and worriedly called the teacher. The teacher was completely surprised. She said emphatically "I love all the kids in my class, and there is no exception. He is such a good boy. I don't have any problem with him. Sometimes I almost forget that he is in class. . ." Later, the mother e-mailed her friend this story, and added ". . .While I was talking with the teacher on the phone, I felt confident that she did not like my son. I don't know why. Maybe she prefers children who require more disciplinary attention. She just ignores him. It is so sad that now he hates her and the school."

Several parents shared with us similar stories, emphasizing the importance of children–teachers' relations. Usually parents complained that teachers did not like the kids when they were naughty, inattentive, and aggressive. Adam's story is an example that due to a mismatch between teachers' expectations and students' behavior. Even pleasant and collaborative students may be neglected by teachers since they do not need constant attention to prevent misbehaving, but these students may feel neglected, rejected, and unappreciated. Several empirical studies documented the teacher's significant contribution to children's development, as well as school academic achievements and social adjustment in different ages from pre-kindergarten children to adolescents (Reio, Marcus, & Sanders-Reio, 2009). For young children, responsive and stimulating teachers and instructional quality aspects in the classroom jointly predicted the children's acquisition of language and pre-academic skills. Research also reported teachers' contribution to children's social competence (Burchinal et al., 2008; Tsigilis & Gregoriadis, 2008). Interactions between family background variables and teacher–child relationships indicated that a closer relationship with the teacher and social processes in classrooms were fundamental for children's academic competence, especially those who were considered at risk for academic difficulties (Burchinal, Peisner-Feinberg, Pianta, & Howes, 2002).

Children's characteristics such as shyness and effortful control also contributed to the quality and frequency of teacher–child interactions. Shy children were less likely to initiate interactions with teachers. These interactions were reciprocal, and shy children initiated fewer interactions with teachers, and these fewer child-initiated interactions predicted lower levels of closeness. The frequency of child- and teacher-initiated interactions contributed to each other; more frequent child-initiated interactions contributed to more frequent teacher-initiated interactions, and more teacher-initiated interactions contributed to fewer child-initiated interactions (Rudasill & Rimm-Kaufman, 2009).

These important relations between children and teachers at the preschool level establish the first formal educational experiences outside the children's homes. This recognition of child–teacher relations does not contradict the appreciation of the prolonged important impact of families. Indeed a continuous influence of the attachment relations throughout development was identified. It was clearly demonstrated that the early attachment experiences of children with mothers and fathers promoted children's abilities to benefit from positive relations with their teachers. Children, who had supporting and responsive homes, were better prepared for the preschool environment and for developing satisfactory relations outside their homes. However, within this relationship consistency some flexibility was identified, emphasizing the important role that teachers may fulfill in promoting significant changes. For example, a longitudinal follow-up study revealed the positive impact of supportive relations with teachers and caregivers outside the home, even for maltreated children whose parents did not establish a secured attachment with them (Manashko, Besser, & Priel, 2009).

Children's behavioral problems may lead to students–teachers conflicts and impair the supportive relations. Teachers' beliefs and perceptions of these problems may predict students' feelings of teachers' support, closeness, or rejection (Hamre, Pianta, Downer, & Mashburn, 2008). Thus, it can be concluded that children's relations with their teachers at preschools have a critical value for all children, but especially for vulnerable children such as children with attention and behavior problems and for children from ethnic minority families. It is not surprising that children who are cared for sensitively and supportively by their parents will continue to benefit from the supportive relations with their teachers. However, even for children at risk, supportive teachers may enhance a change in the children's early abilities to develop meaningful relations. Interestingly, these results are not unique for young children who are considered more flexible in their relation development and personal characteristics, but similar conclusions have been reported for elementary school students and adolescents.

Teacher–Student Relations in Elementary Schools

Students who experienced close relationships with teachers within a supportive school community reported more positive feelings about school and achieved higher levels of social, academic, and behavioral competence. Studies reported that students' perceptions of social relatedness lay a critical foundation for motivated engagement, which in turn promoted academic achievement and positive social adaptation including lower loneliness at school (Gest, Welsh, & Domitrovich, 2005). Social relatedness was conceptualized in a variety of ways, including relatedness to specific social partners such as teachers and peers, and more general perceptions of support and belonging to the school environment versus loneliness and alienation (Furrer & Skinner, 2003). Developmental trends and behavioral predictors for three dimensions of social relatedness were examined in a 6-month longitudinal study of 383 students in Grades 3, 4, and 5 (Gest et al., 2005). Student reports of social relatedness (teacher supportiveness, school supportiveness, and loneliness) and levels of "liking school" indicated that in each of the grades the children felt in the Spring term less positive about the school environment and they liked school less compared to the beginning of the year. A similar decline was reported among students in higher grade levels. It seems that in the beginning of the year students generally had higher expectations that were not fully fulfilled. Yet, their feelings of loneliness were stable during the school year. Several factors predicted their loneliness. It was predicted by teachers' support, by students' aggressive behavior (aggressive children reported higher loneliness), and by the wellbeing indicators at school (lonely children did not like school). Students' perceptions of teacher supportiveness were negatively related to increased loneliness and decreased levels of liking school across the school year. In addition, teacher-rated reports of closeness predicted the maintenance of student's high levels of relatedness. Student's aggression was associated with declines in a student's liking for school only to the extent that it was associated with declines in the student's perception of support from the classroom teacher. These results supported earlier research suggesting that the student–teacher relationship may play a particularly critical role in the overall school adjustment and loneliness of children displaying high levels of aggression (Hamre & Pianta, 2001).

In conclusion, consistency and changes in teachers' closeness to students predicted the wellbeing in school, as well as the students' loneliness. Although relations with teachers and the behavior expressions of closeness change from preschool through elementary school to adolescence, the basic feeling of closeness and relatedness to teachers remains the same, as illustrated by Ron's explanation how his feelings toward school were changed when he moved to high school.

Teacher–Adolescents Relations

Ron was a gifted lonely child during most of the years at elementary school. He was considered a very good student, yet he repeatedly declared that he hated school. Often he made excuses to stay at home and to play with his computer. He did not have a good friend since the second grade when his best friend had moved to another school. His classmates did not like him, and did not include him in games and sports. When he moved to high school, a change was revealed, and his surprised mother said with enthusiasm that he was now "a different boy." From the beginning, the computer teacher realized his creativity and appreciated his gifted abilities. The teacher shared her impressions with other teachers and gradually he felt the teachers' supporting relations and expressions of appreciation. Some teachers asked for his help and he provided it without any hesitation. His reputation in the new school was respected. He was invited to be the leader of the computer group and the editor of the school e-journal. The teacher continuously challenged him with difficult tasks, but at the same time she supported and valued his efforts and success, and clearly showed that she liked him. His parents were astonished and almost wordless when children start asking him for help with regard to their computer problems, and they gradually included him in various social online and offline activities and hung around with him. He told his parents that the move to the high school had changed his life completely. He was perhaps too busy, but had many friends, and his teachers liked and appreciated him.

Ron's story is an example of the positive role that teachers may fulfill for adolescents, especially at this age stage of identity exploration and rapid developmental changes. Research on adolescents further confirmed the importance of positive social interactions and relationships with teachers and peers at school as a foundation for current and future students' adjustment (Wentzel & Wigfield, 2007). In addition, the lack of teachers' nurturance and support of their students was the most consistent negative predictor of academic performance and social adjustment (Wentzel, 2003).

Throughout developmental stages, within an ecological conceptualization, a caring classroom environment in which teachers and peers support and promote the expression of positive social behaviors plays a critical role in enhancing students' adoption and even pursuit of positive social goals. In order to further understand the processes how teachers create a caring classroom environment, researchers proposed to apply adapted models of effective parenting. Wentzel proposed these models of good parenting in order to conceptualize the quality of the relations between students and their teachers (Wentzel, 2002). She examined the applicability of parents' socialization models for the appreciation of teachers' influence on student adjustment in middle schools. Based on reports from 452 sixth graders, the analysis indicated that, similar to research on parenting behavior, when teachers had high expectations of their students and especially expectations for mature and responsible behavior – their students would have higher goals and wider interests. These results on teachers and schools can be considered as a continuation to family studies, in which parental expressions of warmth and approval as well as conscientious protection of children's physical and emotional wellbeing provided secure parent–child relationships. These relations in families as well as in schools would enable children to develop a generalized positive skill of interpersonal relatedness and personal competence. In turn, these positive aspects of self-development further supported the internalization of socially prescribed goals and values, and contributed to a student's sense of belongingness and motivated engagement in appropriate classroom behavior (Wentzel, 2003). Using family research conceptualization, students who perceived their teachers as adults with high levels of caring characteristics tended to pursue appropriate social and academic classroom goals more frequently than students who did not. Similarly, students who liked school had higher academic achievement and a lower incidence of disciplinary conflicts, absenteeism, truancy, and dropping out of school than did those who disliked school. It can be concluded that teachers have an important role in shaping students' feelings about school. Since attachment to school had been shown to affect students' academic performance and social functioning, students' feelings about school were examined for 6th-, 8th-, and 10th-grade students. The results of this study (Hallinan, 2008) showed that students who reported that their teachers cared about them, respected them, and praised them, were more apt to like school than were those who did not.

Attachment at Schools

The attachment conceptualization between children and their teachers as a predictor of children's loneliness and adjustment was examined by several researchers. Initially the attachment conceptualization focused attention on the relations between infants and their caregivers (usually mothers) (Bowlby, 1969). Gradually the concept was generalized to various types of relations (Mikulincer & Florian, 1998) and extended to provide in-depth understanding of the processes underneath teachers'– students' relations (Al-Yagon & Margalit, 2006). According to the attachment conceptualization, children's and adolescents' loneliness was associated with the following three qualities of the teacher–child relationship: closeness, dependency, and conflict (Burgess, Ladd, Kochenderfer, Lambert, & Birch, 1999). Closeness in the teacher–child relationship functions as a form of support, because it represents a warm, affectionate bonding between these two figures. The child approaches the teacher with certain expectations and worries, discussing his or her feelings and experiences, and uses the teacher as a source of support or consolation in times of stress.

In contrast, dependency means that the children exhibit over-reliance on their teachers, clinging to them, demanding to possess the teacher exclusively, requesting their attention and affection. The tendency toward dependency is not infrequent among preschool and early school-age children, but it is expected to decline gradually with age. Dependency has been viewed as different from the children's secure attachment to an adult figure. Secure attachment, as described by Bowlby (1969), permits the child to explore the environment and to seek closeness whenever needed, whereas dependent children are expected to decrease their exploratory behavior, both in the academic and in the interpersonal-social domain in the school. However, the loneliness-dependency association may be reciprocal. Children who feel lonely (due to various sources, such as low parental support, peer rejection, low-quality friendships, academic challenges, etc.) will approach teachers as the significant adults in the school environment. Sometimes teachers will empower children's abilities to cope with challenges and explore solutions to their difficulties by providing them a secure base. In contrast, several teachers may promote increased dependency that will decrease the students' needs for independent solutions and, in addition, contribute to their beliefs in their inabilities to find satisfactory solutions.

A vulnerable balance exists between providing a secure base that will empower children and a sanctuary that will enhance withdrawal from facing their problems, demanding teachers' understanding, insight, and training. Sometimes a developmental and multi-stage approach is requested, with the teachers' abilities to accept the children's needs and expectations for dependency during times of acute and severe crises, and gradually to empower their abilities to see the teachers as a secure base that encourage explorations and experimentations of different solutions. When the teacher–child relationships are characterized by frequent and intense conflicts (discordant interactions and a lack of rapport), the child experiences will be characterized by feelings of distress, anger, anxiety, and loneliness.

Research proposed that children, who reached better social competence due to their positive relations with teachers, will feel less lonely at school. However, in order to reach a clearer understanding of these processes and their contribution to children's loneliness, several studies employed differential approaches to clarify the relations between attachment conceptualization, classroom relations, and loneliness. The growing awareness regarding the important contribution of attachment-based factors to socio-emotional adjustment of individuals across the life span (Mikulincer & Florian, 2001) necessitated a focused consideration of the close relations construct for school-age children, beyond their relations at home and in their families, and to examine children's specific relations with their teachers.

Research (Al-Yagon & Mikulincer, 2004) reported that the secure attachment style of children made a unique and significant contribution to their lower feelings of loneliness, higher Sense of Coherence, and their higher academic functioning. In addition, children's perceptions of their teachers as "a secure base," i.e., considering them as a more available, accepting, and less rejecting figure, also contributed to lower feelings of loneliness, higher Sense of Coherence, and higher academic functioning. In conclusion, the child's appraisal of his or her teacher as a secure base (i.e., available, accepting, and non-rejecting) was related to the teacher's stronger feelings of closeness to the child. More secure attachment patterns in close relationships with teachers were beneficial to children's socio-emotional and academic adjustment.

Furthermore, the comparison of two groups among 266 3rd-graders in Israel (118 children with reading difficulties and 148 children without reading difficulties) (Al-Yagon & Margalit, 2006) identified differences between groups in different aspects of the children's attachment with their teachers. In this study, the children's appraisal of teachers as a secure base examined two unique, yet interrelated aspects: (a) the teachers' availability (assessment of the teacher as available in times of need – i.e., "When I need the teacher's help, she is always there") and as a caring figure who accepts the child's needs, feelings, and behaviors (i.e., "My teacher expresses her appreciation of me even when I fail," "When I am worried or sad, my teacher helps me feel better"); and (b) the teachers' tendency to reject the children (the extent to which the child considers the teacher as a rejecting figure who feels impatient and inattentive to the children's needs i.e., "The teacher makes me feel that I'm unnecessary in the class"; "My teacher tends to complain about me to other adults (for instance, parents, teachers, principal)"). The results of this study showed that children who perceived their teachers as highly rejecting and/or unavailable in times of need reported higher levels of loneliness and a lower Sense of Coherence than did children who perceived their teachers as slightly rejecting or usually available and attentive to their needs.

These diverse attachment patterns with teachers revealed basic individual differences. Children, who developed secured attachment at home before entering school, had a better likelihood to form secure relationships with their teachers. However, research showed that even insecurely attached children were able to develop secure patterns of attachment with their teachers. In order to understand these processes, the characteristics of both partners were examined. The specific current relations' patterns were more influential than the child's earlier global attachment style that was based on the earlier parents–child relations at home. These results underscore the important role that the quality of teachers' care can play in forming supportive child–teacher relationships. The key qualities of these relationships appear to be related to the teacher's ability to provide a sensitive and responsive support. The exploration of teachers' characteristics (Pianta, 1999) provided in-depth understanding of these processes. Teachers who were able to read the child's unique needs, to meet these needs with a sensitive and attentive responding, to convey acceptance and emotional warmth, and to offer the necessary assistance enhanced children's wellbeing.

Two specific factors further extend our understanding of the impact of students–teachers' relations on loneliness, namely, the duration and the variability of the relations with teachers, and especially the conflicts (Burgess et al., 1999). Children's and adolescents' get new teachers every few years and sometimes there are changes from year to year. During the academic year, reciprocal relations are gradually established between students and teachers. Their behavior reflects their mutual expectations, beliefs, and perceptions that interact with the day-to-day occurrences in class. New teachers introduce changes to relations and necessitate new negotiations for student–teacher connections. For several children, these changes may enhance their anxiety and feelings of isolation and loneliness. For example, if a child had a warm, supportive relationship with a teacher during one academic year, he or she may lose it during the next academic year. Children who develop dependency on their teachers may feel desperation, loneliness, and increased anxiety. On the other hand, children who view their teachers as a secure base will be anxious to explore their relations with the new adult figure. In another and quite different situation, changes are welcomed, when the children may otherwise continue to have the same teacher with whom conflictual relationships were established. Thus the new teacher may provide a new promise for developing different relations.

Conflicts between children and their teachers may reinforce feelings of anger, anxiety, and alienation, and all these may predispose the child to withdraw from most school activities and become lonely and socially isolated. Following the teachers' angry expressions, the children that participated in the conflicts became socially isolated. Thus, higher levels of loneliness were reported by children who participated in conflictual interactions with teachers (Ladd & Burgess, 1999). Aggressive children often get into conflicts at schools. However, not all aggressive children are lonely, and the heterogeneity of this group and their interactions with peers and adults, as well as the predictors of their academic achievement, revealed diverse results (Efrati-Virtzer & Margalit, 2009; Galanaki, Polychronopoulou, & Babalis, 2008; Stipek & Miles, 2008). Among aggressive children who reported more conflicts with their teachers, special attention was focused on a special group of aggressive-withdrawn children who had fewer close relations with friends and more conflicts with their teachers. High prevalence of attention difficulties including ADHD and learning disabilities were identified in this group of children, and the conflicts with teachers may have contributed to their difficulties and created interpersonal contexts within which their loneliness may have evolved (Hymel, Tarulli, Hayden Thomson, & Terrell-Deutsch, 1999). Thus, it can be concluded that aggressive children and children with attention and behavior difficulties may be drawn into escalating conflictual relations at school, and may be at risk for developing enhanced loneliness. Children express their loneliness in wide-ranging manifestations, and in order to meet their needs, teachers have, first of all, to be able to identify distressed expressions of children's loneliness at different age groups.

Can Teachers Identify and Help Lonely Children?

The importance of this ability is undeniable, but differences in the children's typical behavior may affect their success. Teachers are especially responsive to aggressive and disturbing children, while most lonely children tend to be withdrawn and reserved, and present difficult challenges to the recognition and appreciation of their distress. After establishing the importance of the relations with teachers, the exploration of this question is critical for ensuring appropriate and sensitive teachers' support to the children. Research found that teachers were able to differentiate not only between prosocial and aggressive behaviors of young children (already at the kindergarten age group), but also between shy (who are sociable) and unsociable children (Arbeau & Coplan, 2007).

Preschool children who were engaged in quiet solitary play were not considered distressed and did not disrupt their classrooms. They were not considered at risk for developing loneliness. Thus, although shy children may have interacted less with peers, they often watched other children without joining the group (i.e., on looking behaviors), and they were not isolated. In contrast, when children displayed overt signs of anxiety and distress, teachers were able to identify their distress and were aware of it. Another group that displayed socially reticent behaviors in early childhood classroom settings had been often associated with psychosocial difficulties, including internalizing problems, lower self-worth, a lack of social competence, loneliness, and peer exclusion (Rubin & Coplan, 2004). Taken together, teachers were able to differentiate between shy children who had a quite temperament, but adequate social competence, and lonely children with internalized difficulties. Similarly (Youngblade, Berlin, & Beslky, 1999), teachers of kindergarten and first-grade children were able to identify aloneness and anxiety and distinguish between lonely children and children who preferred to have time alone, but did not feel lonely.

Inconsistent results were reported for school-age children. Studies (Galanaki & Kalantzi-Azizi, 1999) reported that only 25–30% of the teachers were able to identify the lonely children in their classes, while other studies (Luftig, 1988) informed that most teachers were able to correctly identify loneliness. Our studies (Margalit, 1994) demonstrated that this inconsistency in teachers' sensitivity to children's loneliness reflected the interactions between their personal heterogeneity and students' diverse abilities and difficulties. In addition, many teachers mentioned their anxiety and were reluctant to deal with this issue. They felt more confident to deal with students' learning difficulties than with children's social challenges and frustrations.

In an investigation into teachers' perceptions of their effectiveness in assisting children to avoid loneliness and isolation, many teachers reported that they felt ineffective when they were requested to help lonely children, and they added that they did not feel comfortable when they had to respond to it (Page, 1991). Several teachers even indicated that they did not think that the caring for loneliness was their responsibility. Several teachers did not view it as a worthwhile target for prevention, and most teachers felt unprepared to deal with children's loneliness. Since they considered their major role to be in the academic domains, they suggested referring the lonely children to the mental health professional, such as the school psychologists or the school counselors. This is a sad reality, since teachers play an important role in creating and sustaining children's loneliness. In addition, loneliness was linked to academic achievements, and teachers have many opportunities to prevent and, most importantly, to alleviate this distress. Most children are aware of the teachers' reluctant and anxious reactions to children's loneliness in class (Galanaki, 2007), and they expect teachers to provide meaningful help and support. It is clear that school climate provides critical contextual conditions in which teachers and children interact in ways that reduce or enhance loneliness.

School Climate and Children's Loneliness

School environments vary greatly. The feelings and attitudes that are elicited by a school's environment are referred to as school climate. School climate taps individuals' perceptions of the school as a space for learning and interacting with peers and authority figures (Syvertsen, Flanagan, & Stout, 2009). School climate refers to the quality and character of school life (Cohen, Mccabe, Michelli, & Pickeral, 2009). It reflects norms, goals, values, interpersonal relationships, teaching and learning practices, and organizational structures. In several schools, the supportive, collaborating, and friendly relations among children are encouraged and welcomed, while other environments convey competitive relations, social exclusion, and even intimidating harsh connections among groups. Although it is difficult to provide a single concise definition for school climate, most researchers agree that it is a multidimensional construct that includes physical, social, and academic dimensions. Students' relations with teachers portray only a partial image of this complex construct.

A sustainable, positive school climate fosters children development and learning. The satisfaction of students from their schools was predicted by the extent of students' confidence that their classroom was perceived as a caring, accepting, safe, and supportive environment. These results were confirmed across cultures, as indicated in an examination of school climate in relation to school satisfaction in over 16,000 students aged 11, 13, and 15, in four countries (Finland, Latvia, Norway, and Slovakia; Samdal, Nutbeam, Wold, & Kannas, 1998). Studies also pointed attention to the associations between students' happiness (and unhappiness), and their general views and attitudes toward school, including their overall satisfaction (Suldo, Riley, & Shaffer, 2006). When students believed that they were treated fairly, they were not worried about their safety at school, they had confidence in their teachers' support, and they were satisfied with their life at school. In addition, the students' confidence in their academic competence was also systematically related to their life satisfaction at school, focusing attention on children's at risk for increased loneliness.

The relationship between teachers and students is complex, multidirectional, and changes during development. Family context was found a significant factor in predicting relations with teachers at the beginning of school and lower grades, but not for subsequent development. Gradually, class cohesion, as well as adolescents' perceptions of their teachers, determined the depressive expressions and loneliness of children. In other words, once the adolescent gets used to junior high school, the school context tends to exert more pronounced effects in predicting children's happiness and loneliness (Yi, Wu, Chang, & Chang, 2009). The quality of the student–teacher relationship may be the channel through which the student's loneliness is aggravated or alleviated, reflecting students' individual differences that interact with classroom climate and teachers' preferences. For instance, teachers' emphasis on cooperation, self-esteem enhancement, and the cultivation of a positive social–emotional climate were generally considered to support children' connectedness and decrease loneliness (Galanaki, 2007). The emphasis on a less personalized interaction pattern at school was expected to aggravate loneliness in children because of the little emphasis on cooperation, social problem solving, and dyadic relationships, and on the cultivation of a positive social–emotional classroom climate. However, the complexity of these multifactor interactions has to be recognized. For example, students will generally flourish in a classroom climate that will promote and appreciate school relatedness, and good interpersonal and social relationships. However, in an achievement-focused class environment, an isolated lonely but high-ability student may experience increased wellbeing, acceptance, and self-esteem, and decreased loneliness. In the same class, students with academic challenges may feel socially isolated and generally unappreciated. Thus, the same school climate may interact differently with children's characteristics, such as strengths, challenges, and individualized needs. Learning challenges (as personal factors) often interact with the school climate (as a contextual factor) and may contribute to increased loneliness, in addition to the protective impacts of children's social competence.

Children at Risk of Experiencing Loneliness at School

Special attention was devoted in research to children who face continuous academic difficulties at school, reporting that many of them were at a greater risk for developing loneliness and alienation at school. For example, studies reported that children who had high-prevalence difficulties at school, such as learning disorders, behavior problems, and attention difficulties, were often more lonely than their peers (Margalit, 1994, 2006). The chronic and prolonged academic struggles in different study domains affected their identity formation and were related to their experience of interpersonal isolation in an ongoing and reciprocal manner. Their self-questioning about the roots of their academic challenges and their impact on the developing self-esteem may determine their feelings that they are different from their peers. Many times their emotional experience of social isolation is accompanied with the upsetting jealousy directed toward those children that can reach high academic recognition without extended effort investment and struggles. Dan's example illustrates these processes.

Dan, a fifth-grade student with learning disabilities, said that indeed he could achieve average grades, but he had to invest endless hours in his effort to get them. Some of his classmates studied for examinations just on the last day before tests. He perceived himself unlucky, since he had to work consistently, and could not leave studying for the last minute. Sadly he said that he was not sure if his social isolation was due to less free time to spend with friends, or because his classmates recognized him being different, and reacted to his academic difficulties.

Not only children with learning challenges experience social rejection, but gifted students may also experience social exclusion and identity challenges since they feel different from the group. Historically, research and education of the gifted children has focused attention on cognitive and academic variables, with less attention given to their social and emotional needs, and the social support provided by teachers (Mueller, 2009). Gifted children may similarly be affected by social context, perhaps because they demonstrate a more mature social competence than their chronological peers. Several children may have fewer friends and, in order to feel accepted and make more friends, talented students sometimes deny their academic competence and needs to satisfy social needs. Students, who are able to find intellectual peers, generally feel less pressure to conform and more freedom to pursue their academic interests. The situation can be even more awkward for those students who are extremely talented but have only few friends. As they become less socially adept and more introverted, they will experience increased loneliness (Reis & Renzulli, 2004). They reported feelings of social isolation when they were rejected or alienated from positive persons, places, or things, and when they felt helpless and were not in control of a situation. They used a variety of coping strategies to deal with their loneliness, and preferred individual pursuits and cognitive reframing (Woodward & Kalyan-Masih, 1990). In addition, many gifted children and adolescents are noted for the intensity of their reactions to areas that interest them, and this type of reactivity may be explained as over-excitabilities (i.e., greater capacities to respond to various stimuli). Thus, they may be more susceptible to feelings of boredom with class curriculum when it is neither challenging nor appropriate for their intellectual needs. For example, some gifted children that understand faster ask more questions, hurry through math, and may be terribly disruptive in their classes. Instead of accepting the boredom and waiting for others to catch up, they may create their own intellectual and physical stimulation, which may not correlate with the teachers' expectations and class regulations. Thus, they may feel different, isolated, and distanced from their teachers and classmates (Tieso, 2007).

In addition, several children who felt different and socially isolated expressed lower levels of hope for changing their situation, declaring: "my teacher doesn't like me," feeling secluded and alienated at school. Teachers' attitudes toward children affected their self-perceptions (Lopes, Monteiro, Sil, Rutherford, & Quinn, 2004) as well as their peer attitudes, especially at younger ages. School climate, classroom relations, teachers' beliefs, and teaching styles are important predictive factors that interact with these vulnerable children, contributing to their feelings of alienation. Chapter 5 discusses their social skills' deficits and peer relations; however, the role of their relations with teachers should not be overlooked.

Only a few studies examined child–teacher relations among children with special needs. They highlighted the important role of these relations in explaining students' adjustment (Murray & Greenberg, 2001; Murray & Pianta, 2007; Wenz-Gross & Siperstein, 1998). For example, warm relationships with teachers act as a unique protective factor for children with special educational needs, expressed not only in their increased wellbeing and school satisfaction, but also in reducing the referral rate to special education settings. In addition, a supportive relationship with teachers was positively correlated with social, emotional, and academic adjustment among children with identified and diagnosed difficulties. Special attention was focused on children with learning difficulties in inclusive educational settings and their relations with their teachers. It had to be clarified whether children with special needs felt distanced from their teachers, since they requested increased academic help that the teachers could not provide them, due to limited teachers' time resources in heterogenic classrooms. Another source of this distance could be due to feelings of teachers' rejection of the failing students, and their preferences for the successful students. Diagnosis of the children may support teachers' remoteness, justified by the distinct labeling in heterogenic classrooms with teachers that were trained to work with typical achieving children. In an attempt to distinguish between these possible sources for the students' disappointed perceptions that their teachers were not close to them, we examined students' bonding with their teachers among children who failed in learning to read, before a formal diagnosis of dyslexia was performed and the teachers had more time resources to provide help.

In this study, children with reading difficulties in the third grade viewed their teachers as more rejecting and themselves as more lonely (Al-Yagon & Margalit, 2006). It should be emphasized that, in these schools, special attention, teachers' time allocation and special training was provided for remedial reading to these youngsters, and it was reflected in the students' perceptions. These children viewed their teachers as available to them similarly to their teachers' availability to the typical reading peers. The children were aware that these teachers provided them with adequate instrumental care (i.e., supplying extra help and instruction as needed). However, they concurrently viewed their teachers as more rejecting than did their peers who did not have reading difficulties. These outcomes were surprising in schools that provided special attention and help to students with difficulties. However, the results confirmed the role of children's reading difficulties as a risk factor that may impair the quality of the child–teacher relationship even in educational systems that provided adequate educational support. As a group, these children did not perceive their teachers as providing the expected secure base relations (the basic functions of an attachment figure), and thus may have formed an insecure attachment relationship with the teachers. It seems that these third-grade children differentiated between physical closeness (proximity and availability) of their teachers and emotional closeness, and the latter predicted elevated loneliness. It can be concluded that teachers avoided closeness to children with learning difficulties possibly due to their disappointment from the students' unsatisfactory achievements. These children in turn perceived their teachers as unavailable in times of need and as rejecting and not accepting figures.

Additional reports from teachers in another study with diagnosed children supported the former perceptions. Teachers reported lower levels of emotional closeness to the children with learning disabilities than to the typically developing peers in their classrooms (Al-Yagon & Mikulincer, 2004), and children with diagnosed learning disabilities were significantly overrepresented in teachers' rejection nominations (Cook, Tankersley, Cook, & Landrum, 2000). These results may have further impacts, since teachers' alienation predicted loneliness and extended periods of loneliness may lower these children's self-esteem. This lower self-esteem may then contribute to increased children's loneliness, which in turn may further impede their sense of self-worth and efficacy.

Children with ADHD (Attention Deficit Disorders with Hyperactivity) proposed a unique dilemma due to their over estimation tendencies for presenting their competence. ADHD is a common childhood disorder characterized by a persistent pattern of inattentive and/or hyperactive/impulsive behaviors that are developmentally inappropriate. This group included approximately 3–5% of school children who demonstrated significant deficits in multiple domains including academic achievement, social interactions, and behavior difficulties (Hoza et al., 2004). Yet, often they did not consider themselves as less competent than their peers, regardless of their conflict relations with teachers and peers (Crabtree & Rutland, 2001; Evangelista, Owens, Golden, & Pelham, 2008). It seems that they tended to overestimate their capabilities compared to the perceptions reported by their teachers. This over-estimation has been termed "the positive illusory bias" and it was defined as the disparity between self-report of competence and the actual competence. In an attempt to analyze this illusion, the perceptions were examined. Children with ADHD accurately assessed success and failure of other children. Their assessment of what constituted success and failure was also consistent with that of non-ADHD peers, even when the situations were challenging to interpret. It seems that the children and adolescents fully understood the meaning of success, yet when they had to evaluate their own performance they used their perceptions as a reinforcement to achieve a better self-perception. The positive illusory self-perceptions of children with ADHD may serve a self-protective function, shielding them from feelings of inadequacy.

An additional protective process for students with special needs can be provided by attributions and hopes. When the relations between children's performance, positive attribution style (explaining to themselves why the occurrences are happening to them) and hopes (the identification of future goals and paths to reach them) were examined (Ciarrochi, Heaven, & Davies, 2007), research reported that the positive self-explanations and high-hopeful thinking were related to lower experiences of loneliness for students with learning disabilities in different age groups (Lackaye & Margalit, 2006, 2008). It is impossible to define whether loneliness predicted lower hopes or whether decreased hopeful thinking predicted increased loneliness, since these relations can be considered inter-related and reciprocal.

In an attempt to identify consistency and changes in students–teachers inter-relations for children with special educational needs, the comparison of the two assessments, in the beginning and the end of the school year, revealed a significant change in both teachers' perceptions regarding children with learning disabilities and children's self-perceptions (Margalit, Mioduser, Al-Yagon, & Neuberger, 1997). These children were viewed by their teachers at the end of the year as demonstrating better learning achievements, less internalizing difficulties, and higher levels of social skills. These changes were achieved following a remedial help that was provided in school-based learning centers. Surprisingly, although the children with learning disabilities who obtained higher academic achievements and were doing better academically and socially, they continued to feel lonely and no changes were found in teachers' perceptions. These results drew attention to the consistency of teachers' and self-perceptions of incompetence and distress, even in a group that benefited from educational support. More important, teachers' perceptions at the end of the year were predicted not only by the children's academic achievements and their behavior adjustment, but also by their loneliness experience. Teachers' perceptions showed some changes over time (and some increased awareness of students' feelings of social distress), yet always within a stable set of perceptions.

Summary and Conclusions

In summary, school can be a lonely place for children, and two theoretical models that guided this chapter illustrate the roots of this distress: the Transactional Model of Development (Sameroff & Mackenzie, 2003), and the Ecological and Dynamic Model of Transition (Rimm-Kaufman & Pianta, 2000). The Transactional Model places emphasis on the bi-directional nature of interactions between children and schools. Neither the children nor the educational environments alone account for outcomes. Only the ongoing interplay between children and environments – the transactions between them – may predict outcomes, such as teacher–child relationship quality and feelings of closeness and confidence. The Ecological and Dynamic Model of Transition extends the model's conceptualization by focusing on children's successful transitions and considering them as multi-determined processes of development emerging from combinations of children and educational contextual characteristics. Teachers influence children and children influence reactions from teachers. Gradually these relationships become more patterned over time as participants create expectations and behave in accordance with those expectations.

Teachers can identify children's loneliness, and their perceptions of the children's characteristics including their unique areas of competence and challenges contribute to teachers' patterns of interacting with the children. These modes of adults–children's relating, support, and interpersonal closeness predict children's experience of wellbeing or loneliness at school and their relations to self-perceptions and interpersonal expectations. Children need and long for closeness and affection. The attachment conceptualization provides a theoretical ground for these complex transactional ongoing relations between children and teachers. The children's unique personal characteristics including their giftedness, learning disabilities, and ADHD further provide in-depth clarification to these multifaceted processes. These relations at school are not stable and continue to change along time, reflecting the different attributes and rules of the different school systems such as preschool and high schools. They also reflect children's struggles for identity construction during developmental stages and educational transition. School climate and academic demands extend the complexity of these relations, accentuating the importance of a dynamic conceptualization, and at the same time calling attention to the surprising relative consistency of children's loneliness distress within these multidimensional changing processes. The clarification of peer relations within these interactive contexts will extend the understanding of the sources of loneliness as well as the identification of protective factors.

References

Al-Yagon, M., & Margalit, M. (2006). Loneliness, sense of coherence and perception of teachers as a secure base among children with reading difficulties. *European Journal of Special Needs Education, 21*(1), 21–37.

Al-Yagon, M., & Mikulincer, M. (2004). Socioemotional and academic adjustment among children with learning disorders: The mediational role of attachment-based factors. *The Journal of Special Education*, *38*(2), 111–124.

Arbeau, K. A., & Coplan, R. J. (2007). Kindergarten teachers' beliefs and responses to hypothetical prosocial, asocial, and antisocial children. *Merrill-Palmer Quarterly*, *53*(2), 291–318.

Berguno, G., Leroux, P., McAinsh, K., & Shaikh, S. (2004). Children's experience of loneliness at school and its relation to bullying and the quality of teacher interventions. *The Qualitative Report*, *9*(3), 483–499.

Birch, S. H., & Ladd, G. W. (1997). The teacher–child relationship and children's early school adjustment. *Journal of School Psychology*, *35*(1), 61–79.

Bowlby, J. (1969). *Attachment*. New York: Basic Books.

Burchinal, M. R., Howes, C., Pianta, R., Bryant, D., Early, D., Clifford, R., et al. (2008). Predicting child outcomes at the end of kindergarten from the quality of pre-kindergarten teacher–child interactions and instruction. *Applied Developmental Science*, *12*(3), 140–153.

Burchinal, M. R., Peisner-Feinberg, E., Pianta, R., & Howes, C. (2002). Development of academic skills from preschool through second grade: Family and classroom predictors of developmental trajectories. *Journal of School Psychology*, *40*(5), 415–436.

Burgess, K. B., Ladd, G. W., Kochenderfer, B. J., Lambert, S. F., & Birch, S. H. (1999). Loneliness during early childhood: The role of interpersonal behaviors and relationships. In K. J. Rotenberg & S. Hymel (Eds.), *Loneliness in childhood and adolescence* (pp. 109–134). New York: Cambridge University Press.

Ciarrochi, J., Heaven, P. C. L., & Davies, F. (2007). The impact of Hope, self-esteem, and attributional style on adolescents' school grades and emotional well-being: A longitudinal study. *Journal of Research in Personality*, *41*(6), 1161–1178.

Cohen, J., Mccabe, E. M., Michelli, N. M., & Pickeral, T. (2009). School climate: Research, policy, practice, and teacher education. *Teachers College Record*, *111*(1), 180–213.

Cook, B. G., Tankersley, M., Cook, L., & Landrum, T. J. (2000). Teachers' attitudes toward their included students with disabilities. *Exceptional Children*, *67*(1), 115–135.

Crabtree, J., & Rutland, A. (2001). Self-evaluation and social comparison amongst adolescents with learning difficulties. *Journal of Community & Applied Social Psychology*, *11*(5), 347–359.

Efrati-Virtzer, M., & Margalit, M. (2009). Students' behaviour difficulties, sense of coherence and adjustment at school: Risk and protective factors. *European Journal of Special Needs Education*, *24*(1), 59–73.

Evangelista, N., Owens, J., Golden, C., & Pelham, W. (2008). The positive illusory bias: Do inflated self-perceptions in children with ADHD generalize to perceptions of others? *Journal of Abnormal Child Psychology*, *36*(5), 779–791.

Ewing, A. R., & Taylor, A. R. (2009). The role of child gender and ethnicity in teacher–child relationship quality and children's behavioral adjustment in preschool. *Early Childhood Research Quarterly*, *24*(1), 92–105.

Furrer, C., & Skinner, E. A. (2003). Sense of relatedness as a factor in children's academic engagement and performance. *Journal of Educational Psychology*, *95*(1), 148–158.

Galanaki, E. P. (2007). Teachers and children's loneliness: A review of the literature and educational implications. *European Journal of Psychology of Education*, *22*(4), 455–475.

Galanaki, E. P., & Kalantzi-Azizi, A. (1999). Loneliness and social dissatisfaction: Its relation with children's self-efficacy for peer-interaction. *Child Study Journal*, *29*(1), 1–22.

Galanaki, E. P., Polychronopoulou, S. A., & Babalis, T. K. (2008). Loneliness and social dissatisfaction among behaviourally at-risk children. *School Psychology International*, *29*(2), 214–229.

Gest, S. D., Welsh, J. A., & Domitrovich, C. E. (2005). Behavioral predictors of changes in social relatedness and liking school in elementary school. *Journal of School Psychology*, *43*(4), 281–301.

Hallinan, M. T. (2008). Teacher influences on students' attachment to school. *Sociology of Education*, *81*(3), 271–283.

Hamre, B. K., & Pianta, R. C. (2001). Early teacher–child relationships and the trajectory of children's school outcomes through eight grade. *Child Development, 72*(2), 625–638.

Hamre, B. K., Pianta, R. C., Downer, J. T., & Mashburn, A. J. (2008). Teachers' perceptions of conflict with young students: Looking beyond problem behaviors. *Social Development, 17*(1), 115–136.

Hoza, B., Gerdes, A. C., Hinshaw, S. P., Arnold, L. E., Pelham, W. E., Molina, B. S., et al. (2004). Self-perceptions of competence in children with ADHD and comparison children. *Journal of Consulting and Clinical Psychology, 72*(3), 382–391.

Hymel, S., Tarulli, D., Hayden Thomson, L., & Terrell-Deutsch, B. (1999). Loneliness through the eyes of children. In K. J. Rotenberg & S. Hymel (Eds.), *Loneliness in childhood and adolescence* (pp. 80–106). New York: Cambridge University Press.

Lackaye, T., & Margalit, M. (2006). Comparisons of achievement, effort and self-perceptions among students with learning disabilities and their peers from different achievement groups. *Journal of Learning Disabilities, 39*(5), 432–446.

Lackaye, T., & Margalit, M. (2008). Self-efficacy, loneliness, effort and hope: Developmental differences in the experiences of Students with learning disabilities and their non-LD peers at two age groups. *Learning Disabilities: A Contemporary Journal, 6*(2), 1–20.

Ladd, G. W., & Burgess, K. B. (1999). Changing the relationship trajectories of aggressive, withdrawn and aggressive/withdrawn children during early grade school. *Child Development, 70*(4), 910–929.

Lopes, J. A., Monteiro, I., Sil, V., Rutherford, R. B., & Quinn, M. M. (2004). Teachers' perceptions about teaching problem students in regular classrooms. *Education & Treatment of Children, 27*(4), 394–419.

Luftig, R. L. (1988). Assessment of perceived school loneliness and isolation of mentally retarded and nonretarded students. *American Journal of Mental Retardation, 92*(5), 472–475.

Manashko, S., Besser, A., & Priel, B. (2009). Maltreated children's representations of mother and an additional caregiver: A longitudinal study. *Journal of Personality, 77*(2), 561–599.

Margalit, M. (1994). *Loneliness among children with special needs: Theory, research, coping and intervention*. New York: Springer.

Margalit, M. (2006). Loneliness, the Salutogenic paradigm and LD: Current research, future directions and interventional implications. *Thalamus, 24*(1), 38–48.

Margalit, M., Mioduser, D., Al-Yagon, M., & Neuberger, S. (1997). Teachers' and Peers' perceptions of children with learning disorders: Consistency and change. *European Journal of Special Needs Education, 12*(3), 225–238.

Mikulincer, M., & Florian, V. (1998). The relationship between adult attachment styles and emotional and cognitive reactions to stressful events. In J. A. Simpson & W. S. Rholes (Eds.), *Attachment theory and close relationships* (pp. 143–165). New York: Guilford.

Mikulincer, M., & Florian, V. (2001). Attachment style and affect regulation: Implications for coping with stress and mental health. In G. Fletcher & M. S. Clark (Eds.), *Blackwell handbook of social psychology: Interpersonal processes* (pp. 537–557). Oxford: Blackwell.

Mueller, C. E. (2009). Protective factors as barriers to depression in gifted and nongifted adolescents. *Gifted Child Quarterly, 53*(1), 3–14.

Murray, C., & Greenberg, M. T. (2001). Relationships with teachers and bonds with school: Social emotional adjustment correlates for children with and without disabilities. *Psychology in the Schools, 38*(1), 25–41.

Murray, C., & Pianta, R. C. (2007). The importance of teacher–student relationships for adolescents with high incidence disabilities. *Theory Into Practice, 46*(2), 105–112.

Page, R. M. (1991). Loneliness as a risk factor in adolescent hopelessness. *Journal of Research in Personality, 25*(2), 189–195.

Pianta, R. C. (1999). *Enhancing relationships between children and teachers*. Washington, DC: American Psychological Association.

Reio, T. G., Marcus, R. F., & Sanders-Reio, J. (2009). Contribution of student and instructor relationships and attachment style to school completion. *Journal of Genetic Psychology, 170*(1), 53–71.

Reis, S. M., & Renzulli, J. S. (2004). Current research on the social and emotional development of gifted and talented students: Good news and future possibilities. *Psychology in the Schools, 41*(1), 119–130.

Rimm-Kaufman, S. E., & Pianta, R. C. (2000). An ecological perspective on the transition to kindergarten: A theoretical framework to guide empirical research. *Journal of Applied Developmental Psychology, 21*(5), 491–511.

Rimm-Kaufman, S. E., & Sawyer, B. E. (2004). Primary-grade teachers' Self-efficacy beliefs, attitudes toward teaching, and discipline and teaching practice priorities in relation to the responsive classroom approach. *The Elementary School Journal, 104*(4), 321–330.

Rubin, K. H., & Coplan, R. J. (2004). Paying attention to and not neglecting social withdrawal and social isolation. *Merrill-Palmer Quarterly, 50*(4), 506–534.

Rubin, K. H., & Mills, R. S. L. (1988). The many faces of social isolation childhood. *Journal of Consulting and Clinical Psychology, 56*(6), 916–924.

Rudasill, K. M., & Rimm-Kaufman, S. E. (2009). Teacher–child relationship quality: The roles of child temperament and teacher–child interactions. *Early Childhood Research Quarterly, 24*(2), 107–120.

Samdal, O., Nutbeam, D., Wold, B., & Kannas, L. (1998). Achieving health and educational goals through schools–a study of the importance of the school climate and the students' satisfaction with school. *Health Education Research, 13*(3), 383–397.

Sameroff, A. J., & Mackenzie, M. J. (2003). Research strategies for capturing transactional models of development: The limits of the possible. *Development and Psychopathology, 15*(3), 613–640.

Stipek, D., & Miles, S. (2008). Effects of aggression on achievement: Does conflict with the teacher make it worse? *Child Development, 79*(6), 1721–1735.

Suldo, S. M., Riley, K. N., & Shaffer, E. J. (2006). Academic correlates of children and adolescents' life satisfaction. *School Psychology International, 27*(5), 567–582.

Syvertsen, A. K., Flanagan, C. A., & Stout, M. D. (2009). Code of silence: Students' perceptions of school climate and willingness to intervene in a peer's dangerous plan. *Journal of Educational Psychology, 101*(1), 219–232.

Tieso, C. L. (2007). Patterns of over excitabilities in identified gifted students and their parents: A hierarchical model. *Gifted Child Quarterly, 51*(1), 11–22.

Tsigilis, N., & Gregoriadis, A. (2008). Measuring teacher–child relationships in the Greek kindergarten setting: A validity study of the student–teacher relationship scale-short form. *Early Education and Development, 19*(5), 816–835.

Wentzel, K. R. (2002). Are effective teachers like good parents? Teaching style and student adjustment in early adolescence. *Child Development, 73*(1), 287–301.

Wentzel, K. R. (2003). Motivating students to behave in socially competent ways. *Theory Into Practice, 42*(4), 319–326.

Wentzel, K. R., & Wigfield, A. (2007). Motivational interventions that work: Themes and remaining issues. *Educational Psychologist, 42*(4), 261–271.

Wenz-Gross, M., & Siperstein, G. N. (1998). Students with learning problems at risk in middle school: Stress, social support and adjustment. *Exceptional Children, 65*(1), 91–100.

Woodward, J. C., & Kalyan-Masih, V. (1990). Loneliness, coping strategies and cognitive styles of the gifted rural adolescent. *Adolescence, 25*(10), 977–988.

Yi, C. C., Wu, C. I., Chang, Y. H., & Chang, M. Y. (2009). The psychological well-being of Taiwanese youth: School versus family context from early to late adolescence. *International Sociology, 24*(3), 397–429.

Youngblade, L., Berlin, L. J., & Beslky, J. (1999). Connections among loneliness, the ability to be alone, and peer relationships in young children. In K. J. Rotenberg & S. Hymel (Eds.), *Loneliness in childhood and adolescence* (pp. 135–152). New York: Cambridge University Press.

Chapter 5
Peer Relations and Loneliness Within Different Cultures

In the beginning of the school year, Roni, a 9-year-old shy girl, told her father quietly: "This year I wish to have many good friends." Her father was surprised, and asked, "Don't you already have many friends?" Sara, her older sister who listened to their conversation remarked, "Don't you understand? Kids desperately need best friends." Then quietly she said almost to herself: "This is also my wish for the new year."

Peer relations have been considered an important challenge for boys and girls during different developmental stages. Children's and adolescents' friendships and companionship connections predict their wellbeing. Children with difficulties in establishing satisfactory peer relations, and those with low social status have been considered at risk for experiencing increased loneliness. Thus the quality of interpersonal connections with friends and classmates may be treated both as an index of current developmental adjustment but also as a contributor to future interpersonal competence or difficulties.

Children's relations with other children start in the first years of life, revealing individual differences. The preferences for particular peers emerge already by 3 years of age (Hay, Payne, & Chadwick, 2004). The roots of interpersonal relations and communications can be found in family environment. However, peer relations extend these early connections and modify them. Communication patterns that were modeled in family environments during early developmental stages predicted communication behavior in a variety of social relationships, and the family communication style predicted friendship closeness. Children from families that modeled open communication and frequent discussions learned relational maintenance skill, which influenced their ability to maintain a high level of friendship closeness (Ledbetter, 2009).

During childhood, individuals learn a wide variety of social behaviors, including prosocial and aggressive responses, sex roles, and emotional reactions. Peers may serve as effective models to reinforce socially appropriate or inappropriate behaviors and may help in reducing children's distress in unfamiliar and threatening situations. In addition, spending time with peers provides children with unique opportunities to express and discuss feelings as well as to expand thought processes and share knowledge. They may experiment with age-related task performance and

M. Margalit, *Lonely Children and Adolescents*, DOI 10.1007/978-1-4419-6284-3_5,

social roles (Ladd, 1999). Poor peer relations were viewed either as an early manifestation of emotional difficulties or as a factor leading to such disorders if ignored,
or left untreated (Rubin, Coplan, & Bowker, 2009). The goals of this chapter are
to present the different categories of peer relations and their contribution to children's loneliness. Children's disabilities and difficulties in establishing satisfactory
social connections within different cultural contexts will exemplify the complexity
and multidimensional aspects of having friends and belonging to groups.

Early Social Difficulties

Research reported that social difficulties and problematic peer relations can be identified already at early developmental stages. For example, in a sample of 1,364
children, the frequency of positive and negative peer interactions in childcare peer
groups (children's ages ranging between 24 and 54 months) and the number of hours
spent in groups of different sizes (alone, dyad, small, medium, and large groups) predicted the third graders' peer competence that was expressed in their social skills,
dyadic friendships, and peer-group acceptance (Brownell et al., 2008). Children who
had more positive experiences with peers as infants in childcare centers had better social and communicative skills with peers in third grade, were more sociable,
co-operative, and less aggressive. They had closer friends, and were more accepted
and popular. Similarly, children with more frequent negative experiences with peers
in childcare were more aggressive in third grade, had lower social and communicative skills, and reported having fewer friends. It can be concluded that repeated
early experiences of social threats and rejection, and being considered unpopular
by peers, can have a pervasive, lasting impact on children's wellbeing, especially if
children fail to cope effectively with the emotional impact of these negative experiences (Thomaes, Reijntjes, Castro, & Bushman, 2009). The long-term impact of
peer relations was also demonstrated in research. Young people in their final year of
high school, who feel lonely and disconnected from their peers, carry these risk factors through to life after school, and perceptions of connectedness to peers have
a pronounced and extended impact on individuals' mental health and wellbeing
(McGraw, Moore, Fuller, & Bates, 2008). It is critical to clarify the complex interplay of different types of relationships within children's social networks from early
developmental stages in order to provide an in-depth understanding of the loneliness
distress and also to consider research-based prevention and intervention approaches.

Categories of Peer Relations

Studies on peer relations attempted to acquire answers to several critical questions
such as why some children are well-liked or accepted by peers, whereas others are
rejected or ignored. In addition and more specifically, why several rejected children

feel lonely, whereas others who are similarly rejected do not? Research on social relations focused interest on two specific types of peer relationships:

1. Close friendships
2. Acceptance, popularity, rejection, conflicts, and social status in groups

Loneliness expressed the unsatisfied need for intimate relations with "good and close friends" (emotional loneliness), and/or a reaction to exclusion or rejection by desired social groups (social loneliness). Yet, having friends may paradoxically be related and even contribute to feelings of loneliness, since the quality of friendship relations may contribute or decrease loneliness. The factors and processes that enable children to establish and maintain friendships appear to differ from the factors leading to peers' acceptance and popularity. Some low-status children, who were rated overall as rejected by their peer groups, had best friends and only about two-thirds of the highly accepted children had good friends, and the remaining third of the popular children did not have a close friend. Children's friendship had an influence on children's feelings of loneliness above and beyond the influence of peer group acceptance, further supporting the distinction between friendship adjustment and group acceptance. Children without best friends were more lonely than children with best friends, and this was true regardless of how well-accepted or popular they were (Parker & Asher, 1993).

Friendship Relations

Friendship has been defined at the dyadic level, often as the voluntary and reciprocal relationship between two individuals. Being friendless is harmful to a child's psychological wellbeing and adjustment. Children who are without mutual friends, for instance, tend to report higher levels of loneliness and internalizing problems than those children with friends (Rubin, Fredstrom, & Bowker, 2008). However, loneliness may emerge not only from the lack of a good friend, but also from negative experiences in relational contexts such as unsatisfactory friendship relations. Thus, the developmental implications of friendship relationships cannot be specified without a differential approach that distinguishes between three major aspects of companionship: having friends (the number of good friends), the identity of one's friends (the characteristics of children), and friendship qualities (the characteristics of the relations).

Friendships often provide children with support and with opportunities to learn problem-solving skills. These relations are often important sources of self-knowledge and self-esteem enabling the development of social competence, and providing practice of interpersonal connections (Waldrip, Malcolm, & Jensen-Campbell, 2008). Friends provide one another with cognitive and social scaffolding that differ from the provisions provided by non-friends. Thus, for example, having friends supports good outcomes across normative transitions from kindergarten to school, and from middle school to high school. At least one reciprocal dyadic friendship protects a child who suffers from increases in internalizing and externalizing behaviors and victimization (Asher & Paquette, 2003). Therefore, it seems that adolescents who participate in supportive friendships tend to be generally better adjusted compared to adolescents who do not participate in at least one supportive friendship.

Friendships are manifested through mutual interests and preferences, attraction, closeness, intimacy, and the extent to which these perceptions are stable and shared by both members of the dyads. Even as early as at the preschool stage, children were able to identify other children as their "best friends" and described stable associations with these play companions. Although friendship is a private experience that can best be described through self-reports, often these relations are recognized and reported by significant adults such as parents and teachers, and even by other children. Observations of children's interactions during experimental task performance indicated that they interacted differently with friends than with strangers, showing greater mutuality and more tolerance toward friends, even in times of anger or distress (Coie, 1990). Friendship relations and social acceptance had a clear impact on social judgments and on interpretations of behavior, as revealed by laboratory studies of simulated social conflicts. Children responded differently to a peer's behavior, depending on how much they liked or disliked the person who performed the act. For example, children were told that Dan had brought a toy to the play group, and another child broke it by accident. When children were asked about their reactions, they expressed anger and complained that the child should be more careful. However, they were less angry when it was described as broken by a best friend of the child. They said "it can happen; he did not mean to break it."

The Number of Good Friends

Using a simplistic approach, the process of estimating an individual's number of friends or social network size can be achieved by asking children to name their best friends. However, this measure was found less consistent than expected, and the size of the social network was often difficult to estimate, due to children's tendencies to have differing and in some cases inconsistent relationship styles. In addition, the term "friend" seems to be defined differently by several children at separate times, ranging from descriptions of close, intimate friends to more superficial partnerships at a joint task performance, or even to fellow members of a larger network such as the classroom. Thus, children may provide inconsistent answers, reflecting their individualistic interpretations of the construct. When asked, "How many friends do you have?" children will refer to social networks of different sizes as related to their personal conception of "good" friendships. Some children will name all the children in their class, or all the same gender children in their play group.

An additional approach to estimate the size of the child's network inside schools was achieved by identifying reciprocal choices among the patterns of nominations that children gave in response to questions such as "Who are your best friends?" A child or an adolescent is considered a friend if he or she nominates a peer as a friend and that same peer nominates him or her as well ("reciprocal nominations"). The number of friends has also been evaluated outside the school setting by children's self-reports and adults such as parents and teachers. However, often adults' responses differed from children's responses, reflecting their judgment, attitudes, and different views. For example, Danni, a 7-year-old boy stated to our research assistant that he had many friends, and quickly counted eight names. His mother who was listening to his interview remarked that in fact he was very lonely and without any "real" friend. When she was further asked, she admitted that indeed several children were often hanging around with him, but they were not true friends. With a bitter tone she explained that they were taking advantage of him, copying his homework, and playing with his games. She was confident that in times of need he could not trust any of them. A different example was provided by Molly's mother. She asked for the teacher's help since Molly had complained at home that she was very lonely at school. Sadly, the distressed mother repeated her daughter's words and described her tears. The teacher was taken aback, and she said that she was sure that Molly was very popular at school and was constantly surrounded by several girls inside class as well as at the school courtyard. The teacher promised the mother that she would very gently explore the situation and find out what the girl meant by feeling lonely and without friends, and how she could be helped. She found out that recently Molly had a bitter conflict with her best friend initiated by a minor disagreement (from the teacher's point of view). When Molly did not agree with the friend's preferences, her friend threatened her that she would persuade the other girls to stop talking to her.

Children with a single good friend, or those who are interested in establishing friendship with a specific child, are more vulnerable to conflicts and dominating relations, and may find themselves alone. This may occur as a result of an interpersonal conflict that ends the special friendship, but also when the special friend is away or absent from school. Thus, loneliness has often been linked to the quantity of one's friends and lonely individuals indicating that they have limited companions, spend more time alone, and are excluded from many social activities compared to non-lonely peers.

Developmental differences were also noted. The quantity of friendships was especially considered important for preschool children. Young children who had many friends, interacted more time with those friends and comparatively less time was spent in solitary play or with adults such as teachers, in comparison to children with few friends (Rizzo, 1988). The number of different peers seen by children on a regular basis (who may be identified as friends) increased with age. On the average, preschool children had regular contacts with three to four children, whereas children at the beginning of elementary school regularly met with five to six peers (Ladd, 1999). Friendships generally tended to be relatively stable and to increase in duration with age. Individual differences were noted in the number of friends. Some children had many friends, whereas other had a few or none at all. The number of friends was also related both to contextual conditions (i.e., classroom climate that promoted collaboration) and personal factors (i.e., children with extroverted personality or shyness). Boys and girls differed in the number of different peers with whom they had regular contacts. Girls typically had fewer friends than boys, their friendship relations were slowly developed, and they differentiated between friends and acquaintances more clearly. In order to predict developmental outcomes, in addition to the number of friends, the behavioral characteristics and attitudes of children's friends have to be considered as well as qualitative features of these friendship relationships (Hartup, 1996).

Friends' Characteristics and Qualities of Relations

The children's characteristics predict the quality of friendships. Many children become friends with those who resemble them racially, behaviorally, emotionally, attitudinally, and developmentally. Friends' selection may not simply be "another child like me." Rather, it may well be "some child who is like me, who likes me, and who meets my needs." For example, a shy/withdrawn child may befriend and continue a relationship with a similarly behaved child who provides supportive companionship and is comfortable doing so in the periphery of the social scene (Rubin et al., 2008).

Conflicts and jealousy in friendship relations contributed to maladjustment and harmed children's wellbeing (Bukowski, Adams, & Santo, 2006). Students with disruptive behavior, similar to students with withdrawn behavior, were often less competent in initiating companionship, experiencing lower levels of the mutuality, responsiveness, and positive behaviors that characterize positive friendship relations. In addition, friendships with peers who were low in aggression could serve a positive protective role for children who were victims of bullying. For example, relations with aggressive friends may be considered a risk factor, since victimization by peers could lead to increased feelings of loneliness and depression that interfered with attention and concentration in the classroom activities (Kochenderfer-Ladd & Wardop, 2001). Aggressive friends increased the distress and also contributed to the development of maladaptive attitudes toward school. Friendships with aggressive peers were also likely to be low in features that promoted school adjustment (i.e., warmth, trust, intimacy) (Berndt, 2002; Schwartz, Gorman, Dodge, Pettit, & Bates, 2008).

Research has indicated that positive friendship relations that provided closeness, intimacy, trust, support, and companionship may be considered a protective factor for children at risk for developing depression due to maltreatment or abuse (Powers, Ressler, & Bradley, 2009). Positive effects of friendships seem to reduce adolescents' emotional distress and depressive symptoms while increasing their positive involvement in classroom activities. Developmental differences were noted in the friendship identifications. Younger children were more concerned with the activities they shared with their friends. Common activities also provided foundations for friendships in middle childhood and adolescence. Gradually additional companionship characteristics gained importance in the descriptions of best friends during adolescence, such as intimacy, self-disclosure, trust, loyalty, and commitment (Newcomb & Bagwell, 1995).

The quality of friendship predicted children's happiness, while conflicts with friends predicted loneliness (Demır & Weitekamp, 2007). High-quality friendships had positive effects on children: fostering their self-esteem, improving their social adjustment, and increasing their ability to cope with stressors. For example, among early adolescents, having friendships with more positive features were related with greater involvement in school, higher self-perceived social acceptance, and higher general self-esteem (Berndt, 2002). Within the qualities of friendship, research emphasized the importance of the following provisions provided through these relations: companionship and recreation; help and support; intimate exchange and validation of self-worth.

Companionship, i.e., doing things with a friend and spending time together, was one of the most important quality dimensions of friendship (Demır & Weitekamp, 2007). The friendship relationship provided children with play opportunities, companionship, recreation, and spending enjoyable time together. When children were asked to define "what is a friend?" most children described leisure and recreation time in specific and nonspecific terms. A friend was described as someone with whom they liked to spend time, to play different games, or even with whom to "hang around" without having any specific plans. They reported staying connected with friends most of their time, using various technological means such as cells and internet, sending texts, and playing computer games from a distance, in addition to face-to face meetings. Malls were considered a place in which to spend time, meet new children, and hang out with friends. Connections between loneliness and motivation for mall shopping were documented (Kim, Kim, & Kang, 2003).

Many children proposed that friends were children who provided assistance, help, and guidance, when the need arose, in line with the old proverb, "A friend in need is a friend indeed." The actual meaning of help may change, revealing different needs, cultural, age and individual differences, from providing materialistic resources to offering emotional support. Children with special needs, who were more aware of their consistent difficulties, accentuated this friendship characteristic, revealing their increased needs for support and that they sometimes felt unequal to their friends. For example, during interviews (Margalit, 1994), the friend's role as a source of help was described by more than half of the group of children with special needs as a very important provision in their friends. They often expected to get help and were less aware of the need for providing help to others.

Intimate exchange was described by several children at different ages, relating to different contents. Generally, a friend was identified as a child that you could trust, with whom children and adolescents share secrets and private concerns, disclosing personal information and feelings. Even preschool children sometimes described their friends as children who would stay with them, spend enjoyable and distressed times, and share "secrets." Children in various ages reported that they tell their friends "things that they would not tell others." To the probing researcher questioning a preschool group of children and asking for an example, several children answered simply – "secrets of nothing," and explained that the contents of the secrets included the day-to-day events that were not truly secretive, yet the sharing and the closeness were the important segments of this intimate social interaction. Intimacy has been described as closeness to another person and as openness in describing and sharing thoughts and feelings. Children and adolescents often declare that "best friends tell each other everything," or disclose their most personal thoughts and feelings. These personal self-disclosures are the hallmark of an intimate friendship (Berndt, 2002). Thus, a close friend serves as an important source of emotional support and a safe environment for self-exploration and identity formation. Youngsters' ability to build trust and experience intimacy depends on their capacity to appropriately self-disclose (i.e., to share feelings, thoughts, and desires) and develop an affective bond with a friend (Parker & Asher, 1993). Individual differences were noted among the children, and those with high trust beliefs tended to form closer peer relationships and felt less lonely (Rotenberg, MacDonald, & King., 2004). From early school grades children expressed trust in friends, and thus early identification of those children who were at risk of poor psychosocial development because of low trust and limited friendships could help those children before loneliness became a chronic distress (Betts & Rotenberg, 2008).

Friends' characteristics and the overall friendship quality were also important to intimacy development. Moreover, higher personal Sense of Coherence and secured attachment with family predicted that these youngsters would pursue intimacy in their relationships with friends, disclosing secrets, and supporting others when they were sad. In order to form intimate friendships, adolescents had to be mature enough and able to balance their identity and autonomy needs and share inner feelings and fantasies with close friends without worrying about the risk to the self's identity (Bauminger, Finzi-Dottan, Chason, & Har-Even, 2008).

Lower friendship's qualities enhanced loneliness, since children and adolescents may experience low social support when facing emotional problems (Selfhout, Branje, & Meeus, 2009). Friendship styles of girls' and boys' had different qualities and characteristics revealing their unique needs for intimacy and autonomy (Rose & Rudolph, 2006). Girls' friendships were characterized by dyadic relations that consisted of high levels of personal disclosure, support-seeking and -giving. Boys' relationship styles were typically involved in larger groups' relationships and lower levels of disclosure or closeness (Rose, Swenson, & Robert, 2009). Yet, regardless of gender differences, the friendship relations were related to children's self-perceptions.

Trust among friends was an additional important quality that contributed to intimacy (Betts, Rotenberg, & Trueman, 2009). Trust is a complex phenomenon that requires individuals to interpret the behavior of others and the ability to infer the intentions of others in potentially ambiguous situations. Generalized trust reflects the propensity to believe that an individual's or a group's word, actions, honesty, and ability to maintain confidentiality can be relied upon in a range of social contexts. Generalized trust is a central quality for the formation, maintenance, and survival of relationships (Erikson, 1963). The relations between loneliness and generalized trust were complicated. The expectations of children who wished for a high trust may not have been fulfilled when others broke promises or did not keep secrets as expected. Therefore, because these children's expectations were not met they may have experienced elevated levels of loneliness (Betts et al., 2009). Thus, children who have a very high trust and a naive approach toward others were left vulnerable to betrayal by their peers (Rotenberg, Boulton, & Fox, 2005). Low trust was often related to fewer friends because children with very low trust beliefs may hold a suspicious, cynical, attitude toward their peers. Trustful friendships support the validation of self-perceptions.

Children confirm their self-worth by their importance to their friends. Self-validation and perceiving others as reassuring, agreeing, encouraging, listening, and otherwise helping to maintain one's self-image as a competent and worthwhile individual (answering items in questionnaires such as "points out things that I am good at" and "compliments me when I do something well"), predicted not only positive self-perception but also happiness (Demır & Weitekamp, 2007). Adolescents, for example, who viewed their friendships as positive or supportive, often reported higher general self-worth (Ladd, 1999). The protective value of supportive friendship was especially demonstrated for adolescents at risk who were victimized, and often suffered from internalizing problems (Waldrip et al., 2008). A supportive friend was for them as an important buffer against social maladjustment when group-level peer acceptance and the size of the friendship networks were small.

In conclusion, high-quality friendships can be considered protective factors that positively affect children: fostering their self-esteem, improving their social adjustment, protecting them from loneliness, and increasing their ability to cope with stressors. Moreover, friendship quality was consistently related with indicators of life quality and social adjustment. Children who had positive friendships reported greater involvement in school, higher self-perceived social acceptance, and higher general self-esteem. However, several negative qualities of friendship such as jealousy, conflicts, aggression, and victimization should not be ignored since they may extend the impact of developmental risks.

Negative Aspects in Friendships

Without ignoring the important value of good friends for enhancing an inoculation against loneliness, the relations with friends can also trigger negative emotions emerging from competing relations, loyalty dilemmas, and exclusivity demands. In consequence, children and adolescents may develop perceptions of betrayal and violations of expectations even within close relationships (Parker, Walker, Low, & Gamm, 2005). In addition, the time and emotional commitments that partners make to outside peers may initiate dissatisfaction and even anger. In particular, if young adolescents perceive outsiders as threatening the quality, uniqueness, or survival of their friendship relations, feelings of jealousy may pose challenges to the partner, initiating and enhancing deep feelings of isolation and loneliness experiences. The study of young adolescents who experienced jealousy to friends revealed extended individual differences that contributed to different levels of loneliness and dissatisfaction with their peers and friends (Parker et al., 2005). Several negative social experiences were interconnected and should not be discussed in isolation. Jealousy was often connected with distressful feelings of a small or limited network of friends, and being the target of victimization were related in overlapping ways with feelings of loneliness. Therefore it is particularly important to focus attention on the unique additive contribution of jealousy to the experiencing of loneliness.

In a comprehensive survey of studies (Parker, Saxon, Asher, & Kovacs, 1999), a large number of children who were well-adjusted by traditional markers (i.e., many high-quality friendships, being well liked), surprisingly reported that they experienced loneliness. The study of jealousy provided a partial answer to this paradox, since for vulnerable individuals, friendships were sometimes sources of subjective distress, disillusionment, and jealousy. Girls reported greater jealousy over friends than did boys, yet jealousy contributed similarly among boys and among girls to problems of social rejection and loneliness. Younger adolescents expressed greater jealousy than older ones. In addition, the link between jealousy over friends, conflicts, and aggression was consistent. It seems that jealousy triggers frustrations and angry reactions to the distressed experiences expressed in many conflicts.

An additional source of loneliness emerging in friendship relations is the existence of conflicts among friends. Conflicts often occur among children, and represent different points of view, attitudes, and interests. Even best friendships, from time to time, may have conflicts with each other, reflecting disagreements and different motivations. For example, children typically think of themselves as equal to their friends, and complain when their friends try to boss them around or dominate them. Sometimes children are engaged in rivalry and competitions to avoid feelings of inferiority. When asked about ideal friendships, children describe friendships based on collaboration and emphatic relations. Yet, when asked to describe actual friendships, children usually report the co-occurrence of many conflicts, dominance attempts, and rivalry. Indeed, conflicts among friends are quite common and special attention should be focused not only on the prevalence of conflicts, but especially on conflict resolution patterns – the degree to which these disagreements within the friendship relations are resolved with an emphasis on their efficient and fair resolution.

The types of conflicts that children experience, their affective impact, and the ease and readiness with which these conflicts are resolved affect not only the quality of friendships, but also children's adjustment and feelings of isolation. For example, kindergarten boys who had many conflicts with friends during the school year reported by the end of the year that they did not like school, they reduced their engagement in classroom activities, and experienced increased loneliness. Similarly, older children (seventh graders) whose friendships included many conflicts in the beginning of the school year reported increased disruptive behavior at school after several months (Berndt, 2002). It can be concluded that friends who frequently get into conflicts with each other, or who often try to dominate or assert their superiority over one another, are in fact practicing a repertoire of negative social interactions that may generalize to interactions with other peers and adults. Naturally, the children's negative behaviors provoke negative reactions from classmates and teachers. Those negative reactions encourage the students to disengage from classmates and classroom activities, leading to social exclusion and loneliness. Many of these children expressed hatred of their school.

It can be concluded that students with supportive, intimate friendships became increasingly involved with school, while those who considered their friendships to be conflict-ridden and rivalries became increasingly disruptive and troublesome. Perceived conflicts in friendships predicted increasing forms of school maladjustment, especially among boys, including school loneliness and avoidance as well as school liking and engagement (Hartup, 1996). Considering the concurrent and long-term impacts of friendship relations, their stability requests a special consideration.

Stability and Changes in Friendship Relations

Short-term instability in children's and adolescents' networks is fairly common. The notion of stability refers to the maintenance of a relationship over time, whereas the instability, fluidity, and change are multiple terms used to define modifications observed in friendship bonds (Hardy, Bukowski, & Sippola, 2002). Hardy et al. (2002) assessed adolescents' peer relationships using six time points and reported friendship instability during the transition to middle school. Another study assessing friendship stability on a monthly basis, revealed that approximately one-third of adolescents' nominated friendships' changes over the course of 5 months, being either newly formed or lost from 1 month to another (Chan & Poulin, 2007).

Two types of instability have been observed in friendship relations. The first type of friendship instability is the termination of relationships, which assumes a temporary or permanent withdrawal from peer interactions. The breakup of a friendship (even if it is voluntary) provokes distress and pain due to the separation and lost bonding and social support. The second type of instability is the formation of new friendships. Despite the typical expectation that friendship formation may promote emotional wellbeing, this is a demanding emotional process that may initiate anxiety before trust and intimacy are developed. Chan and Poulin (2009) focused attention on the early adolescence period (i.e., between 11 and 13 years), since fluctuations in youths' social relations may be more pronounced during this period of transition to high school along with numerous developmental changes at the cognitive, social, and biological levels. They reported that adolescents who experienced many changes in their networks (either losing old friends or making new ones) experienced lower quality in their friendship network, less support, and higher levels of loneliness. It is not clear if the friendship instability affected the loneliness, or the lonely relationship's style contributed to the instability. Probably these processes interacted reciprocally affecting one-another. Maybe, when the adolescents start to display depressive and lonely behaviors, others may provide support and reassurance at first, but gradually withdraw from interactions. As the lonely child receives mixed messages of approval and rejection from others, he/she may perceive his/her relationships as unstable (Chan & Poulin, 2009).

During development and school transitions, children gradually interact with larger and more complex educational systems and increased developmental challenges (i.e., the move from the intimate small preschools to elementary school with growing academic demands; the transition from elementary to junior high schools). For most children and youth, such transitions involve dramatic shifts, as they move from small, self-contained groups and classrooms to larger, heterogeneous education systems with heightened demands for independent academic performance and gradually reduced levels of teachers' close support (Aikins, Bierman, & Parker, 2005). Additionally, the typical junior high school peer group is not only much larger than the elementary school peer group, but also more autonomous, with reduced adults' monitoring. The complexity of the relations between stability of friendships and loneliness were demonstrated in various studies.

In a short-term longitudinal study that examined the impact of personal and interpersonal characteristics (i.e., friendship and future personal expectations) on youth adaptation across the transition to junior high school (Aikins et al., 2005), the friendship and personal characteristics differentially predicted the transition outcomes. Friendship characteristics were predictive of later friendship quality, contributing to school adjustment, and they predicted loneliness only indirectly. Youth who had skills to form satisfactory friendships' relations prior to the transition, were able to develop positive social connections in junior high school and to demonstrate adaptive behaviors that promoted adjustment and resulted in lower loneliness than those youth whose friendship skills were less well-developed. In turn, youngsters with high-quality friendships (i.e., greater intimacy, openness, and warmth) were more likely to maintain these relationships over the transition. Given the emerging salience of dyadic friendships for social-emotional development during the adolescent years, the stability of quality friendships and the provisions they afforded, served as important protective resources for social and emotional support during the transition, significantly influencing both friendship and school adjustment. Similarly, lower expectations and hopes predicted higher levels of post-transition emotional distress, increased loneliness, and lower levels of school adjustment. However, a group of children that felt lonely after transition, even when they reported high-quality friendships, focused attention on the complexity of the processes.

In another study (Oh et al., 2008), the unexpected positive impact of the transition was also demonstrated. The lack of friendship relations for children when they made the transition into middle school and unstable best friendship involvement during their last year of elementary school were considered significant risk factors. However, when the social withdrawal of the children was followed from the final year of elementary school, across the transition to middle school, and then to the final year of middle school (fifth-to-eighth grades), individual differences were revealed. Indeed most participants (85%) maintained a low-stable trajectory of social withdrawal. However, approximately 8% of the sample exhibited a decreasing trajectory of social withdrawal from middle childhood through early adolescence, suggesting that not all withdrawn children maintained their risk status. These children experienced less exclusion after the transition to middle school, and they became more sociable and established new friendships. In contrast, approximately 7% of the sample demonstrated an increasing pattern of social withdrawal and loneliness over time, pointing at the needs for wider and dynamic understanding of the joint impacts of positive and negative adjustment predictors.

Enemies and Antipathies

Most studies explored the different aspects of friendship relations, and the study of children's enemies has often been neglected. Many children share with parents that there is a child in their class (or school) who hates them and they hate him or her. This child, who is viewed as an "enemy," may affect the life quality in many ways. A study that investigated the role of mutual dislike dyads in the development of aggressive behavior across the middle childhood years, documented the association of school antipathies with higher levels of aggression among boys in the late elementary years (Erath, Pettit, Dodge, & Bates, 2009). In another study that examined the factors that predicted loneliness for elementary school children in Israel, the existence of identified enemies (mutual dislike dyads) at school predicted loneliness among boys and girls alike, in addition to their self-perceptions and the conception of friendship qualities (Margalit, Tur-Kaspa, & Most, 1999). It seems that the existence of mutual antipathies was not an isolated risk factor, but had a cumulative impact in addition to other risk factors. A follow-up of the same group of children during a school year revealed that children with learning difficulties felt lonelier at the end of the year then in the beginning of the year, had fewer friends and more enemies. In the beginning of the year about 50% of the group of children with academic difficulties revealed that they had one or more enemies at school. By the end of the year a larger group of children reported that they had an enemy at school that contributed to their unhappiness and dissatisfaction. Their classmates without academic challenges showed an opposite trend, revealing fewer enemies and more friends toward the end of the year. In the beginning of the year 41% of the children reported having one enemy or more, but at the end of the year only 27% had mutual antipathies (Tur-Kaspa, Margalit, & Most, 1999).

Parents are aware of the children's suffering. Surprisingly, very little is known about the prevalence of mutual antipathies among children and adolescents as well as when and why these negative relationships emerge. The few studies clearly indicated that mutual antipathies were common experiences for boys and girls in different age groups, different cultures, and different timing during the school year (Parker & Gamm, 2003; Tur-Kaspa et al., 1999). Not surprisingly, adolescents involved in many mutual antipathies were not as well accepted by the peer group as adolescents with few mutual antipathies. Moreover, they also experienced more victimization and bullying by peers. These findings supported a distinction between involvement in mutual antipathy and general peer group rejection (Parker & Gamm, 2003). Poorly accepted and victimized preadolescents often reported higher levels of loneliness and social dissatisfaction at school. However, the number of mutual enemies in Parker's study was related to victimizing and to peer's acceptance. It seems that the number of enemies was not the critical aspect in this study for predicting loneliness, but the quality of the mutual negative relations affected their behavior outcomes. Bullying research exemplifies the significant role of the quality of peer negative relations in predicting children's loneliness.

Bullying and Victimizing

Bullying is an act of repeated aggressive behavior in order to intentionally hurt another child and involves a real or perceived imbalance of power with the more powerful children or groups attacking those who are less powerful. Two types of bullying have been identified: direct and relational bullying. The former refers to physically aggressive acts such as kicking/pushing/hitting, whereas the latter refers to name calling, teasing, socially isolating others, spreading false rumors, social exclusion, peer manipulation, and rumor spreading (Woods, Done, & Kalsi, 2009). In fact, bullying often refers not to a static situation, but to a dynamic process of negative relations and hostile interactions. Many times, children's bullying behavior begins as relationship aggression and later develops into more subtle forms of physical aggression. For example, it may be that initially the lonely child is teased, but this teasing gradually develops into ridiculing the child's appearance or expressing ethnic origin's remarks, reaching overt physical and/or verbal aggression. Bullying can be related to many stigmatization sources. For example, children who are obese are at an increased risk of being victimized by their peers. Negative views toward obese individuals may be expressed through children's friendship selections and expressed levels of overt (i.e., pushing, hitting) and relational (i.e., spreading rumors, weight-based teasing) forms of aggression, resulting in increased loneliness (Gray, Kahhan, & Janicke, 2009). It may be that peers resort to malicious gossip about the lonely child, which in turn may escalate into sustained physical aggression. Victimization, conversely, is defined as the receipt of these behaviors.

Victimization behavior has been defined as deliberate, repeated negative actions toward children and adolescents with the victims' awareness to the imbalance of power. Children who were victims reported higher levels of loneliness, had fewer best friends than non-involved individuals, and had more difficulties in maintaining friendships' relations. Their friends were also less adjusted socially, tended to be introverted and lonely, and sometimes they were also victimized. Bullies appear to know quite well which children and adolescents to bully, and who are the children with large networks of friends who might provide help when the victim child is attacked. Even if these friends are not powerful individually, together they may exert enough social influence to make a bully refrain from attacking (Scholte et al., 2009).

Relational victims appeared to be at risk of both loneliness and emotional problems, and this was true for both males and females alike. Friendship qualities moderated the association between direct victimization and loneliness. Low loneliness was experienced by victimized children who had high levels of friendship quality. However, loneliness was experienced by victims who had low levels of friendship quality.

Once the child has experienced bullying, he or she is faced with the choice of either attempting to resolve the conflict on his/her own, or informing teachers and asking for help. Teachers who fail to intervene effectively and allow the bullying to continue are also contributing to the child's continued experience of loneliness (Berguno, Leroux, McAinsh, & Shaikh, 2004). Self-perceptions and the perceptions of friends also have an important role in these dynamic relations between peer victimization and loneliness (Ladd & Troop-Gordon, 2003). Children, who had positive views of themselves and their friends, were less vulnerable to the impacts of victimization and less lonely. Several studies hypothesized a unidirectional account of the influence of peer victimization on children's experiences of loneliness, while others suggested a bi-directional influence, assuming that victimization contributed to loneliness, but at the same time loneliness also contributed to victimization. In addition, cognitive deficits in social competence and the quality of interpersonal relations extended the understanding of the connections between bullying and loneliness, emphasizing its multidimensional dynamic nature. Several contextual factors such as family cohesion, the quality of the school environment, and the levels of adults' monitoring in school for aggressive behavior also predicted the development of loneliness following victimizing (Wienke Totura et al., 2009).

The results of these studies clearly showed the importance of the schools' strategies in targeting children's bullying and aggression. There is a need for empowering students' self-perceptions, encouraging the formation of friendships and collaborations among children, and involving parents in supporting learning of social problem-solving. In addition, the structuring of classroom environments is critical for decreasing bullying and for enhancing appropriate skills for dealing with bullies by the whole class, especially when bullies function as groups or cliques.

Clique Affiliation

Beginning in middle childhood, children tend to form exclusive peer affiliations called "cliques" (Kwon & Lease, 2009). Children in a clique are likely to share similar social information and experiences, and often keep frequent, intense, and exclusive interactions (Gest, Farmer, Cairns, & Xie, 2003). Clique members are often similar in many social and behavioral characteristics, including grades, academic motivation, school adjustment, aggression, externalizing and internalizing problems (Kiuru, Nurmi, Aunola, & Salmela-Aro, 2009). They are also perceived by peers as highly similar, even when the basis of that similarity is not explicitly specified. Children's involvement in a clique contributes differently to their social and emotional adjustment and loneliness depending on the type of clique to which they belong (Kwon & Lease, 2007). When competent cliques are perceived to be highly cohesive, they may affect clique members favorably as each member becomes more strongly associated with the positive reputation (i.e., prosocial, smart, fun) of their clique, and they experience lower levels of loneliness (Kwon & Lease, 2009). This is usually considered a protective factor (Rubin et al., 2009). Nevertheless, when friends shared similarities in cliques' maladaptive characteristics, such as bullying and aggression, friendship appeared to be a risk rather than a protective factor for adjustment. If the child's mutual friends were socially withdrawn, he or she was more likely to show an increase in social withdrawal (Oh et al., 2008). Similarly, children belonging to groups with a norm for bullying were also found to display more bullying behaviors than those who belonged to groups with an anti-bullying norm (Duffy & Nesdale, 2009).!!!

In conclusion, friendships in childhood and adolescence provide many important provisions such as affection, good company, and fun; the emotional security and helpfulness among friends meet their varied needs for advice as well as for instrumental aid. Friendship relations enable sharing of interests, hopes, and fears and provide opportunities for intimate disclosure. Friends are thought to bolster feelings of self-worth and promote the growth of social skills and inter-personal sensitivity (Rubin et al., 2008). Mutual enemies are considered a risk for children's pronounced loneliness and distress. However, friendship with aggressive children may be considered a risk factor for development, while friends who are not aggressive can provide an adaptive socializing influence and promote the resilience even for victimized children. The drive to initiate and sustain friendship bonds is so fundamental to the human experience, that even adolescents, who develop friendship bonds with deviant, delinquent, or abusive peers belonging to aggressive cliques, report lower levels of loneliness than their friendless adolescent peers (Asher & Paquette, 2003). Needless to say that friendship with a well-behaved classmate can enhance the development of skills that facilitate behavioral and cognitive engagement in the classroom. Likewise, non-aggressive friends may encourage positive attitudes toward school by providing social support and companionship for victimized children (Schwartz et al., 2008). Thus, satisfactory friendship relations predicted lower levels of loneliness and was also related indirectly to popularity. Popularity among children strongly influenced friendship, which, in turn, affected loneliness. It appears that popularity is important for setting the stage for relationship development, but it is the quality of dyadic friendship experiences that most directly influence feelings of loneliness (Nangle, Erdley, Newman, Mason, & Carpenter, 2003).

Social Status: Acceptance, Rejection, and Popularity

Peers played an essential role in the socialization of interpersonal competence, and the skills acquired during social interactions affected the individual's long-term adjustment. The concept of peer status refers to a group's acceptance of a child and is defined as the degree to which the child is liked or disliked by group members (Ladd, 1999). Different status classifications were defined by research (Coie, Dodge, & Coppotelli, 1982), and the most common were the popular group (children who were nominated frequently as a best friend and were rarely disliked by their classmates) and the rejected group (children who were nominated infrequently by classmates as a best friend and are disliked by their peers). The concept of peer status refers to the child's interrelations with the entire group and it is different from the concept of friendship that refers to a specific relationship between children's dyads. Research on children's loneliness often explored the influence of acceptance versus rejection by peers (Asher & Paquette, 2003).

Peer acceptance in school was typically assessed using sociometric measures in which children either nominated schoolmates they liked or didn't like (i.e., "Whom do you like to study/play with? With whom do you not like planning a project?"). An alternative method was to apply a rating scale in order to indicate how much they like each of their peers. A consistent association was found between acceptance by peers and loneliness. Children who were poorly accepted reported experiencing greater loneliness. This finding remained consistent whether loneliness was measured in classroom, lunchroom, playground, or physical education contexts, suggesting that there was no safe haven at school for poorly accepted children (Asher & Paquette, 2003). Rejected children experienced more loneliness than other children in different age groups ranging from kindergartners through elementary-school children to adolescents. Even young children before entering school recognized when they had peer relationship difficulties and shared their unhappiness associated with their rejection. Furthermore, these associations had been found in research in many different countries and among boys and girls alike.

Sociometric status was related in schools with social and academic competencies. Children identified as members of a popular group tended to do well academically and behaved in socially competent ways, whereas children who were identified as belonging to the rejected group (i.e., those who were highly disliked by their peers) tended to have poor academic records and behaved in socially inappropriate ways. Middle-school children in the popular group tended to be more prosocial while those in the rejected group tended to be more aggressive (Wentzel, 2003). Yet, no difference in loneliness levels was found between average children and popular children, suggesting that children do not need to be exceptionally popular or well-liked to avoid feeling lonely (Cassidy & Asher, 1992). However, rejection contributed to loneliness even among young children and they expressed feelings of intense and extreme loneliness and difficulties in developing age-appropriate social skills (Schmidt, Demulder, & Denham, 2002).

A survey of longitudinal studies disclosed the relative stability of rejection and popularity among groups of children (Zettergren, 2007). Earlier peer rejection was identified as the strongest predictor of children's rejection at middle school, and children who experienced rejection or low friendliness at the start of middle childhood, perhaps in association with early behavior problems, would be at heightened risk for rejection and low levels of friendliness throughout the developmental stage

(Pedersen, Vitaro, Barker, & Borge, 2007). A wide range of children's difficulties and deficits (i.e., poor sociability, social skills' deficits, and communicative unresponsiveness) as well as aggressive and attention-deficit disorders contributed to the rejection (Lee, 2009), as well as children's appearance, athletic abilities, and academic competence (Vannatta, Gartstein, Zeller, & Noll, 2009). It was also related to various factors such as atypical behavior (i.e., aggression, disruption, and solitary behavior), appearance, and verbal differences (DeRosier & Mercer, 2009).

In order to reach an in-depth understanding of the rejection, distinct subgroups of rejected children were identified: aggressive-rejected children and withdrawn-rejected children. The withdrawn-rejected group consistently reported greater loneliness than the aggressive-rejected group, although during elementary school both groups reported higher levels of loneliness than children with an average degree of acceptance by their peers (Asher & Paquette, 2003). An additional factor that may have accounted for variability in rejected children's feelings of loneliness was overt victimization (Storch & Masis-Warner, 2004).

Peer relations have concurrent and longitudinal impacts. For example, rejection from peers was associated with a number of adjustment difficulties in children and adolescents (Rubin, Bukowski, & Parker, 1998). A follow-up study revealed increased rejection for rejected children, while the popular children became more popular (Zettergren, 2007). A longitudinal study that followed children from kindergarten through 5th graders (Buhs, Ladd, & Herald, 2006) reported that early peer rejection was associated with declining classroom participation, increasing school avoidance, and social exclusion. In another longitudinal study that followed 524 children (students of the second grade) and their teachers in Italy for a 2-year period, the relations between peer rejection and academic achievement were confirmed. Children who were rejected by their peers demonstrated consistently worse academic performance than did children who were not rejected, whereas children who were regularly accepted by their peers performed better in school than did their peers who were rejected one or more times. Several children, who became rejected during this period, exhibited an academic decline, while others who became accepted showed improvement (Greenman, Schneider, & Tomada, 2009). The exploration of the children's emotional world provided an additional understanding of the stability of the distressful relations. Children who were rejected at the early stages of school developed expectations of continued rejection regardless of changes in classes, and these expectations contributed to their social anxiety, anger, and loneliness (London, Downey, Bonica, & Paltin, 2007). Children's feeling of relatedness to classmates promoted their readiness for academic effort investment and higher achievements, while loneliness, social isolation, and negative mood consistently emerged following conflicts and peer exclusions (Reynolds & Repetti, 2008).

It can be concluded that (a) children who were less well-accepted by their kindergarten classmates were at greater risk for peer maltreatment in subsequent grades; (b) chronic peer maltreatment throughout the primary school years, including sustained peer exclusion and peer abuse, forecasted later school disengagement; and (c) the association between peer group rejection in kindergarten and children's achievement during the middle-grade school years was mediated by their exposure to chronic peer exclusion and decelerating classroom participation. These observed linkages supported the observation that early peer rejection was a precursor of at least two forms of chronic peer maltreatment (exclusion, abuse), and these forms of chronic maltreatment predicted children's school engagement. Having a friend at an early age seemed to protect a child from the risk of further maladjustment such as aggression and rejection (Criss, Pettit, Bates, Dodge, & Lapp, 2002). However, in middle childhood and adolescence, the protective features of peer relations reflected the growing complexity of social networks that characterized the world of peers (Hay et al., 2004).

The negative experiences of rejected children shape their attitudes toward other people in a way that amplifies antisocial behaviors such as aggression and or social withdrawal. Their social difficulties seem to result not only from their peers' negative attitudes toward them, but reciprocally they may also emerge from the way they interpret social situations and from their emotional reactions and strategies for dealing with these situations (Ladd, Herald-Brown, & Reiser, 2008). Coie's model of peer rejection was based on the assumption that children's social behavior was the primary cause for rejection by peers (Coie, 1990). Although non-behavioral factors such as appearance (Meriaux, Berg, & Hellstrom, 2010, disabilities, and athletic competence also had an important impact on peers' evaluations, the model proposed that children disliked peers because of the way in which they interacted with peers. Rejected children were more overtly and relationally aggressive than their peers (Putallaz et al., 2007).

Peer rejection in first grade was often related to aggressive behavior and contributed directly to subsequent conduct problem behavior in the fourth grade (Miller-Johnson, Coie, Maumary-Gremaud, Bierman, & Bierman, 2002). Withdrawal and shy behavior was also related to children's rejection, yet the risk posed by withdrawn behavior for peer rejection and future loneliness was related to their developmental stages. Low relations were documented during the early grade school years, but higher connections were identified during the middle grade school years when, perhaps, peers began to judge and criticize withdrawn behavior as atypical or deviant (Ladd, 2006). As children grew older, those prone to engage in withdrawn behavior became increasingly marginalized from the mainstream of social interaction and, accordingly, began to experience stronger feelings of alienation, anxiety, and loneliness. Furthermore, by middle childhood and thereafter, withdrawn behavior became a less mature way of coping with the social demands of peer environments, and children who were engaged in such behaviors were at greater risk for peer criticizing and distancing. The behavior of the children and the dynamics of the group – interacted differently not only at different ages, but also at various stages of the rejection development (Coie, 1990).

The process of acquiring social status was conceptualized as having different dynamics than the process of maintaining a stable identity as a rejected child. At the stage of entry into peer interactions, the most important determinant was the child's behavior, which was constantly evaluated by the peers and compared to expected standards. At this stage, the children's characteristics were more important and the group dynamic was less significant in explaining the initial stages of the rejection process. However, after the children gained a reputation as rejected and disliked by a significant number of peers, the group dynamic became more important. As the children continued to experience rejection, their feelings about themselves changed, decreasing their social confidence and promoting their inadequate social skills. Surveys of longitudinal studies (Asher & Paquette, 2003) disclosed that once children got a reputation of rejected children in their group, they faced a growing difficulty in finding steady play partners. They had limited opportunities to interact with popular children, tended to interact mostly with peers who had a similar lower status, or to spend more time alone. Sometimes they played with younger and/or unpopular children. They got reduced social support not only from peer groups but also from teachers. Many rejected children tended to withdraw from the group, and had difficulties in initiating and maintaining satisfactory interpersonal relations.

Social withdrawal is a complex term that includes several groups of children who are reluctant to join their peers. Some children have been considered shy and have difficulties joining others. They watched the group from afar, remained unoccupied in social company, and hovered near the other children, but were not engaged in social interactions (Coplan, Girardi, Findlay, & Frohlick, 2007). Some children may be motivated to approach others and be engaged in social interaction; however, their social motivation is attenuated by fear and anxiety, resulting in avoiding others (Coplan, Findlay, & Nelson, 2004). Rubin proposed two separate developmental processes of children's withdrawal and fewer interactions with peers (Rubin et al., 2009). The first process was termed "active isolation." It represented the process whereby some children spend time alone because their peers actively rejected and isolated them. The causes of their active isolation were varied and included the display of unacceptable behavior such as aggression, uncontrolled impulsivity, and social immaturity, as well as having disabilities, special appearance, belonging to a minority group, and inclinations that vary in some aspects from those of the majority of the peer group. These children were often viewed by teachers as impulsive and aggressive, and were disliked by their peers. Yet, longitudinal studies revealed that active isolation had a wide range of developmental variability. The second process – "social withdrawal," referred to the group of children who isolated themselves from the peer group due to internal factors such as anxiety, insecurity, negative self-esteem, and self-perceived difficulties in social skills and social relationships. Longitudinal studies revealed the stability of this behavior style, with increased risk for developing loneliness, negative self-perceptions of social competence, depressive mood, and internalizing and/or externalizing behavior difficulties.

Shy-withdrawn children are often rejected since they rarely initiate contact with peers, take longer than typical children to initiate conversation, and speak less frequently than their non-withdrawn counterparts. When these children do interact with peers, they appear to be less socially competent than typical children. Peers reject socially withdrawn children whose behavior is different from age-specific norms and expectations for social interaction and group involvement. Thus, the association between social withdrawal and peer rejection steadily increases with age

(Ladd, 2006). The withdrawn children and young adolescents were often viewed at high risk for peer victimization, experiencing repeated and consistent physical and verbal abuse from their peers and classmates, maybe since they were considered easy targets, often presenting themselves as physically and emotionally weak. Language impairments increased the likelihood of subsequent children's social anxiety. Among children with lower pragmatic language skills, shyness at the start of the school year predicted increased self-reported social anxiety and loneliness, as well as teacher-rated social withdrawal at the end of the school year (Coplan & Weeks, 2009).

Many withdrawn and shy children experience social difficulties, yet those who were able to form and maintain close friendships even within a small social network were less lonely. They tended to have at least one mutual and stable best friend. Rubin et al. (2009) reported that approximately 65% of socially withdrawn 10-year-olds had a mutual best friendship, and approximately 70% of these best friendships were maintained across the academic year, similarly to their non-withdrawn 10-year-old peers. Still, a detailed examination of the quality of their friendship relations revealed that many socially withdrawn children and young adolescents appeared to have friends who were experiencing similar psychosocial difficulties. Thus, sometimes withdrawn young adolescents rated their friendship relations as unsatisfactory, lacking in helpfulness, guidance, and intimate disclosure; the best friends of these withdrawn young adolescents rated their friendships as providing less fun and help than did the best friends of non-withdrawn adolescents.

For some children, the social withdrawal and peer rejection were stable. A follow-up over the 4-year period revealed that these children were noted as having unstable friendships and periods of friendlessness. However, decreases in social withdrawal were sometimes evident for those young adolescents who experienced decreases in rejection and victimization as they made the transition from elementary to middle school (Oh et al., 2008). In conclusion, complexity of peer relations, the negative impacts of rejection as well as social withdrawal were related to loneliness, yet at the same time focusing attention on the complexity of intervening personal and interpersonal factors. Studies of loneliness experienced by children with special educational needs presented them as a group at risk for peer rejection and increased loneliness, and exemplified the complexity of the intervening factors.

Social Status of Children with Special Needs

Students with special education needs were often at risk for peer rejection and limited companionship. Bryan's pioneering studies (Bryan, 1974, 1976) initiated the research focused on the social difficulties experienced by students with learning disabilities. Research reported that the students' difficulties were related not only to the children's academic achievements (i.e., reading and mathematics), but also to

their social difficulties expressed in children's social status (rejection and reciprocal nomination) and distressed expressions related to their interpersonal functioning
(Bryan, 1999; Chapman, 1988). Many students with learning disabilities received
low social ratings from peers and were identified as rejected or isolated in their
classrooms (Bryan, 2003; Margalit et al., 1999).

In a longitudinal study that followed children with learning disabilities from
the third grade through fall of the sixth grade, even when students with learning
disabilities were matched to their typically achieving peers in terms of group academic functioning and characteristics, they were viewed as lower in social status
among their classmates, and these effects were maintained over time (Estell et al.,
2008). Even children with learning disabilities who were educated in different educational environments (environments that emphasized the importance of the group
and collective such as the schools in the Israeli kibbutz versus environments that
emphasized individualistic orientation such as the schools in the Israeli cities) were
less competent socially, less accepted, and more rejected by peers. They experienced
similar high levels of loneliness when compared to typically achieving children
(Margalit & Ben-Dov, 1995).

Yet, it remained unclear if the children's experience of difficulties predicted their
social isolation or whether their belonging to a special group of children that were
labeled and diagnosed as children with special needs contributed to their loneliness. In order to clarify this dilemma, a study that examined the self-perception and
social interactions of children with reading difficulties that were not diagnosed as
learning disabled revealed that the experience of difficulties was by itself enough
to predict their adjustment difficulties and loneliness. As a group, these children
with reading difficulties reported higher levels of loneliness than their classmates
(Al-Yagon & Margalit, 2006). Similar high levels of loneliness were reported for
school-age children who revealed behavior difficulties at school, yet were not diagnosed or identified as revealing specific disabilities nor identified as belonging to
special education categories (Efrati-Virtzer & Margalit, 2009). We have performed
several studies, exploring the loneliness experience of children with different difficulties from high prevalence disabilities to severe disabilities at various age groups
and documented their loneliness as related to social difficulties as well as to their
competence in age-related challenges (Margalit, 2006). Yet, two unique groups of
children with difficulties were not lonelier than their classmates.

Children with attention-deficit disorder with hyperactivities were the first group
that provided a distinct social evaluation. Regardless of the fact that they were often
rejected by peers and had fewer quality friendships; they did not report increased
loneliness. Indeed research consistently showed that they had difficulties in initiating and maintaining friendship connections. Their teachers rated the children's
friendships as marginal to non-existent, and with lower qualities. They attributed
the children's feelings of isolation to their interpersonal style and described them:
"They are prone to being loners..."; "They are rejected, but they also isolate
themselves..." (Taylor & Houghton, 2008). Yet, the students presented a different
perspective, considering themselves as socially integrated in their classes similar to
their classmates, with 'lots of friends,' and revealing their positive illusory bias"

(Owens, Goldfine, Evangelista, Hoza, & Kaiser, 2007; Taylor & Houghton, 2008). This tendency to deny loneliness and social difficulties had an unexpected self-protective value for these children, and promoted their resilience (Heath & Glen, 2005; Wiener, 2004).

A second group of children with disabilities and difficulties who were not lonely and were not rated lonely by peers and adults were a resilient group. In many studies that we performed we were able to identify about 30% of the sample who were not different from their classmates in their social competence and loneliness experience. The positive self-perception of this group was not a positive illusory bias, but a realistic judgment. Regardless of their academic challenges, they were able to capsulate their difficulties and to perform socially as well as their peers. Their adjusted performance reflected their efficient coping strategies and sometimes even compensation tendencies (see Chapter 7 on coping strategies).

In conclusion, children with special needs were often rejected by peers, had fewer friends, and expressed their loneliness. The self-perceptions of lower competence, their anxiety and social exclusion time had again predicted their loneliness. These children received intensive academic help in order to meet their learning needs, but their loneliness distress and social difficulties were often ignored and neglected, even though the relations of social difficulties with the school failure and decreased motivation were documented. In addition, not all of the children considered themselves lonely children. The value of positive self-perceptions, as an expression of resilience and effective coping with challenges, even when it was not validated and reflected an illusory bias, was recognized as a protective factor. More attention to the school culture is needed in order to meet these social needs, and since loneliness reflects the individual's perceptions of his/her relations with others in his or her community, cultural differences have also to be clarified.

Social Relations and Loneliness in Different Cultures

Loneliness is experienced in different cultures, and the universality of the experience does not deny the recognition for cultural uniqueness disclosed in cross-cultural research (DiTommaso, Brannen, & Burgess, 2005). The term "cross-cultural" has been related to groups from diverse cultures and geographical settings, and also refers to different ethnic groups sharing the same environment such as visiting students who spend time in another culture. Even though loneliness studies explored personal and interpersonal factors (i.e., difficulties and preferences), loneliness qualities were further clarified by attitudes and expectations that differed across socio-cultural contexts. Expressions of the social distress disclosed distinctive cultural conventions that characterized different traditions. For example, differences were noticed between the loneliness in societies that value the group cohesion versus those that appreciate individualization, autonomy, and privacy. Thus, the loneliness experience may be related differently not only to personal characteristics but also to contextual conditions.

Studies that examined patterns of peer relations, social behaviors, peer-group affiliation, family functioning, and loneliness experiences recognized similarities but also identified differences across stereotypes and attitudes' variations in different cultures such as the Turkish, Chinese, Indian, Greek, and South American (Chen & Wellman, 2005; Prakash & Coplan, 2007; Rokach, Orzeck, Moya, & Exposito, 2002; Uruk & Demir, 2003; Valdivia, Schneider, Chavez, & Chen, 2005). Socially withdrawn children were at risk for developing loneliness in different cultures. For example, socially withdrawn elementary school-aged children in New Delhi (India) reported greater loneliness and depressive symptoms than their comparison group with average behavior (Prakash & Coplan, 2007). They were rated by teachers as more anxious and were more likely to be rejected by peers.

The relations between loneliness and social capital aspects (such as perceptions of the local community, social support, and social networks) were not simple or direct (Fealy, 2006; Lauder, Mummery, & Sharkey, 2006; Lauder, Sharkey, & Mummery, 2004). However, higher levels of loneliness were associated with western cultural orientations that emphasized individualism and independence. For example, the comparisons between North America and Spain revealed higher levels of loneliness for the first group. In addition, those who lived in North America were more painfully blaming their own contribution to their loneliness (Rockach, Orzeck, Moya, & Exposito, 2002). Additional comparisons of the loneliness experience between Canadians and Czechs further validated the impact of cultures. Collectivistic cultures such as the Czech emphasized relatedness and conformity to the group in thought, feeling, and action. Individualistic cultures such as the Canadian encouraged an independent social representation of the person and focused attention on inner experiences. Thus, emotional experience such as loneliness was perceived and experienced more intensely in individualistic (Canada) rather than in collectivistic (Czech) cultures (Rokach & Bauer, 2004). Similarly, comparisons of the loneliness experienced by American and Korean students revealed that American young adults experienced intense loneliness in comparison with Korean young adults (Seepersad, Choi, & Shin., 2008).

Surprisingly, the comparisons of loneliness experienced by children in several cultures revealed that children who were socialized under different social and cultural backgrounds might experience, to a similar extent, similar feelings of loneliness and social dissatisfaction (Chen et al., 2004). Multinational studies were performed in Canada, Brazil, China, and Southern Italy. Canada represents a North American individualistic culture, whereas China represents a typical Asian group-oriented or collectivistic culture. Brazilian and Southern Italian societies are both a mixture of diverse values and traditions, characterized by personalized considerations (i.e., people are expected to consider the needs and views of others with whom they share relational bonds, but not necessarily the interests of the society or larger groups) and concern for individual autonomy. The comparisons of loneliness reported by children in these four samples did not differ in the mean scores of self-reported loneliness. Yet, the results indicated that in each society, multiple factors including personal and relational aspects were associated differently with children's feelings of loneliness. The diverse patterns of relations between loneliness and social functioning (such as aggression and shyness-sensitivity), suggested that the broad socio-cultural contexts affected the nature of children's loneliness.

For example, the attitudes toward aggressive behavior differentiated between cultures, with different consequences to companionship and loneliness. Indeed aggressive behavior was generally discouraged in Western individualistic cultures, yet aggressive children and adolescents may have received social support from peers and sometimes were perceived as popular in their youth cultures. Thus in Western cultures, aggressive children often did not experience higher levels of loneliness (Rubin, Chen, & Hymel, 1993). They tended to overestimate and misinterpret their own competence relative to peers' evaluation (Hymel, Bowker, & Woody, 1993). Moreover, they viewed themselves just as positively as average children viewed themselves. Aggressive children may have received support from peer networks and may even have been viewed as "stars" in some peer groups (Salmivalli, Kauliaine, & Lagerspetz, 2000). As a result, despite their social and behavioral problems, aggressive children often had biased self-perceptions, overestimated their social competence, and did not report psycho-emotional distress. They may have lacked self-awareness or tended to deny negative traits, and thus they didn't feel lonely. They also may have formed social networks with other aggressive peers (Xu & Zhang, 2008). Belonging to social networks might work as a buffer against their feelings of loneliness.

A different link between aggression and loneliness was documented in Chinese children. In Chinese schools, aggressive, disruptive, and defiant behaviors are prohibited and considered a threat to group harmony. These schools required the children to evaluate themselves in the group regarding their behaviors and whether they had made improvement over time. Peers and teachers provided feedback on the child's self-evaluations. This social interactive process made it difficult for aggressive children to develop inflated or "biased" self-perceptions of their competence and social status. Consequently, aggressive children in China displayed their pervasive social and psychological difficulties including low social status, poor quality of peer relationships, negative self-perceptions, and feelings of loneliness and depression (Chen et al., 2004). Similarly, in the structured Korean school context, which requires task-oriented and task-persisted behaviors, acting out behavior and expressions of aggression were viewed as a problem behavior and related to loneliness (Shin, 2007). Self-regulation and compliance to the group norm were more emphasized in peer interactions in Chinese culture, and this emphasis was reflected in the robust negative relations between aggression, peer relationships, and loneliness in Chinese groups.

Withdrawn and shyness as children's characteristics had even more diverse implications in different cultures. Shy children in North America were more likely to experience problems in peer interactions than in China, which in turn may have lead to negative feelings about their social world and loneliness (Chen et al., 2004). Children who displayed shy-inhibited behaviors were viewed in Western cultures as socially incompetent and immature (Fox, Henderson, Marshall, Nichols, & Ghera, 2005). They experienced lower peer acceptance and poor social adjustment (Rubin et al., 2009). Over time, these children tended to develop negative self-perceptions, received ongoing negative social feedback, and became aware of their social difficulties and exclusion. Similarly, in India, withdrawn children reported greater loneliness and more depressive symptoms (particularly girls), and were rated by teachers as having more internalizing problems (i.e., anxiety) (Prakash & Coplan, 2007). These socially withdrawn children in India were more likely to be rejected by peers.

Unlike their counterparts in the West and in India, shy children in China were accepted by peers and performed well socially and academically in childhood and adolescence and they did not feel lonely. Similarly, shyness was viewed as less problematic in some Asian cultures, such as Indonesia and Korea, than in North America. Shyness was also found to lead to less negative outcomes in Swedish youth than in American youth (Chen & French, 2008). It can be concluded that within collectivistic cultures, a strong emphasis was placed on group cohesion; consequently, shy-reserved behavior may have been more accepted and appreciated than in Western cultures that supported individualistic beliefs and norms. Yet, since collectivism may be expressed differently within different cultures, these differences may affect societal norms and expectations regarding social behaviors and loneliness. Additionally, researchers have suggested that shyness may not be a unitary factor, and, therefore, it is necessary to differentiate between subtypes of this behavior (Hart et al., 2000). The quality of peer relations in the different cultures was especially influential. Sometime shy and withdrawn children, who had good friends in different cultures, were not lonely.

A closer examination of social competence in the different cultures revealed that social initiative and behavioral control represented two major dimensions. Cultural norms and values with respect to these two dimensions affected the exhibition, meaning, and development of specific social behaviors such as sociability, shyness-inhibition, cooperation-compliance, and aggression defiance, as well as the quality and function of social relationships and alienation (Chen & French, 2008). In Western individualistic cultures, acquiring autonomy and assertive social skills is an important socialization goal. The lack of active social participation and initiative is considered a maladaptive functioning. The culture promotes self-enhancement, in which a positive view of the self is seen as a necessity for an individual's psychological wellbeing and adaptation to societal demands. The social initiative may not be highly appreciated or valued in group-oriented or collectivistic societies, such as in many East Asian and Latin American societies, because it may not facilitate cohesiveness in the group. To maintain interpersonal and group harmony, individuals need to restrain personal desires in an effort to address the needs and interests of others. In cultures such as China, children were encouraged to comply with external demands, and social and behavior expectations. However, regardless of cultural differences (comparisons of bullying and friendship networks and loneliness in several countries – China, England, Finland, Ireland, Italy, Japan, Portugal, and Spain), loneliness was reported by children in the different cultures, gender, and age groups, and was related to the children's interpersonal reality, social networks, and difficulties such as being bullied (Junttila & Vauras, 2009).

In a longitudinal study children were followed from the first grade to the 6th grade in a middle-sized town in Sweden (Nyberg, Henricsson, & Rydell, 2008). High levels of internalizing and externalizing behavior as well as poor social competence in the first grade predicted loneliness and low peer acceptance in sixth grade. Peer acceptance of the older group emerged as a complex, multifaceted aspect, with concurrent, independent predictions from both externalizing and internalizing problem behaviors as well as social competence. Loneliness, on the other hand, was distinctively associated for this age group with high levels of concurrent internalizing problems. Thus, early internalizing problems in the Swedish culture predicted loneliness, but the early manifestation of externalizing and aggressive behavior by itself was not enough to predict loneliness. Only when it was associated with peer rejection, did they jointly predict later loneliness.

A unique loneliness consideration in early developmental stages can be found in Japanese preschools, emerging from social motives and the desire to fit in society. A key pedagogical goal of Japanese preschool teachers was to provide young children with opportunities to develop empathy, which required the ability to be aware of the feelings of others (Hayashi, Karasawa, & Tobin, 2009). The concept of loneliness was introduced by teachers because this construct provoked responses of empathy and fueled young children's desires for sociality. Expressions of loneliness provoked empathic responses of inviting the lonely child to join the group. Teachers used stories and metaphors to increase the use of the concept (i.e., lonely doll), since they believed that children needed specific and focused learning opportunities to express their loneliness and to act in ways that invited empathic, caring responses. They assumed that if children felt lonely but were not acquainted with socially appropriate ways of showing and expressing it as well as if they needed help but hide their helplessness, they reduced the possibility of empathic, prosocial responses from others. Learning to express loneliness in Japanese preschools was therefore considered a crucial developmental task for young children. Children in preschools had ample opportunities to experience loneliness, as well as situations that would enable them to express social needs. Nevertheless, they needed experimenting and training to respond to others' needs, modeled by teachers and encouraged by peers.

In order to examine whether peer relationships were associated with loneliness in Korean children (Shin, 2007), a sample of fifth- and sixth-grade students was examined. Consistent with previous findings in Western contexts, children's involvement and experiences in peer relationships had implications on their social exclusion and loneliness. Children who were accepted by peers, able to form friendships or had high positive friendship quality tended to be relatively protected from loneliness in compared to other children. Furthermore, Korean children who were characterized by aggressive tendencies experienced low peer acceptance and few friends. Low-achieving children had difficulties being accepted by peer groups and also in forming dyadic friendships with peers in class.

Low-achieving children in several cultures, such as Korea, also experienced social difficulties. They were less accepted by peer groups and also disclosed difficulties in forming dyadic friendships with peers in the class. Thus, low-achieving children reported higher levels of loneliness because of relational difficulties and negative friendship quality. Due to cultural emphasis on academic achievement, poor-achieving Korean children were likely to obtain a negative social reputation in peer groups. Consequently, children who did poorly in school in cultures that value academic competence may have been at risk for peer difficulties, which in turn influenced their feelings of social isolation and alienation at school. Even when these low-achieving children had friends, the number of friends did not compensate for feelings of loneliness for these low-achieving children. It has been suggested that since many times they formed friendship relations with children who were similar to them in behavioral characteristics as well as academic achievement, the academically incompetent Korean children tended to affiliate with similar children in school, so the friends' characteristics such as academic reputation may not have buffered children's loneliness, and the friendship quality was low and did not meet their needs (Shin, 2007).

Cultural differences were also expressed in the behavior of boys and girls. For example, Korean girls reported greater adjustment problems when they bullied others, whereas Korean boys reported greater problems when others bullied them, indicating that Korean boys and girls felt uneasy when their roles did not correspond to cultural norms (Yang, Kim, Kim, Shin, & Yoon, 2006). Korean girls who were characterized by shy disposition were usually accepted by peers; therefore, withdrawal style was unlikely to be associated with feelings of loneliness for girls (Shin, 2007). Different contextual conditions resulted in different profiles of competences, and the rejected children in a developing rural village had significantly lower academic scores than popular children. However, these rejected children were not rated by their teachers as having significantly more problems involving withdrawal or aggressive and antisocial behaviors (Jimerson, Durbrow, & Wagstaff, 2009).

The choice of leisure activities such as sport participation was also related to cultural preferences. Team sports were highly valued in different countries such as Australia. It was expected that this cultural appreciation of sport would have an impact on the wellbeing of boys with mild-coordination difficulties (i.e., developmental coordination disorder – DCD). These boys reported lower rates of participation in these sport activities and higher rates of dropping-out as they grow older, relative to boys who were well-coordinated. They were rejected by the team and not selected to the group of players (Poulsen, Ziviani, Cuskelly, & Smith, 2007). By 11–12 years of age, boys with motor impairments participated more in individual or dyadic sports than team sports and at 15 years of age, adolescents with motor impairments not only had low social–physical activity participation, but low participation in all social leisure-time activities, whether physical or non-physical, and these decreased leisure activities predicted increased experiences of loneliness and low global life satisfaction (Poulsen, Ziviani, Johnson, & Cuskelly, 2008). This research documented a reciprocal ongoing process of loneliness development, where boys with poor motor abilities, who had initially lower participation in physical activities in a culture that valued sport activities for boys as signs of their gender identity, had reduced opportunities to practice their motor skills, and this further led to activity deficits and a growing gap in their skill-learning, that contributed to the development of loneliness and peer rejection.

In collectivistic societies, people derive much of their sense of personal identity from their membership in larger collective units, such as their communities,
extended families, or nations. The developing countries of Asia, Africa, and Latin
America are considered collectivistic, and the social participation and close friendship are emphasized and valued there. In societies and families that emphasize
social connections and group relations, children grow up expecting high levels of
social support. This can lead to disappointments and loneliness for individuals who,
due to personal characteristics or social deficiencies, do not achieve the high levels of rewarding social interactions. In addition, for some children who need time
for themselves, too many social contacts and social expectations may contribute
to children's loneliness and alienation. Most English-speaking countries – Canada,
Great Britain, the United States, and Australia – represent the individualistic societies, emphasizing personal autonomy and valuing their prerogative to choose their
friends. It can be concluded that even though loneliness is universal, yet it also
reflected the uniqueness of different cultures. Thus, the specific nature of children's
loneliness reflects the joint impacts of children's personal characteristics and the
different environments in diverse cultures, as presented in Fig. 5.1.

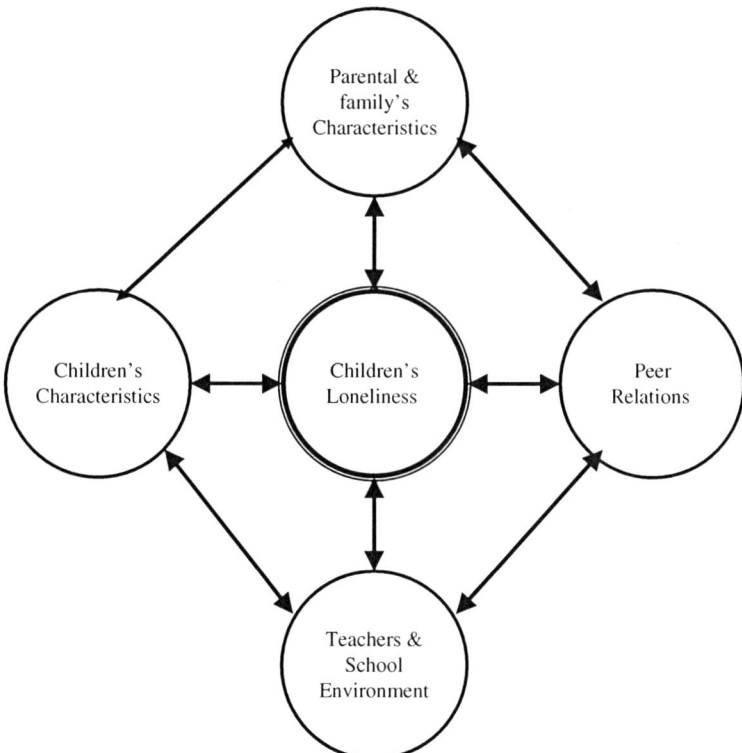

Fig. 5.1 Loneliness as the outcome of interacting personal and contextual characteristics

Summary and Conclusions

In conclusion, socio-cultural contexts, different attitudes, and social expectations toward social relations have important roles in predicting loneliness. Children actively and continually construct meaning in their environments and interrelations. Teachers' attitudes toward children affect peer relations, especially at younger ages. School climate, classroom relations, and teaching styles are important predictive factors for children's interactions with peers and the development of friendship relations and rejections. Teachers' attitudes, their perceptions of children's competence, effort, behavior, and success may further contribute to the children's experience of social isolation, jointly with the children's unique characteristics. Contextual variations reflect differences in cultural values that guide people's desires to an optimal network of social relationships, as well as sensitize individuals to the extent to which loneliness is associated with stigma and prejudices (Scharf & de Jong Gierveld, 2008). In addition, the expressions of loneliness may differ across cultures. Comparative research clearly demonstrated universality of the loneliness experience and children who were socialized under different social and cultural backgrounds similarly experienced feelings of loneliness and social dissatisfaction. Even if cultures of interdependence trends protected children from being alone, they may not have protected children from feeling lonely. These results were rather surprising, given the dramatic differences among these societies in the cultural norms and values concerning social interactions and personal relationships.

Even though, the psychological cultural meaning attributed to loneliness as well as to any given social behavior is, to a large extent, the function of ecological contexts within which they are produced (Rubin et al., 2009). If a given behavior is viewed by the community as acceptable, then parents and teachers will attempt to encourage its development and enable its expressions; if the behavior is perceived as maladaptive or pathological, then they will attempt to discourage its development and manifestation. Children are actively engaged in social interactions, creating friendships, developing groups, and participating in constructing peer cultures. Children play an active role in selecting and adopting different segments of the existing culture while ignoring other portions and also participate in adopting cultural norms and values for social evaluations and group activities. Thus, the social processes are dynamically bidirectional and transactional in nature. Through these processes, personal characteristics, socialization processes, and cultural factors, children's social behaviors, and social relationships are collectively shaped. Overall, the experience of loneliness is significantly affected by cultural heritage, especially when the cultures under question are different economically, geographically, religiously, and socially. Many basic psychological processes operate across cultures: the kinds of goals we seek, the kinds of problems we face, and the kinds of capabilities we have as a result of simply being human. But the expression of loneliness and the intensity differ among cultures and genders (DiTommaso et al., 2005). Social competence is a complex construct, including peer perceptions and self-perceptions. In addition, the differences between individualistic cultures and group-oriented cultures are influenced not only by the existing conceptions, but also by the dramatic ongoing social changes in several countries that may affect the development of a global youth culture (Chen & French, 2008).

Research found that the combination of sociometric popularity and self-perceived social acceptance jointly predicted social adjustment (McElhaney, Antonishak, & Allen, 2008). However, the dynamic contribution of self-perceptions and feeling of competence to social relations with individuals and with the peer group structured social satisfaction and distress. For example, when adolescents felt socially confident and comfortable with their peers, they did well regardless of their actual sociometric ratings. Additionally, those adolescents who were liked by their peers also fared well, regardless of their own perceptions of their social standing. Finally, the adolescents who demonstrated the worst social outcomes over time were those who lacked both a strong sense of their own social acceptance, and were also rated as unpopular by their peers. This complexity has a unique value for planning intervention programs, as will be further discussed in Chapter 8. The contribution of cultures to social adjustment and loneliness cannot ignore the new emerging culture of the Internet. The entrance of technology in everybody's life challenged the conventional concepts of contexts and interpersonal relations, as will be discussed in Chapter 6.

References

Aikins, J. W., Bierman, K., & Parker, J. G. (2005). Navigating the transition to junior high school: The influence of pre-transition friendship and self-system characteristics. *Social Development, 14*(1), 42–60.

Al-Yagon, M., & Margalit, M. (2006). Loneliness, sense of coherence and perception of teachers as a secure base among children with reading difficulties. *European Journal of Special Needs Education, 21*(1), 21–37.

Asher, S. R., & Paquette, J. A. (2003). Loneliness and peer relations in childhood. *Current Directions in Psychological Sciences, 12*(3), 75–78.

Bauminger, N., Finzi-Dottan, R., Chason, S., & Har-Even, D. (2008). Intimacy in adolescent friendship: The roles of attachment, coherence, and self-disclosure. *Journal of Social and Personal Relationships, 25*(3), 409–428.

Berguno, G., Leroux, P., McAinsh, K., & Shaikh, S. (2004). Children's experience of loneliness at school and its relation to bullying and the quality of teacher interventions. *The Qualitative Report, 9*(3), 483–499.

Berndt, T. J. (2002). Friendship quality and social development. *Current Directions in Psychological Science, 11*(1), 7–11.

Betts, L. R., & Rotenberg, K. J. (2008). A social relations analysis of children's trust in their peers across the early years of school. *Social Development, 17*(4), 1039–1055.

Betts, L. R., Rotenberg, K. J., & Trueman, M. (2009). The early childhood generalized trust belief scale. *Early Childhood Research Quarterly, 24*(2), 175–185.

Brownell, C., Belsky, J., Booth-LaForce, C., Bradley, R., Campbell, S. B., Clarke-Stewart, K. A., et al. (2008). Social competence with peers in third grade: Associations with earlier peer experiences in childcare. *Social Development, 17*(3), 419–453.

Bryan, T. (1974). Peer popularity of learning disabled children. *Journal of Learning Disabilities, 7*(10), 621–625.

Bryan, T. (1976). Peer popularity of learning disabled children – Replication. *Journal of Learning Disabilities, 9*(5), 307–311.

Bryan, T. (1999). Reflections on a research career: It ain't over till it's over. *Exceptional Children,* *65*(4), 438–448.

Bryan, T. (2003). The applicability of the risk and resilience model to social problems of students with learning disabilities: Response to Bernice Wong. *Learning Disabilities Research and Practice, 18*(2), 94–98.

Buhs, E. S., Ladd, G. W., & Herald, S. L. (2006). Peer exclusion and victimization: Processes that mediate the relation between peer group rejection and children's classroom engagement and achievement? *Journal of Educational Psychology, 98*(1), 1–13.

Bukowski, W. M., Adams, R. E., & Santo, J. B. (2006). Recent advances in the study of development, social and personal experience, and psychopathology. *International Journal of Behavioral Development, 30*(1), 26–30.

Cassidy, J., & Asher, S. R. (1992). Loneliness and peer relations in young-children. *Child Development, 63*(2), 350–365.

Chan, A., & Poulin, F. (2007). Monthly changes in the composition of friendship networks in early adolescence. *Merrill-Palmer Quarterly, 53*(4), 578–602.

Chan, A., & Poulin, F. (2009). Monthly instability in early adolescent friendship networks and depressive symptoms. *Social Development, 18*(1), 1–23.

Chapman, J. W. (1988). Cognitive-motivational characteristics and academic achievement of learning disabled children: A longitudinal study. *Journal of Educational Psychology, 80*(3), 357–365.

Chen, W., & Wellman, B. (2005). Charting digital divides: Comparing socioeconomic, gender, life stage, and rural-urban Internet access and use in eight Countries. In W. Dutton, B. Kahin, R. O'Callaghan, & A. Wyckoff (Eds.), *Transforming enterprise* (pp. 467–497). Cambridge, MA: MIT Press.

Chen, X., & French, D. C. (2008). Children's social competence in cultural context. *Annual Review of Psychology, 59,* 591–616.

Chen, X., He, Y., Oliveira, A. M. D., Coco, A. L., Zappulla, C., Kaspar, V., et al. (2004). Loneliness and social adaptation in Brazilian, Canadian, Chinese and Italian children: A multi-national comparative study. *Journal of Child Psychology and Psychiatry and Allied Disciplines, 45*(8), 1373–1384.

Coie, J. D. (1990). Toward a theory of peer rejection. In S. R. Asher & J. D. Coie (Eds.), *Peer rejection in childhood* (pp. 365–401). Cambridge: University Press.

Coie, J. D., Dodge, K. A., & Coppotelli, H. (1982). Dimensions and types of social status: A cross-age perspective. *Developmental Psychology, 18*(4), 557–570.

Coplan, R. J., Findlay, L. C., & Nelson, L. J. (2004). Characteristics of preschoolers with lower perceived competence. *Journal of Abnormal Child Psychology, 32*(4), 399–408.

Coplan, R. J., Girardi, A., Findlay, L. C., & Frohlick, S. L. (2007). Understanding solitude: Young children's attitudes and responses toward hypothetical socially withdrawn peers. *Social Development, 16*(3), 390–409.

Coplan, R. J., & Weeks, M. (2009). Shy and soft-spoken: Shyness, pragmatic language, and socio-emotional adjustment in early childhood. *Infant and Child Development, 18*(3), 238–254.

Criss, M. M., Pettit, G. S., Bates, J. E., Dodge, K. A., & Lapp, A. L. (2002). Family adversity, positive peer relationships, and children's externalising behavior: A longitudinal perspective on risk and resilience. *Child Development, 73*(4), 1220–1237.

Demır, M., & Weitekamp, L. A. (2007). I am so happy 'cause today I found my friend: Friendship and personality as predictors of happiness. *Journal of Happiness Studies, 8*(2), 181–211.

DeRosier, M. E., & Mercer, S. H. (2009). Perceived behavioral atypicality as a predictor of social rejection and peer victimization: Implications for emotional adjustment and academic achievement. *Psychology in the Schools, 46*(4), 375–387.

DiTommaso, E., Brannen, C., & Burgess, M. (2005). The universality of relationship characteristics: A cross-cultural comparison of different types of attachment and loneliness in Canadians and visiting Chinese students. *Social Behavior and Personality, 33*(1), 57–68.

Duffy, A. L., & Nesdale, D. (2009). Peer groups, social identity, and children's bullying behavior. *Social Development*, *18*(1), 121–139.

Efrati-Virtzer, M., & Margalit, M. (2009). Students' behaviour difficulties, sense of coherence and adjustment at school: Risk and protective factors. *European Journal of Special Needs Education*, *24*(1), 59–73.

Erath, S. A., Pettit, G. S., Dodge, K. A., & Bates, J. E. (2009). Who dislikes whom, and for whom does it matter: Predicting aggression in middle childhood. *Social Development*, *18*(3), 577–596.

Erikson, E. (1963). *Childhood and society* (2nd Rev. ed.). New York: Norton.

Estell, D. B., Jones, M. H., Pearl, R., Van Acker, R., Farmer, T. W., & Rodkin, P. C. (2008). Peer groups, popularity, and social preference: Trajectories of social functioning among students with and without learning disabilities. *Journal of Learning Disabilities*, *41*(1), 5–14.

Fealy, G. M. (2006). Commentary on Lauder W, Mummery K & Sharkey S (2006) Social capital, age and religiosity in people who are lonely. *Journal of Clinical Nursing*, *15*(6), 797–799.

Fox, N. A., Henderson, H. A., Marshall, P. J., Nichols, K. E., & Ghera, M. M. (2005). Behavioral inhibition: Linking biology and behavior within a developmental framework. *Annual Review in Psychology*, *56*, 235–262.

Gest, S. D., Farmer, T. W., Cairns, B. D., & Xie, H. (2003). Identifying children's peer social networks in school classrooms: Links between peer reports and observed interactions. *Social Development*, *12*(4), 513–529.

Gray, W. N., Kahhan, N. A., & Janicke, D. M. (2009). Peer victimization and pediatric obesity: A review of the literature. *Psychology in the Schools*, *46*(8), 720–727.

Greenman, P. S., Schneider, B. H., & Tomada, G. (2009). Stability and change in patterns of peer rejection: Implications for children's academic performance over time. *School Psychology International*, *30*(2), 163–183.

Hardy, C. L., Bukowski, W. M., & Sippola, L. K. (2002). Stability and change in peer relationships during the transition to middle level school. *Journal of Early Adolescence*, *22*(2), 117–142.

Hart, C. H., Yang, C., Nelson, D. A., Robinson, C. C., Jin, S., Win, P., et al. (2000). Peer acceptance in early childhood an subtypes of social withdrawal behaviour in China, Russia and the United States. *International Journal of Behavioural Development*, *24*(1), 77–81.

Hartup, W. W. (1996). The company they keep: Friendships and their developmental significance. *Child Development*, *67*(1), 1–13.

Hay, D. F., Payne, A., & Chadwick, A. (2004). Peer relations in childhood. *Journal of Child Psychology and Psychiatry*, *45*(1), 84–108.

Hayashi, A., Karasawa, M., & Tobin, J. (2009). The Japanese preschool's pedagogy of feeling: Cultural strategies for supporting young children's emotional development. *Ethos*, *37*(1), 32–49.

Heath, N. L., & Glen, T. (2005). Positive illusory bias and the self-protective hypothesis in children with learning disabilities. *Journal of Clinical Child and adolescent Psychology*, *34*(2), 272–281.

Hymel, S., Bowker, A., & Woody, E. (1993). Aggressive versus withdrawn unpopular children: Variations in peer and self-perceptions in multiple domains. *Child Development*, *64*(3), 879–896.

Jimerson, S. R., Durbrow, E. H., & Wagstaff, D. A. (2009). Academic and behavior associates of peer status for children in a Caribbean community findings from the St Vincent Child Study. *School Psychology International*, *30*(2), 184–200.

Junttila, N., & Vauras, M. (2009). Loneliness among school-aged children and their parents. *Scandinavian Journal of Psychology*, *50*(3), 211–219.

Kim, Y. K., Kim, E. Y., & Kang, J. (2003). Teens' mall shopping motivations: Functions of loneliness and media usage. *Family and Consumer Sciences Research Journal*, *32*(2), 140–167.

Kiuru, N., Nurmi, J. E., Aunola, K., & Salmela-Aro, K. (2009). Peer group homogeneity in adolescents' school adjustment varies according to peer group type and gender. *International Journal of Behavioral Development*, *33*(1), 65–76.

Kochenderfer-Ladd, B., & Wardop, J. L. (2001). Chronicity and instability of children's peer victimization experiences as predictors of loneliness and social satisfaction trajectories. *Child Development, 72*(1), 134–151.

Kwon, K., & Lease, A. M. (2007). Clique membership and social adjustment: The contribution of the type of clique to children's self-reported adjustment. *Merrill-Palmer Quarterly, 53*(2), 216–242.

Kwon, K., & Lease, A. M. (2009). Examination of the contribution of clique characteristics to children's adjustment: Clique type and perceived cohesion. *International Journal of Behavioral Development, 33*(3), 230–242.

Ladd, G. W. (1999). Peer relations and social competence during early and middle childhood. *Annual Review of Psychology, 50*, 333–359.

Ladd, G. W. (2006). Peer rejection, aggressive or withdrawn behavior, and psychological maladjustment from ages 5 to 12: An examination of four predictive models. *Child Development, 77*(4), 822–846.

Ladd, G. W., Herald-Brown, S. L., & Reiser, M. (2008). Does chronic classroom peer rejection predict the development of children's classroom participation during the grade school years? *Child Development, 79*(4), 1001–1015.

Ladd, G. W., & Troop-Gordon, W. (2003). The role of chronic peer difficulties in the development of children's psychological adjustment problems. *Child Development, 74*(5), 1344–1367.

Lauder, W., Mummery, K., & Sharkey, S. (2006). Social capital, age and religiosity in people who are lonely. *Journal of Clinical Nursing, 15*(3), 334–340.

Lauder, W., Sharkey, S., & Mummery, K. (2004). A community survey of loneliness. *Journal of Advanced Nursing, 46*(1), 88–94.

Ledbetter, A. M. (2009). Family communication patterns and relational maintenance behavior: Direct and mediated associations with friendship closeness. *Human Communication Research, 35*(1), 130–147.

Lee, E. (2009). The relationship of aggression and bullying to social preference: Differences in gender and types of aggression. *International Journal of Behavioral Development, 33*(4), 323–330.

London, B., Downey, G., Bonica, C., & Paltin, I. (2007). Social causes and consequences of rejection sensitivity. *Journal of Research on Adolescence, 17*(3), 481–506.

Margalit, M. (1994). *Loneliness among children with special needs: Theory, research, coping and intervention*. New York: Springer.

Margalit, M. (2006). Loneliness, the Salutogenic paradigm and LD: Current research, future directions and interventional implications. *Thalamus, 24*(1), 38–48.

Margalit, M., & Ben-Dov, I. (1995). Learning disabilities and social environments: Kibbutz versus city comparisons of loneliness and social competence. *International Journal of Behavioral Development, 18*(3), 519–536.

Margalit, M., Tur-Kaspa, H., & Most, T. (1999). Reciprocal nominations, reciprocal rejections and loneliness among students with learning disorders. *Educational Psychology, 19*(1), 79–90.

McElhaney, K. B., Antonishak, J., & Allen, J. P. (2008). "They like me, they like me not": Popularity and adolescents: Perceptions of acceptance predicting social functioning over time. *Child Development, 79*(3), 720–731.

McGraw, K., Moore, S., Fuller, A., & Bates, G. (2008). Family, peer and school connectedness in final year secondary school students. *Australian Psychologist, 43*(1), 27–37.

Meriaux, B. G., Berg, M., & Hellstrom, A. L. (2009). Everyday experiences of life, body and well-being in children with overweight. *Scandinavian Journal of Caring Sciences, 24*(1), 14–23.

Meriaux, B. G., Berg, M., & Hellstrom, A. L. (2010). Everyday experiences of life, body and well-being in children with overweight. *Scandinavian Journal of Caring Sciences, 24*(1), 14–23.

Miller-Johnson, S., Coie, J. D., Maumary-Gremaud, A., Bierman, K., & Bierman, K. (2002). Peer rejection and aggression and early starter models of conduct disorder. *Journal of Abnormal Child Psychology, 30*(3), 217–230.

Nangle, D. W., Erdley, C. A., Newman, J. E., Mason, C. A., & Carpenter, E. M. (2003). Popularity, friendship quantity, and friendship quality: Interactive influences on children's loneliness and depression. *Journal of Clinical Child & Adolescent Psychology, 32*(4), 546–555.

Newcomb, A. F., & Bagwell, C. L. (1995). Children's friendship relations: A meta-analytic review. *Psychological Bulletin, 117*(2), 306–347.

Nyberg, L., Henricsson, L., & Rydell, A. M. (2008). Low social inclusion in childhood: Adjustment and early predictors. *Infant and Child Development, 17*(6), 639–656.

Oh, W., Rubin, K., Bowker, J., Booth-LaForce, C., Rose-Krasnor, L., & Laursen, B. (2008). Trajectories of social withdrawal from middle childhood to early adolescence. *Journal of Abnormal Child Psychology, 36*(4), 553–566.

Owens, J., Goldfine, M., Evangelista, N., Hoza, B., & Kaiser, N. (2007). A critical review of self-perceptions and the positive illusory bias in children with ADHD. *Clinical Child and Family Psychology Review, 10*(4), 335–351.

Parker, J. G., & Asher, S. R. (1993). Friendship and friendship quality in middle childhood. *Developmental Psychology, 29*(4), 611–621.

Parker, J. G., & Gamm, B. K. (2003). Describing the dark side of preadolescents' peer experiences: Four questions (and data) on preadolescents' enemies. *New Directions for Child & Adolescent Development, 2003*(102), 55–72.

Parker, J. G., Saxon, J., Asher, S. R., & Kovacs, D. (1999). Dimensions of children's friendship adjustment: Implications for studying loneliness. In K. J. Rotenberg & S. Hymel (Eds.), *Loneliness in childhood and adolescence.* (pp. 201–224). New York: Cambridge University Press.

Parker, J. G., Walker, A. R., Low, C. M., & Gamm, B. K. (2005). Friendship jealousy in young adolescents: Individual differences and links to sex, self-esteem, aggression, and social adjustment. *Developmental Psychology, 41*(1), 235–250.

Pedersen, S., Vitaro, F., Barker, E. D., & Borge, A. I. H. (2007). The timing of middle-childhood peer rejection and friendship: Linking early behavior to early-adolescent adjustment. *Child Development, 78*(4), 1037–1051.

Poulsen, A. A., Ziviani, J. M., Cuskelly, M., & Smith, R. (2007) Boys with developmental coordination disorder: Loneliness and team sports participation. *American Journal of Occupational Therapy, 61*(4), 451–462.

Poulsen, A. A., Ziviani, J. M., Johnson, H., & Cuskelly, M. (2008). Loneliness and life satisfaction of boys with developmental coordination disorder: The impact of leisure participation and perceived freedom in leisure. *Human Movement Science, 27*(2), 325–343.

Powers, A., Ressler, K. J., & Bradley, R. G. (2009). The protective role of friendship on the effects of childhood abuse and depression. *Depression and Anxiety, 26*(1), 46–53.

Prakash, K., & Coplan, R. J. (2007). Socioemotional characteristics and school adjustment of socially withdrawn children in India. *International Journal of Behavioral Development, 31*(2), 123–132.

Putallaz, M., Grimes, C. L., Foster, K. J., Kupersmidt, J. B., Coie, J. D., & Dearing, K. (2007). Overt and relational aggression and victimization: Multiple perspectives within the school setting. *Aggression and School Social Dynamics, 45*(5), 523–547.

Reynolds, B. M., & Repetti, R. L. (2008). Contextual variations in negative mood and state self-esteem: What role do peers play? *The Journal of Early Adolescence, 28*(3), 405–427.

Rizzo, T. A. (1988). The relationship between friendship and sociometric judgments of peer acceptance and rejection. *Child Study Journal, 18*(3), 161–191.

Rockach, A. T., Orzeck, T., Moya, M. C., & Exposito, F. (2002). Causes of loneliness in north America and Spain. *European Psychologist, 7*(1), 70–79.

Rokach, A., & Bauer, N. (2004). Age, culture, and loneliness among Czechs and Canadians. *Current Psychology, 23*(1), 3–23.

Rokach, A., Orzeck, T., Moya, M. C., & Exposito, F. (2002). Causes of loneliness in North America and Spain. *European Psychologist, 7*(1), 70–79.

Rose, A. J., & Rudolph, K. D. (2006). Review of sex differences in peer relationship processes: Potential trade-offs for the emotional and behavioral development of girls and boys. *Psychological Bulletin, 132*(1), 98–131.

Rose, A. J., Swenson, L. P., & Robert, C. (2009). Boys' and girls' motivations for refraining from prompting friends to talk about problems. *International Journal of Behavioral Development, 33*(2), 178–184.

Rotenberg, K. J., Boulton, M. J., & Fox, C. L. (2005). Cross-sectional and longitudinal relations among children's trust beliefs, psychological maladjustment and social relationships: Are very high as well as very low trusting children at risk? *Journal of Abnormal Child Psychology, 33*(5), 595–610.

Rotenberg, K. J., MacDonald, K. J., & King, E. V. (2004). The relationship between loneliness and interpersonal trust during middle childhood. *Journal of Genetic Psychology, 165*(3), 233–250.

Rubin, K. H., Bukowski, W., & Parker, J. G. (1998). Peer interactions, relationships, and groups. In N. Eisenberg (Ed.), *Handbook of child psychology* (pp. 619–700). New York: Wiley.

Rubin, K. H., Chen, X., & Hymel, S. (1993). Socioemotional characteristics of aggressive and withdrawn children. *Merrill-Palmer Quarterly, 39*(4), 518–534.

Rubin, K. H., Coplan, R. J., & Bowker, J. C. (2009). Social withdrawal in childhood. *Annual Review of Psychology, 60*, 1–31.

Rubin, K. H., Fredstrom, B., & Bowker, J. (2008). Future Directions in. . .;Friendship in childhood and early adolescence. *Social Development, 17*(4), 1085–1096.

Salmivalli, C., Kauliaine, A., & Lagerspetz, K. (2000). Aggressive and sociometric status among peers: Do gender and type of aggression matter? *Scandinavian Journal of Psychology, 41*(1), 17–24.

Scharf, T., & de Jong Gierveld, J. (2008). Loneliness in urban neighbourhoods: An Anglo-Dutch comparison. *European Journal of Ageing, 5*(2), 103–115.

Schmidt, M., Demulder, E., & Denham, S. (2002). Kindergarten social-emotional competence: Developmental predictors and psychosocial implications. *Early Child Development & Care, 172*(5), 451–462.

Scholte, R., Overbeek, G., ten Brink, G., Rommes, E., de Kemp, R., Goossens, L., et al. (2009). The significance of reciprocal and unilateral friendships for peer victimization in adolescence. *Journal of Youth and Adolescence, 38*(1), 89–100.

Schwartz, D., Gorman, A. H., Dodge, K. A., Pettit, G. S., & Bates, J. E. (2008). Friendships with peers who are low or high in aggression as moderators of the link between peer victimization and declines in academic functioning. *Journal of Abnormal Child Psychology, 36*(5), 719–730.

Seepersad, S., Choi, M. K., & Shin, N. (2008). How does culture influence the degree of romantic loneliness and closeness? *Journal of Psychology, 142*(2), 209–220.

Selfhout, M., Branje, S., & Meeus, W. (2009). Developmental trajectories of perceived friendship intimacy, constructive problem solving, and depression from early to late adolescence. *Journal of Abnormal Child Psychology, 37*(2), 251–264.

Shin, Y. (2007). Peer relationships, social behaviours, academic performance and loneliness in Korean primary school children. *School Psychology International, 28*(2), 220–236.

Storch, E. A., & Masis-Warner, C. (2004). The relationship of peer victimization to social anxiety and loneliness in adolescent females. *Journal of Adolescence, 27*(3), 351–362.

Taylor, M., & Houghton, S. (2008). Difficulties in initiating and sustaining peer friendships: Perspectives on students diagnosed with AD/HD. *British Journal of Special Education, 35*(4), 209–219.

Thomaes, S., Reijntjes, A., de Castro, B. O., & Bushman, B. J. (2009). Reality bites-or does it? Realistic self-views buffer negative mood following social threat. *Psychological Science, 20*(9), 1079–1080.

Tur-Kaspa, H., Margalit, M., & Most, T. (1999). Reciprocal friendship, reciprocal rejection and socio-emotional adjustment: The social experiences of children with learning disorders over a one-year period. *European Journal of Special Needs Education, 14*(1), 37–48.

Uruk, A. C., & Demir, A. (2003). The role of peers and families in predicting the loneliness level of adolescents. *Journal of Psychology, 137*(2), 179–193.

Valdivia, I. A., Schneider, B. H., Chavez, K. L., & Chen, X. (2005). Social withdrawal and maladjustment in a very group-oriented society. *International Journal of Behavioral Development, 29*(3), 219–228.

Vannatta, K., Gartstein, M. A., Zeller, M., & Noll, R. B. (2009). Peer acceptance and social behavior during childhood and adolescence: How important are appearance, athleticism, and academic competence? *International Journal of Behavioral Development, 33*(4), 303–311.

Waldrip, A. M., Malcolm, K. T., & Jensen-Campbell, L. A. (2008). With a little help from your friends: The importance of high-quality friendships on early adolescent adjustment. *Social Development, 17*(4), 832–852.

Wentzel, K. R. (2003). Sociometric status and adjustment in middle school: A longitudinal study. *The Journal of Early Adolescence, 23*(1), 5–28.

Wiener, J. (2004). Do peer relationships foster behavioral adjustment in children with learning disabilities? *Learning Disabilities Quarterly, 27*(1), 21–30.

Wienke Totura, C. M., MacKinnon-Lewis, C., Gesten, E. L., Gadd, R., Divine, K. P., Dunham, S., et al. (2009). Bullying and victimization among boys and girls in middle school: The influence of perceived family and school contexts. *The Journal of Early Adolescence, 29*(4), 571–609.

Woods, S., Done, J., & Kalsi, H. (2009). Peer victimisation and internalising difficulties: The moderating role of friendship quality. *Journal of Adolescence, 32*(2), 293–308.

Xu, Y. Y., & Zhang, Z. X. (2008). Distinguishing proactive and reactive aggression in Chinese children. *Journal of Abnormal Child Psychology, 36*(4), 539–552.

Yang, S., Kim, J., Kim, S., Shin, I., & Yoon, J. (2006). Bullying and victimization behaviours in boys and girls at South Korean primary schools. *Journal of American Academy of Child and Adolescence Psychiatry, 45*(1), 69–77.

Zettergren, P. (2007). Cluster analysis in sociometric research: A pattern-oriented approach to identifying temporally stable peer status groups of girls. *The Journal of Early Adolescence, 27*(1), 90–114.

Chapter 6
Loneliness and Virtual Connections

When we met Dorin, she was a 10-year-old girl living in Boston. If you entered her room in one of the early autumn evenings, you could probably see her doing homework while listening to "noisy" music and, at the same time, sending texts on her cell to a group of friends. Her computer was on and she was also communicating with another group of friends, while searching on a forum for friends and checking if she got any answers to her comments. She was able to move quickly from one activity to another. To her annoyed mother, Dorin stated that her attention was focused all the time on her homework. Yet, she did not want to miss her friends, and these activities (including the music) helped her to concentrate on schoolwork. She complained that her father did not understand that she stayed focused while communicating, and he also limited her use of the cell. Dorin is not different from many children around the world who express their strong motivation to stay continuously in contact with peers, using a rich variety of technology-supported devices.

It has to be clearly stated that this online communication is not separate from the overall youth social interactions. Several young people have become super-communicators who are using a host of technology options for connecting with family and friends (Heim, Brandtzaeg, Kaare, Endestad, & Torgersen, 2007). The worried concerns of many parents, educators, and mental health professionals are focused on the growing involvement of children and youth in communicative technology and its paradoxical connection with their consistent loneliness. Children are connected most of their free time using various means. They talk on their cells, send text messages, write and send photos to social sites, play online group games, and new communication means are developing all the time and attracting children's motivation to participate. These activities reflect their strong urge to stay connected with many people such as close friends, classmates, family members, and individuals that they met on the Internet (and they also call them "friends"). They play games together, share music, and keep a very active online social life. One of the most under-researched aspects of childhood loneliness is the dilemma whether these activities buffer or promote loneliness? Do they enhance social connectedness, provide training in social relatedness, or contribute to growing alienation and social exclusion?

The Internet as a social medium enables communication and prompts interpersonal relationships, extending the boundaries of time and space and freeing individuals from the constraints of geography and the isolation related to poor social skills during face-to-face interactions. Research reported that communicating with others over the Internet, not only helps to maintain close ties with one's family and friends, but also facilitates the formation of close and meaningful new relationships. Information and communication technology has become a central part of the everyday life of children, adolescents, and adults. Their homes are saturated with media. Many young people carry miniaturized, portable media with them wherever they go. Children and adolescents are the primary audience for popular music, TV, movies, video games, and print media (each of these industries produces extensive amount of contents targeted primarily at kids); they typically are among the early adopters of the new generation of cells and the innovative versions of personal computers and are a primary target of much of the content of the communication applications (Roberts, Foehr, & Rideout, 2005). Before discussing the contribution of the communication technology to personal identity and interpersonal links, the prevalence of usages is presented without ignoring the recognition for its quick transformations and development.

Prevalence of Internet's Usages

Among children and adolescents, the Internet has become a fundamental social context for their development. The vast majority of children in the United States and Canada have accessed the Internet (Jones, 2009). The spreading of Internet use is comparable or slightly lower in other developed countries. Many children access the Internet at least once a week from school, home, or libraries; surveys from the past few years indicate that up to one-half of the children spend more than 1 h on the Internet per day (Roberts et al., 2005; Varnhagen, 2007).

Even the youngest children in our society have a substantial amount of experience with various types of electronic media. In a typical day, 83% of children aged 6 months to 6 years use some form of screen media, including 75% who watch television, 32% who watch videos or DVDs, 16% who use a computer, and 11% who play either console or handheld video games. Children between the ages of 4 and 6 years are engaged in screen activities more often than the younger age group (ages 3 years and under). For example, 43% of 4–6-year-olds use a computer several times a week or more, and 24% often play video games (Rideout & Hamel, 2006). These proportions are spreading quickly, and more and younger children are using the Internet.

Adolescents use various types of technology more often than younger children. Over 65% of online American youth are using social networks and have a profile on an online social network site (i.e., MySpace, Facebook) (Lenhart, 2009). Social networks are spaces on the Internet where users can create a personal profile, displaying personal information and enabling others to connect to that profile and to generate personal contents. The users post new and varied information to their profiles and use tools embedded within social networking websites to contact other users and to express their emotional reactions. Social networking sites comprise several different communications tools that have been popular with youth – these include chat rooms, instant messaging, and blogging. They upload pictures and videos on blogs. Communication can occur in real time using chat room and instant messaging capabilities or can be posted for users to read at their leisure as in e-mail and on message boards (Mitchell & Ybarra, 2009). Children in different cultures use different sites and communication devices. For example, inner-city adolescents are more likely to use My Space and suburban adolescents are more likely to use Instant Messengers; moreover, suburban teens are more likely than inner-city teens to be the early adopters of both My Space and Instant Messengers. This urban–suburban difference revealed another dimension of a second digital divide (Zhao, 2009), demonstrating the gaps between different ecologies, but recognizing the common trends of constantly growing proportions of young participants in the Internet culture.

Social network sites are embedded in children's and adolescents' lives in many ways. Most children and youth are using technology to connect with people they already know, to keep up with friends, and to make plans. However, many teens use them to make new friends (Lenhart, 2009). Research (Rideout & Hamel, 2006) reported that adolescents use a wide variety of Internet applications such as instant messaging, bulletin boards, chat rooms, and blogs to connect with their peers and to explore typical adolescent issues such as sexuality, identity, and partner selection. For many families, media-use has become part of the fabric of daily life, revealing a great deal of variation, from children who spend an extraordinary amount of their time with that medium to those who spend no time at all. Social networking sites allow teenagers to explore their identities, make new friends and continue to develop long-standing relationships, explore their sexuality, voice their opinions, and be creative – all normal aspects of adolescent development.

Similar reports were provided in different cultures. For example, in Taiwan, junior and senior high school students' experiences in online relationships revealed a similar situation (Chou & Peng, 2007). About 46% of students used the Internet not only to interact with friends known in real life, but also to form new relationships. Students reported that, on average, their first experience with making online relationships was when they were about 12–13 years old (about grades 7–8). They used a variety of Internet applications such as Internet communication software (i.e., MSN, Yahoo Messenger, ICQ) (70.6%), online games (66.2%), chat rooms (53.2%), e-mail (37.0%), websites for making friends (30.4%), and websites for trading goods (8.3%). Students spent an average of 2.38 h (143 min) per day on the Internet after school, using more than half of it for communicating online with their friends. In different countries net-friends were a part of middle-school students' social life, and the Internet became an easy way to form and maintain companionship (Chou & Peng, 2007). Thus, the mall, the school yard, or the neighborhoods' play grounds were no longer perceived as the obvious meeting point, and the Internet environment gained importance in the life of the young generation. In fact, teenagers are growing up in a media-saturated society in which the Internet is simply another environment akin to home and school, with the MySpace site as analogous to their favorite store at the mall where they hang out (Mitchell & Ybarra, 2009).

Among youth who use MySpace, Facebook, or other social network sites, 41% reported that they send messages to friends every day via those sites. More than one in four (28%) of online teens had blogs (mostly girls) (Lenhart & Madden, 2007). Youngsters participated in conversations, and nearly half (47%) of online teens posted photos where others could see them, and 89% of those teens who posted photos said that people commented on the images at least "some of the time." Adolescents who posted videos reported that nearly three quarters (72%) of the video posters received comments on their videos, demonstrating that these contents were created not only for self-satisfaction, but also to initiate audience's reactions and communication with others (Lenhart & Madden, 2007). Recently the communicative behavior of a teenager was described in order to illustrate its uniqueness (Deresiewicz, 2009). She sent 3,000 text messages during 1 month. It means that she sent 100 messages a day, or about one every 10 waking minutes, morning, noon, and night, weekdays and weekends, class time, lunch time, and homework time. So on average, she was never alone. Can a similar overflow of unlimited connectivity for many adolescents mean the end of solitude for them?

In conclusion, the new technology has increased the overall frequency of adolescents' social interaction with others. In addition, many of these super-communicator children and adolescents have kept on the more traditional face-to-face meetings. Nearly two-thirds (63%) of the teens now have a cell phone, and for teens who have them, they are the premier communication method for talking and sending texts with friends. Among teens with cell phones, 55% say they use them to talk with friends every day. Teens are generally also intense users of instant messaging technology, and use it in addition to other online spaces and tools to play with and manage their online identities and social connections. Often they are engaged in several media activities simultaneously, demonstrating superb abilities for multifunction (Roberts et al., 2005). Several youngsters develop compulsive Internet behaviors. Since one of the major motives driving individuals' Internet use is to relieve psychosocial problems (i.e., loneliness), individuals who are lonely or do not have good social skills are at a greater risk for developing strong compulsive Internet-use behaviors resulting in negative life outcomes (i.e., harming other significant activities such as work, school, or significant relationships) instead of relieving their original problems (Kim, LaRose, & Peng, 2009). Such negative outcomes may isolate individuals from social activities and lead them into increased loneliness. However, since this is a new emerging culture, it requires a different new conceptualization of the meaning of social relations, as well as different understanding of effective attention and cognitive processing, treating distractions and information processing differently (Fox, Rosen, & Crawford, 2009).

It seems that children and adolescents are constantly and endlessly connecting with others. The outsiders, who eavesdrop to their conversations and/or read their online messages, will recognize three major themes in their activities:

(1) Staying connected;
(2) Disclosing/sharing personal contents; and
(3) Promoting and examining the quality of their friendship relations.

The goals of the communication were to fulfill individuals' interpersonal needs for relatedness. Need fulfillment and goal-directed communication behavior were central premises of usages and gratifications. Communicating with other people was one of the most important uses of the Internet (Pornsakulvanich, Haridakis, & Rubin, 2008). People communicated to satisfy various psychological needs for forming, maintaining, and developing interpersonal connections. Children and adolescents wished to belong, to be part of a desired group, to have relationships with others, and to be loved by others (Baumeister & Leary, 1995). They communicated to fulfill their needs for social inclusion, acceptance, affection, and control. These needs produced different communication motives, which in turn interacted with cultural impacts and were expressed through varied communication choices, strategies, and behaviors. For example, the examination of the motives for the employing of social network sites revealed the wide range of personal characteristics and individual differences (Barker, 2009). Adolescents with a positive self-esteem not only utilized the sites to communicate with peer group members, but also had additional goals such as entertainment and passing time. Those who reported negative self-esteem described a more instrumental interest in the use of the sites for social compensation, and for seeking the companionship that they wished for and could not find. Gender differences were also reported and males were more likely to seek social compensation and social identification as well as to find out about their identity within the "social" world (Barker, 2009). Blogs are an example of online communication choices that revealed the complexity of this developing culture and the wide range of personal needs and individual differences.

Blogs

Blogs represent a new medium for computer-mediated communication and offer insight into the ways in which adolescents communicate and present themselves online, especially in terms of self-expression and peer-group relationships. The construction of their developing identity is affected by these activities. "Blog" is an abbreviated version of "web-log," which is a term used to describe web sites that maintain ongoing information. A blog is fundamentally a continuously updated web page, with entries ("posts") and often many authors contribute to the blog (Wilkins, 2008). A personal blog is frequently updated, featuring diary-type commentary and links to articles on other web sites. Blogs are made publicly accessible on the web, and they have the following distinctive technological features (Huffaker & Calvert, 2005):

(1) Ease-of-use, as users do not need to know web programming languages;
(2) Ways to archive information and knowledge;
(3) Expectations for an audience to comment or provide feedback;
(4) Links to other "bloggers" that enable them to form online communities.

Among the different types of blogs, personal diary-type records have the most user groups in many countries. This personal record reflects the inner world of a blogger through self-disclosure, a process by which an individual shares his or her feelings, thoughts, experiences, or information with others. Usually children and adolescents disclose their personal information, preferences, and relatedness as expressions of trust, and usually within the process of developing emotional closeness and intimate relations. Self-disclosure is a process whereby an individual gains acquaintance, obtains net-friends, or even develops intimate relationships with others. Therefore, self-disclosure may help bloggers not only to maintain existing personal relations, but also to extend their social networks, both of which are considered important to promote their wellbeing. Bloggers are characterized as individuals who are open to new experience, tend to discuss details of their personal lives, and are likely to use other forums for online social interactions in addition to the blog (Guadagno, Okdie, & Eno, 2008). The use of blogs may support the children's and adolescents' struggle for structuring their self-identity. Since no technical expertise is needed to create or maintain blogs, it is accessible even to children who may archive photos and use different existing signs, symbols, and animation. In addition, the ability to archive the records creates a way to scaffold on previous personal impressions and expressions; thus, the constructing identity can be a continual process for children and adolescents, and one to which they can refer.

Finally, since blog software offers a link to other bloggers, as well as receiving feedback of others, this can foster a sense of peer-group relationships and social support within a virtual community, another important aspect for the children's identity formation. The following research example demonstrates the impact of using blogs. Teenage girls reported that they built and maintained their friendships relations by sharing their thoughts, disclosing freely their frustrations, happiness, disappointments, and occasional despair with friends via blogging (Bortee, 2005). In another study, a follow-up of bloggers who were surveyed to examine their psychosocial development over time, the bloggers' social integration, reliable alliance, and friendship satisfaction were all significantly increased in comparison to non-bloggers, suggesting that blogging had beneficial effects on wellbeing, specifically in terms of perceived social support (Baker & Moore, 2008). The results of a recent study (Ko & Kuo, 2009) that consisted of a large sample (596 bloggers ages 16–22) further confirmed these earlier results, revealing that the self-disclosure of bloggers significantly and directly affected a blogger's perception of social integration, and promoted the bloggers' subjective wellbeing, pleasure perception, positive emotions, and higher life satisfaction (Diener, Lucas, & Oishi, 2002). In conclusion, bloggers shared their inner thoughts of their moods/feelings with others through writing, gained greater social support, and improved their social integration. Further analyzing of the blogging contents revealed that descriptions of "moods/feelings expression" appeared most frequently. Ninety three percent of the participants mentioned that they expressed their feelings of pressure in their blogs, indicating that they were able to share their inhibitions and depression with others through their writing. When youngsters shared their inner thoughts and their moods with others, they gained greater social support and improved their social bonding with their group. Most of the bloggings' audiences came from their classmates and friends in real life (classmates 88.76%, friends 77.68%), indicating that journal bloggers' self-disclosure may have helped them improve existing relations in real life. Thus, self-disclosure through blogging may have served as the core of building intimate relationships with existing friends, resulting in improved interpersonal communication and overall quality of life (Ko & Kuo, 2009).

It has to be clearly stated that blogging did not exchange face-to-face relations. Studies indicated, in contrast to earlier reservations, that blogging did not diminish or reduce substantial relations in real life. On the contrary, it provided help, supported the bloggers' existing relations through improved social bonding, and overall enhanced their wellbeing. In addition, the audiences interacting with bloggers were not only existing friends. Lurking strangers (32.55%) and online friends (38.76%) also sent supporting comments, suggesting that self-disclosure behavior could help individuals to expand their social networks. Blogs may therefore become a viable way of seeking emotional support from others, strengthening self-identity, the sense of belonging, and improving intimacy and connection with others. By sharing experiences, thoughts, and moods through self-disclosure, the heightened social integration and bonding predicted subjective wellbeing. Thus, as the writing of a blog was merged into the user's daily life, it provided extension of substantial relations as well as supporting relations with others, and enabling emotional expression (Ko & Kuo, 2009). However, parents and educators have to be aware of the existing risks of communicating with strangers, and help children develop protecting measures and codes of behavior. The impact of blogging and children's loneliness was not the focus of research, but the potential impact of blogging have to be considered in intervention planning, as will be discussed in Chapter 8. Games' playing and cell usages provided additional clarifications to the roles of this changing culture in shifting social relations and identity development by opening new opportunities for satisfactory collaborations.

Playing Games Is a Social Activity

Playing games has been widely depicted as the most preferred computer activity reported by children in different cultures and with different abilities and socialization success. Almost all children play computer games from a very early age, and playing games has become a universal interpersonal activity and a way of socializing. Only few children reported that they didn't play games. Many children and adolescents played games with others at least some of the time, and gaming as a social activity was among the key components of their overall social experiences.

They mostly played games with friends and people they knew. Still, sometimes they played with individuals that they met online regularly, or only a few times. They played games in a wide variety of ways, including with others in person (several children played together on the same computer), with others online (kids they knew and kids that they had never met offline), and by themselves, comparing their achievements with others and with their earlier scores. These games challenged their skills, stimulated curiosity, and contained fantasy. Even very young children gradually developed fluent gaming skills through continuous playing, and developing successful strategies to overcome difficulties, applying skills such as planning, learning to predict sequences, and focusing their concentration on improving their scores. It was exciting and provoking to follow even children with attention deficit disorders who had pronounced and diagnosed difficulties in concentrating on their homework, but by using creative strategies when they were playing computer games they were able to compensate tendencies for distraction and their short attention span. In the early days of personal computers' entrance to homes and schools, we pointed out that playing computer games was a serious subject that could be useful for achieving the following two major goals: to enrich the leisure activities especially of children with difficulties and to promote effective problem-solving instruction through highly motivating activities (Margalit, 1990). Almost 20 years later, the gaming world has passed many transformations and developments, yet the debates related to the games' advantages and risks continue to engage parents and educators, and have remained the center of research dilemmas.

The growing body of research into the experience and effects of video games indicated that the enjoyment of playing was a complex, dynamic, and multifaceted phenomenon (Klimmt, Rizzo, Vorderer, Koch, & Fischer, 2009). The feelings of suspense were the major motivational component, and they contributed to video game enjoyment. Players' uncertainty about their success or failure in resolving the games' tasks while they were confronted with several challenges (i.e., an attacking monster, or a sinking transport ship), affected their persistent activities, and shaped their imagination, excitement, effort, and enjoyment. Because players pursued short-term and long-term life goals, they experienced high relevance of such necessities to act and to struggle, as these general goals were symbolically related to the goals in these games (i.e., surviving, competing, winning, or controlling challenges).

The connections between violent computer games and children's aggressive feelings and behavior were widely examined (for a detailed survey see Barlett, Anderson, & Swing, 2009), and they are beyond the goals of this chapter. Yet, adolescents and children experienced differently the same games when they were played alone or with others (a multiplayer game in a collaborative social context), and the difference was especially noted in violent and excitation provoking games. When compared with a solo play, the collaborative violent games led to a significant decrease in the personal arousal while leading to a slight increase for playing in non-violent tasks. Even when the physiological arousal was measured and compared (and not provided by self-report) in a multiplayer online gaming, the social contexts modified and buffered the effects of violent game tasks on personal arousal (Lim & Lee, 2009). Thus, it can be concluded that social contexts of game playing can shape the psychological experiences in multiplayer online games. In addition, the global consideration and evaluation of the gaming activity is meaningless if it will not reflect the abilities to provide different experiences to different children, answering to different personal motivations and needs, reflecting the rich variety of the game characteristics such as the different topics of the games, the different modes of playing (solo or a multiplayer game), the different styles of playing (prolonged periods or short periods when the child enters the game, performs a move, and at the same time continues doing other activities), speeded or not, etc.

For example, the browser games are a specific type of digital games that players can typically use free of charge. Large communities of players can interact in such browser games; for instance, they can form alliances or participate in mass war campaigns, or develop a city. The time structure of playing browser games differs from other types of games because players typically log on the game several times a day, make some decisions (i.e., initialize the production of new military units, reallocate economic resources) that produce results only after some time has passed, then leave the game world, planning to return later for the next brief visit. Browser gaming is thus rather an "easy-in, easy-out" type of game play. Youngsters participated in a survey and reported that multiplayer games were enjoyed by them primarily because of the social relationships involved in game play and the specific time and flexibility function. The gaming was considered by them as a stage for making friends, meeting other children, and elaborating social relationships through joint-game characteristics (Klimmt, Schmid, & Orthmann, 2009).

A recent study (Frostling-Henningsson, 2009), reported that gaming is foremost motivated by social reasons providing the gamers with a possibility of cooperation and communication. The participants emphasized in their interviews that the social aspects of playing the online game were the most important factor in playing. They also declared that the online gaming provided them with the opportunities to do things and try out behaviors that would be impossible to do or try in real life. It gave them more excitement and experiences than could be provided in real life. Playing games was also considered as a way of developing interpersonal relationships: pursuing old connections and initiating completely new ones. During interviews, youngsters explained that through gaming, they learned how to cooperate with others, to understand each other, and to develop teamwork. Nevertheless, adults need to be sensitized to the repeated findings that several children and adolescents often communicate with complete strangers. About one-third of teen gamers aged 15–17 reported that they had played with people they had met online, and even 22% of younger gamers aged 12–14 reported that they had played with complete strangers (Lenhart et al., 2008). The cultural comparisons of the gaming behavior of American adolescents with Spanish adolescents (Hart et al., 2009) demonstrated similarities in playing patterns between the groups, with gender differences. Boys played video games far more than girls. In addition, no relations were documented between the extent of game playing and reports of school's achievements, social activities, or distress in areas of daily functioning.

In summary, playing video games was embedded within the life experiences of many youngsters, enabling new experiences of social interactions and collaboration, and the social interactions enhanced their enjoyment. About 75% of youngsters played games with others, but occasionally they also played by themselves. These networking possibilities may have increased the distressed experience of social isolation among lonely children who played computer games mostly alone, knowing that their peers played with friends. The relations between game playing and self-esteem were inconsistent. For several children playing games was associated with a lower behavioral self-concept and lower self-esteem (Jackson et al., 2009), but not for others. It was also not clear whether video game playing had a detrimental impact on self-concept perceptions, or whether children with a lower self-concept played more games as a compensation. Yet, there were clear relations between the following factors: game playing, self–perceptions, and social relations. The common motivation and excitement of children to participate in gaming, regardless of their levels of self-concept and social competence may trigger considerations of future possibilities to use the principles of the gaming construct (Gentile & Gentile, 2008) for enhancing social connectivity and for reducing loneliness.

Special attention has to be focused on those individuals who often feel lonely – and their loneliness is more pronounced on the background of a society that is connecting and interacting most of their time, even during video games. These trends challenge future intervention directions to expand the social-skills learning to the growing virtual possibilities for promoting social relations. The connectivity by cells furthers these social exclusion experiences, adding identity formation aspects.

Cell Phone Identity

The cell phone has become an essential part of the way of life among youngsters in many countries, as well as a way of forming and expressing their identity, and of distinguishing themselves from others. Children and adolescents express themselves with and through their cell phones, caring about its shape and color, and carrying it in smart bags. It has become a symbol of identity that supports independence in their communications, both within and outside the home. An extensive survey that was performed in Spain demonstrated the similarities in the usages of cells in different cultures (Sanchez-Martinez & Otero, 2009). This study included 1,328 adolescents aged 13–20 years in nine secondary schools of the Community of Madrid that were followed during the period January to April 2007. Almost all children (96.5%) had their own cell phone (80.5% had one, and 15.9% had two or more). Some 54.8% took it to school and 46.1% kept it on during class; 41.7% used it intensively. They expressed their identity by the ring-tone, special toys connected to the cell, and color as well as design preferences. Most boys used the new technologies to explore different possibilities and to play games, while girls used them mostly for communication. Similar patterns were reported in additional countries. For example, results from 595 adolescents in Korea (Ha, Chin, Park, Ryu, & Yu, 2008) showed that the youngsters had a tendency to identify themselves with their cellular phones. They were strongly attached to their cells, perhaps because it supported their developing identities and independence, as well as providing them with an effective communication method. Frequent changing of ring-tones and unnecessary (in the adults' eyes) use of a cellular phone were signs of an individual's psychological identification with their phone and an effort to present their distinctiveness. Among usage patterns, the most popular activities were sending and receiving text messages. Adolescents believed that this type of communication enabled them to make broader and deeper friendship connections and they felt more comfortable to connect by cells than through face-to-face interactions.

Nowadays, if you sit on a bus, in New York or in Tel Aviv, or in many other public places, you may listen (sometimes unwillingly) to many private conversations of individuals of all ages. Several conversations deal with private issues in public places, ignoring the presence of the passers by audience. Many times you may listen unintentionally to "Hi – By" short conversations (kids inquiring what the other kids are doing, saying or writing where they are, and then finishing the conversation). These conversations seem to reflect the need to stay updated and connected with your network peers or family members most of the time. In this culture, children and adolescents who don't participate in the ongoing connections' maintenance may feel alienation and excluded. A 17-year-old boy who came to visit my office at Tel Aviv University with his parents asked to check his messages on my computer. Very quickly he went through many messages, reading the short notes very superficially, and informing me that if many kids would not contact him all the time (!) he "would feel neglected, miserable, ignored, and lonely." After he left, I could not stop thinking that the extended social skills in virtual environments of many kids are probably not a source of extended distress to lonely children.

Online Communication and Loneliness

Technology-supported communication is currently an important part of the youth culture and children are connected to other children using different means. However, relations between social connections and personal loneliness remain a puzzle. Research provided inconsistent answers to the question whether the Internet is detrimental to one's psychological health and promotes loneliness, or whether, it might enhance one's wellbeing by extending and enriching different new opportunities for less demanding and more available social connections. In the early developmental stages of the Internet, researchers proposed that extensive use of the Internet had negative effects on individuals, and a risk for increased loneliness (Kraut et al., 1998). However, after 3 years of follow-up, the same researchers stated that almost all of the previously reported negative effects had dissipated (Kraut et al., 2002). Instead, higher levels of Internet usages were positively correlated with measures of social involvement and psychological wellbeing. More recent studies confirmed that the Internet usages contributed positively to psychological wellbeing (Whitty & McLaughlin, 2007). A similarity between socialization online and offline was also documented, and similar communication patterns were identified between Internet interactions and face-to-face contacts. A similar style was employed for the telephone and cells' connections (Baym, Zhang, & Lin, 2004). In an attempt to examine the relations between the communication usages and loneliness, it was reported that loneliness was not related to the total time spent online, nor to the time spent on e-mail messages (Subrahmanyam & Lin, 2007). Likewise, no relations were found between instant-messaging use and self-concept perceptions, and in addition, the amount of time spent online was not related to measures of loneliness, social anxiety, depression, or daily-life satisfaction (Gross, 2004). The conclusions from these studies call for an alternative and more differential approach to the understanding of the impact of this online culture.

A differential approach was proposed to the conceptualization, and the impacts of different activities (i.e., e-mailing, chatting, messaging, playing games, and surfing) were compared (Punamaki, Wallenius, Holtto, Nygard, & Rimpela, 2009). The results of the study pointed attention to the diverse results. For example, boys used technologies mostly for entertainment and excitement, and girls typically for communication. Entertainment usage of Internet was associated in this study with poor peer and parental relations. Intensive Internet surfing was related with poor maternal relations, especially evident in daughter–mother communication. Intensive game playing was associated with poor friendship quality among girls and younger children, and intensive Internet surfing with high loneliness among girls. It should be noted that the results could be treated like pieces of a puzzle, which overall demonstrated that the online communication and gaming had individualized meaning adapted to personal characteristics and needs. These differential results did not confirm the negative impacts of various online activities. They were considered an expression of compensatory dynamics of the Internet activities. The new technology options provided excitement and feeling of belonging to lonely and rejected children who may have sought for alternatives to their prolonged disappointments and frustrations. Yet, the intensive escape to online entertainment opportunities may be considered a developmental risk if it will replace their future commitment to establish friendship relations or enhance their alienation from their family and peer relations. Thus, instead of struggling with face-to-face relations' formation difficulties with friends and family, they will invest their time and involvements in virtual environments of game playing and surfing.

The inconsistent results regarding the impact of the Internet activities emerged from two major sources: children's interpersonal profiles and the varied technological usages. For example, in one of the studies, increased Internet use and greater video-game playing and Internet communication were associated with decreased psychological wellbeing (Jackson et al., 2008). In another study (Gross, Juvonen, & Gable, 2002) adolescents who communicated primarily with school friends using instant messaging, reported their closeness to their partners and increased wellbeing. In contrast, adolescents who reported feeling socially isolated, communicated with more people that they did not know well. The usages of instant messages to perform relational maintenance functions revealed a rich variability in using different strategies to maintain different types of social connections with different partners (good friends, acquaintances, and family members), promoting different types of relationships. Many participants supported the communication by using emotional signs, and they felt more freedom to express emotions using these symbols than face-to-face communication. Overall, online communicating was effective in maintaining and supporting interpersonal connections for individuals who had social connections, supporting closeness to partners who were located in physically distant locations (Ramirez & Broneck, 2009). Studies of children and adults in different cultures also provided inconsistent results. For example, in Turkey, Internet usage did not have a significant connection with loneliness (Eldeleklioglu, 2008). These conclusions request more in-depth examination of the group of children who reported more loneliness following their Internet involvement.

A detailed study of the group of depressive and lonely children aged 10–17 extended the understanding of the connections between online activities and negative affect. These children who reported significant depressive symptoms spent more time on the Internet and used it more often for social communications than those reporting fewer or no depressive symptoms (Ybarra, Alexander, & Mitchell, 2005). These children reported that they established close personal relationships with individuals they had met on the Internet more often than did children who were not as troubled (Wolak, Mitchell, & Finkelhor, 2003). It is not clear whether children, who use e-communication, especially with people that they don't know well, experience more loneliness following the connections. These children may be initially lonelier and use the e-connections to compensate their social isolation. However, even if these lonely youngsters, who don't have satisfactory networks, used the Internet connections as a substitute, these relations did not satisfy their connections' needs. An additional issue that should alert adults is the desperate needs of these lonely children who, instead of remaining socially isolated and lonely, reach out to online friends in an attempt to change their social distress. Indeed there are many risks in these connections, yet their advantages have to be recognized as well. Through these e-communications children found others who convey empathic concern, focused conversation on emotional disclosure, and prompted personal narratives. As a result, online communication could be expected to provide them with an incomparable opportunity to gain insight into their difficulties in addition to emotional support. However, studies that documented the relations between loneliness and usages of Internet for communication did not disclose its effectiveness (Ceyhan & Ceyhan, 2008), and it was impossible to determine whether loneliness was a symptom of excessive Internet use, or whether heavy Internet use was a symptom of loneliness. Since the loneliness experience was persistent regardless of the expected beneficial impact of self-disclosure through e-communication, a more differential exploration has to be adopted.

It is not fully clear what lonely individuals prefer with regard to social connections. Examinations revealed that many lonely individuals preferred online social interactions to face-to-face interactions. They reported that online interactions were less threatening and more rewarding for them than participating in actual meetings (Caplan, 2003, 2005; Morahan-Martin & Schumacher, 2003). They valued their relationship with online partners, and declared that they could turn to virtual friends in times of need (Subrahmanyam & Lin, 2007). Those participants, who reported receiving less support from their parents, were more likely to become good friends with an online acquaintance. Most online relationships of adolescents remained in the online realm. The majority of these adolescents had not met their online partners in person, and also did not wish to meet with them. Only a few youngsters reported that they had become good friends with an online acquaintance, and that they probably would approach these acquaintances in an emergency.

An additional dilemma that troubled the researchers was related to the quality of the online friendships. If the Internet relations with people you met only online could be judged as more superficial, this answer provided a solution to the persistent loneliness regardless online networks. Studies did not confirm this assumption. These relations were valued and considered an important source of social support. In our Internet studies mothers, for example, clearly stated that they shared with their online friends contents that they did not communicate to face-to-face friends, since they were confident that "only the online friends who were mothers facing similar challenges could truly understand them" (Margalit & Raskind, 2009).

The fact that a small number of the children reported meeting their online acquaintances in person and speaking with them on the telephone revealed the value of these connections to several children. Yet, this finding focused further attention on the vulnerability of lonely children and adolescents to dangers of meeting with strangers. It also portrayed the vital needs of these individuals for social connections, and their consideration of the online connections as a valued option. These online relations can be treated as different connections. Yet, maybe instead of treating the Internet communication as a separate entity in children's life, trying to explore its' unique impact, and to evaluate its value as deep or superficial, an alternative approach can be proposed. The Internet has to be treated as "a new cultural devise" that children use to achieve the same social and cultural goals' within their wide range of social activities, revealing their abilities and difficulties (Matei & Ball-Rokeach, 2001). Thus, research questions such as "what lonely children did differently online than their classmates" have to be explored, since the quality and range of activities may propose directions to develop help in the children's struggle with the continuous social isolation (Whitty & McLaughlin, 2007). Several activities were identified. Those who scored higher on loneliness used the Internet not only for communication, but more often for entertainment and also to obtain information about the entertainment world. It seems that the Internet represented a safe, low-risk social environment for lonely individuals, and an escape from the anxiety provoking outside world.

Studies focused on the outcomes and the understanding how lonely individuals felt following online communication. In order to clarify the dilemma if the communication online promoted loneliness or if the lonely individuals who communicate online felt better afterward, an experimental study was performed. The study explored the loneliness levels of individuals after participating in an online chatting. The results confirmed that the loneliness levels increased after online chatting, and individuals chatting online experienced higher levels of loneliness than those chatting face to face. A differential impact was also demonstrated. The computer-mediated communication continued and even increased the loneliness of the group of individuals with initial high levels of loneliness. In the second group of individuals whose loneliness levels were low, both comparisons did not reveal significant differences (between online/face-to-face communication, and between before/after communication) (Hu, 2009). The results of this study showed that the e-communication did not provide a satisfactory solution to the communicating needs of lonely individuals, and in fact even provoked the users' frustrations and resulted in increased loneliness. However, these results have to be treated with caution, since they examined only a single and unique method of communicating – online chatting that requires special skills such as quick responding.

The deficient social skills of lonely individuals probably affected their participation in the chatting. There is a need to compare different characteristics of different communication approaches that may compensate for the difficulties of lonely individuals. In different types of online communication, such as e-mail or blogs, individuals have more time to deliberate, construct, and revise their messages before sending them. For lonely individuals it seems easier to build a more positive image through "selective self-presentation" that enables them to control their emotions and to include more positive, socially oriented information. Overall, the online connections of lonely individuals have distinctive characteristics, and they will be further discussed in context of coping and emerging options for social support and intervention. In addition, lonely youngsters who wish to participate in their youth culture are not pleased with the e-mail alternatives, since most youngsters use the online chatting options, emphasizing the needs for intervention planning to promote e-communication literacy of lonely youngsters guided by the current and changing youth culture. An additional consideration is proposed by the focus on the characteristics and provisions proposed by virtual friendship.

Virtual friends are currently an inseparable and integral part of children's and adolescents' social lives; they use a variety of applications and spend relatively large amounts of time online communicating with them on a daily basis. Generally children's attitudes toward their virtual friends were positive (Chou & Peng, 2007). They appreciated the benefits emerging from these relations, such as increased chances of self-exposure and self-promotion, escape from pressures (homework, parental, school, etc.), more chances to experiment with their "ideal self," more chances to fulfill their imaginations, and the belief that such relationships were fun and convenient. Consistently, research reported that lonely children and adolescents reported communicating with children that they met on the Internet and considered them as best friends. Yet, regardless of the increased social connections, they continued to report their loneliness.

Differentiated conceptualizations proposed that the Internet primarily benefited children and adults with better social competence that could develop satisfactory social relations in the same way online or offline, confirming the "rich-get-richer" assumption (Vergeer & Pelzer, 2009). Accordingly, children who had social difficulties, and who often experienced the loneliness distress, were at a greater risk to become lonelier. The online relations may propose an alternative solution to their social needs and at the same time an opportunity to experiment and enhance their deficient social competence. Indeed children differ in their social and psychological characteristics, which may affect how they use media to fulfill their psychological needs, and the resulting impacts. For example, those individuals who have difficulties in face-to-face interaction (i.e., communication avoidance) may communicate better in computer settings than in face-to-face settings. There is a need to explore the differential impact of online activities not only as related to the varied characteristics of the Internet activities, but also as a function of personality characteristics and unique needs of the individuals.

The relations between adolescents' friendship formation and their individual differences including personality characteristics, such as introversion/extraversion, were explored (Peter, Valkenburg, & Schouten, 2005). Introversion has been defined as an individual's tendency to prefer his/her own company to large social events and quiet reflection to social interaction. Extraversion captures the person's inclination to seek company and social interaction (Hamburger & Ben-Artzi, 2000). Both groups developed online friendship, yet the processes and motives were different, revealing their different characteristics. Extraverted adolescents tended to communicate online more frequently, to share personal contents and this, in turn, facilitated the formation of their wide range of online friendships. Introverted adolescents were more strongly motivated to communicate online in order to compensate for their deficient social skills and to make friends. Among introverted adolescents, a stronger motive for social compensation was expressed and resulted in more frequent online communication and online self-disclosure. This model proposed that the antecedents of online friendship formation were complex, and different personal motives for online communication reflected children's and adolescents' personality differences, leading to the friendship formation (Peter et al., 2005). The relations between loneliness and the number of virtual friends revealed that participants who have a large number of online friends and also have low self-evaluations of their physical attractiveness, reported a lower level of loneliness through Internet-based interpersonal relationships (Ando & Sakamoto, 2008). Thus, a differential approach to the understanding of relations between personal characteristics and online connections requests an in-depth awareness to additional interacting processes. The fulfillment of several basic needs such as the need for self-disclosure and for social support provided further clarification of the varied relations between children's loneliness and online communication.

Self-Disclosure

A large body of experimental and anecdotal evidence suggested that computer-mediated communication and general Internet-based behavior could be characterized as advancing high levels of self-disclosure (Joinson, 2007). Self-disclosure has been considered a major component in the processes of relationship formation and maintenance and often exists between intimate friends and relatives. Self-disclosure was defined as the act of revealing and sharing personal information to another person (including thoughts, feelings, and experiences) (Derlega, Metts, & Sandra,

1993; Swenson & Rose, 2009). The ability to disclose personal contents provides the individual with an emotional relief from the need to keep secrets, as well as with the expectation for empathy and supportive understanding by the partner to the disclosure.

The Internet enables a different type of self-disclosure, not with friends, but with strangers who may keep anonymity, yet are expected to provide understanding and support. Individuals tend to share more openly private and personal contents during online communication, and adolescents write to social sites and describe private contents that they may be hesitant to disclose even to best friends. In some ways this behavior is similar to the behavior patterns of individuals who share intimate contents with strangers that they meet on a train, expecting never to see them again. Online relationship and self-disclosure promote closeness due to the interaction between anonymity (i.e., reduced public self-awareness) and heightened private self-awareness (the individual is often working alone from private spaces). During the message writing, the reduced social cues may be considered an advantage for individuals who tend to avoid face-to-face interactions. Several participants remarked that writing in a forum was for them similar to talking openly to themselves, and yet they also received support and validation that their experience or distress was experienced by others who understood them. Participants, who used online communication for self-fulfillment and disclosed personal information to others, afterward felt closer to their online partners and felt satisfied with their relations. In addition, the communication partners often used similar self-disclosure and expressed appreciation and emotional support more than the participants' face-to face partners (Tidwell & Walther, 2002).

In some ways, online communication functions similarly to expressive writing that was considered as a beneficial therapeutic approach for providing emotional relief (Radcliffe, Lumley, Kendall, Stevenson, & Beltran, 2007). The expressive writing paradigm (Pennebaker & Beall, 1986) encouraged participants to write uninhibitedly about an emotional topic. The existence of a possible audience enhanced the positive impact of this emotional writing (Joinson, 2001). In line with the research on expressive writing, the very act of writing out narratives of one's thoughts and feelings to an audience, i.e. an online support group, may promote positive reappraisals of the emotional distress and alleviate loneliness (Caplan & Turner, 2007).

In conclusion, meaningful relationships can be formed online, because of, and not despite of, its communication limitations. In this medium, people often reveal themselves far more intimately than they would be inclined to do without the intermediation of screens and pseudonyms (Joinson, 2007). Their self-disclosure has supplementary beneficial impacts due to additional major segments – the writing of personal narratives and the expectations of supportive, anonymous, yet paradoxically, very friendly audience. It can be concluded that personal dispositions, communication motivation, and self-disclosure predict communication satisfaction. They were able to express their "true selves" on Internet rather than in face-to-face interaction settings and were more likely to form close relationships with individuals that they had met on the Internet (Bargh, McKenna, & Fitzsimons, 2002). The fact that social networking sites such as YouTube and Facebook are the two most visited sites on the Internet pointed attention to their importance. Generally, online communication provides social satisfaction to lonely children and adolescents. However, a special group of lonely individuals who suffered from social and communication deficits, such as communication avoidance and loneliness, expressed their dissatisfaction with their online relationships and continued loneliness (Pornsakulvanich et al., 2008). This group demonstrated the need to keep a close awareness of the variability in human needs for social connections and intervention. The online communication for these individuals did not provide the expected relief. They need a planned intervention that will provide meaningful and sensitive answers to their unique needs for relationship closeness and network relations, and their reluctance from immersing into closeness. The mere presentation of options for online communication will not provide meaningful answers to the varied loneliness needs and self-identity struggles.

Identity, Pretence, and Social Competence Online

The Internet can offer adolescents many opportunities to experiment with their identities (Stern, 2004; Subrahmanyam, Smahel, & Greenfield, 2006). Several characteristics of online communication such as the reduced auditory and visual cues stimulate online-identity experimentations. These reduced cues may encourage adolescents to emphasize, change, or conceal certain features of their self. The Internet communication often happens in online social communities that are separate from those in real life. Such communities, in which social repercussions for offline life were reduced, may have encouraged identity experiments (Turkle, 1995). Individual differences were noted in the reactions for reduced cues as enhancing dyadic relations and/or belonging to a group in which anonymity could improve collaboration performance as a function of shared social identity (Tanis & Postmes, 2008). However, comparisons between identity presentations on different social sites indicated that the online world was not monolithic, and online self-presentations varied according to the nature and characteristics of the settings (Zhao, Grasmucka, & Martin, 2008). In order to exemplify how children present their identities and distress, a research on children with learning and behavior difficulties will be described.

The identity presentation of children with special needs online provided an in-depth understanding of youngsters who were at increased risk for developing loneliness due to their academic deficiencies. In order to "listen" to the authentic voices of these children (Raskind, Margalit, & Higgins, 2006) and to understand how these children figured out their academic and social difficulties, e-mail narratives of children who communicated on a public website designed for children with learning and attention problems were examined. Children with learning disabilities are the largest group of children with special needs. In every class there are, on average, 2–3 children with learning and attention difficulties. Their academic needs are widely and internationally recognized. The children considered the website as a safe environment that enabled them to share private aspects of their identity and reveal freely their thoughts, feelings, and attitudes toward life with such difficulties. The study consisted of 164 children (108 girls and 56 boys), with a wide age range (9–18) who wrote 4,903 letters to the social site during 3 years. The analyses of the messages revealed themes that reflected self-perceptions and identity explorations.

The children presented their identity by providing information about their age (i.e., "I'm 10"); their gender and clinical definition (i.e., "I have a LD (learning disability) and I am a girl"); and their location in terms of state or city (i.e., "I live in . . ."). Several children provided a more extended physical description (i.e., "I am short, really short"); disclosed information about their families (parents, brothers, sisters, a dog); revealed personal preferences regarding youth culture (teen idols, music, movies, TV, clothing, favorite colors); and discussed hobbies. Many messages contained information about themselves, preferred games, and their areas of competence and interest: "I am really into sports." The children's characteristics included their belonging to a group of children with learning problems, and they expressed their dissatisfaction from this part of their identity. For example, they wrote questions that bothered them such as "How did I get learning disabilities, why?" Children shared their attitudes toward themselves "Did u feel u were stupid." Several children disclosed their loneliness with comments such as "Sometimes it feels like I am the only one with a LD" and "I have no friends." Loneliness and social exclusion were the most important issues in their self-perception. They provided details on their social isolation, asking for help and advice ("Why don't they want me in their team." "This girl . . . keeps teasing me."). The children's descriptions of the cruelty of their peers were vivid and emotional. For example, "They never sit with me at lunch" and "Nobody plays with me during recess." The analysis of the messages revealed the children's identity and their difficulties. Children shared openly their challenges, and they described in details their loneliness, social rejection, and bullying. The online communication was effective not only as a way to share and express their distress, but also to "meet" online with children who shared similar difficulties and to get their support, understanding, and encouragement. Several children wrote that they felt better after corresponding with children who shared similar difficulties, yet others did not seem relieved. This example from our study was provided to exemplify children's self-disclosure and identity struggles related to their social alienation. It should be emphasized that children with learning disabilities, dyslexia, and ADHD are part of the typical school community. In schools, most attention focused on their academic difficulties, and their loneliness and social difficulties were often neglected (Margalit, 2006).

A considerable percentage of adolescents used the Internet to experiment with alternative identities and participants reported a wide range of pretence contents (Gross, 2004; Huffaker & Calvert, 2005). For example, they presented themselves by creating home pages – web sites with a focus on self-presentation (Stern, 2004). Children who wrote private homepages explored the dilemma "who am I," or "Who I want to be." They sometimes proposed different personalities and styles in the anonymity of the online environment, including the possibility to have a large audience (Turkle, 1995). Subsequently, authors can receive feedback from their home page visitors. Altogether, the process of home page construction can be viewed as a creative and gradual process, much like the process of identity formation itself. Personal home pages allow the children who created them greater social control than face-to-face encounters because the children and adolescents can decide what to include or omit in their self-descriptions, and what to embellish or underemphasize. They also allow the youngsters to repeatedly "reinvent" themselves, since home pages may be updated as often as they desire, and may be produced anonymously. The personal home pages can enable adolescents to feel free to express ideas and concerns, and to explore the reactions of their audience. A series of studies that examined adolescents' personal home pages revealed (Stern, 2004) that girls and boys provided personal, intimate, and immediate narratives. Emotional and relational lives were highlighted, and the home pages were abounded with stories about themselves, presenting descriptions of loneliness and disappointments, but also of hopefulness and their future dreams. Of the 233 home pages that were analyzed in this study, 70% were created by boys and 30% by girls. They explained who they were to themselves and others. Sometimes their descriptions did not reflect reality, but rather their wishes and pretence.

Pretence online is not rare, and can be considered as an identity experimentation. Early surveys reported that almost a quarter of adolescents who used instant messaging indicated that they had pretended to be someone else (Lenhart, Rainie, & Lewis, 2001). Additional surveys reported that about 50% of the Internet users pretended to be different than they were or had different characteristics (i.e., taller, long blond hair, etc.). Pre-adolescents and early adolescents experiment more often with their online identity than older adolescents (Gross, 2004; Valkenburg & Peter, 2007). Boys and girls do not differ in the frequency in which they experiment with their identity online, but they do differ significantly in the types of online identities that they pretend to be (Valkenburg, Schouten, & Peter, 2005). Only few studies reported research on the consequences of online identity experiments. Research usually focused on two outcome variables: offline social competence and the self-concept unity.

Studies examined the relations between online identity experiments and offline social competence (Caplan, 2005; Engelberg & Sjoberg, 2004; Harman, Hansen, Cochran, & Lindsey, 2005) and provided inconsistent results. Two studies found negative relationships between online communication and offline social competence. Individuals, who lacked self-presentational skills, preferred online social interactions over face-to-face communication. Individual differences also contributed to the gap between online and offline behavior, revealing loneliness (Caplan, 2005; Engelberg & Sjoberg, 2004). Online identity experiments may provide adolescents with many opportunities to communicate with people of different ages and cultural backgrounds and present themselves as they wish. These experiments may provide them with opportunities to learn how to relate to a wide variety of people. Still, studies expressed worries related to the wider and tempting options of positive unrealistic self-presentation (Harman et al., 2005). Several adolescents who used the Internet to experiment with identities gradually related more to their online identities than their true offline self, and may have, as a result, become less socially competent in offline situations. In order to investigate the effects of adolescents' online identity experiments on their social competence and self-concept unity (Valkenburg & Peter, 2008), an online survey was conducted among 1,158 Dutch adolescents. Eighteen percent of the adolescents who used the Internet for online communication indicated that they experimented with their identity when being online. The results of this study showed that engaging in online identity experiments had an indirect positive effect on adolescents' social competence. Adolescents who more often experimented with their identity on the Internet, more often communicated online with people of different ages and cultural backgrounds. This communication had a positive effect on adolescents' social competence. Yet their identity explorations were also related to loneliness, social anxiety, and lower self-concept. Several adolescents established relationships that originated online, and afterward these connections were developed to offline connections (Lenhart & Madden, 2007). In this culture of identity exploration, special attention has to be devoted to the special group of lonely adolescents. They also used the Internet to experiment with their identities, while in their offline lives, these lonely adolescents typically were engaged in fewer social interactions, had fewer opportunities to experiment with their identity development, had fewer close friends, and had more difficulties disclosing themselves than their non-lonely peers (Gross et al., 2002).

A survey among 687 adolescents (Peter & Valkenburg, 2006) examined the impact of Internet communication and the role of background variables (i.e., age, gender, social anxiety, loneliness, need for affiliation) in explaining the differences in personal relationships. They reported that younger, socially anxious, and lonely adolescents valued more strongly the controllability characteristics of Internet communication and perceived it as broader, deeper, and more reciprocal than older peers who were less anxious.

The Internet, with its abundant opportunities for online identity experiments, may especially provide help to lonely adolescents in their search for identity development and their ongoing struggles for connectedness. Yet, the inconsistent results of several studies indicated the varied needs of these youngsters for help and supportive training to achieve online communicative competence in order to take advantage of these interpersonal opportunities. Indeed the Internet may provide adolescents with additional prospects to connect with people and to practice their social and communicative skills. Yet, the unique needs of several youngsters, such as lonely children and children with social deficits, for extended tutoring and support should guide future planning attempts. Since the Internet is becoming part of the children's life and day-to-day experiences, a longitudinal study that will follow children who adopted the technology may reveal its long-range impact.

The impact of communication during several months was examined with a longitudinal design, a large sample of early adolescents, and a differential methodological approach that enabled considering different risks, technological options, and personal differences (Eijnden, Meerkerk, Vermulst, Spijkerman, & Engels, 2008), The results showed the value of avoiding global answers. Adolescents who were frequently engaged in instant messaging and chatting had a higher risk of compulsive Internet use after 6 months. The use of e-mails resulted differently. It did not request reactions in real time, was not associated with compulsive Internet use as revealed 6 months later. Lonely youngsters were less engaged in instant-messenger use than individuals who were low in loneliness. This finding is in contrast to the expectation that lonely teenagers would be attracted more to the applications of online communication, than their less lonely counterparts. Instead, lonely teenagers seemed to withdraw from several online options such as instant communication. It seemed that their social difficulties were more pronounced in immediate technologies. Accordingly, it was suggested that feelings of loneliness evoked an avoidant coping style in which communication with others was further evaded (Seepersad, Choi, & Shin, 2008). A downward spiral model proposed that the avoidance tendencies as a coping with loneliness style provoked increased loneliness and extended more avoidance behavior (Eijnden et al., 2008). The fact that these youngsters often used activities online that were less appreciated and not often used by their peers (i.e., e-mail messages) supplemented their social difficulties and their increased isolation and loneliness. Research also documented the tendencies of lonely youths to cope with their loneliness in an avoidant way, and to prefer the use of the Internet for entertainment functions rather than for communication (Seepersad, 2004). Thus, studies supported the "poor-get-poorer" assumption (i.e., it seems plausible that lonely and socially isolated adolescents, more than their socially integrated peers, communicate online to meet new people), and a negative association was found between online communication with strangers and psychosocial wellbeing among adolescents (Valkenburg & Peter, 2007). Thus, the online communication might evoke feelings of depression, at least among socially isolated youngsters, because these youngsters rely on Internet communication to obtain social relations and support and are often disappointed (LaRose, Eastin, & Gregg, 2001).

Overall, contradictory results were reported with regard to the impact that online communication has to the wellbeing of lonely and socially isolated individuals. Children are motivated to maintain social connection with others, and they are engaged in a variety of behaviors to form social connections and to alleviate the pain of temporary social disconnections. Those who have limited social connections with others may try to compensate this by creating alternative connections with non-human agents such as their cells and computers. This may occur by anthropomorphizing non-human agents such as non-human animals, stuffed dolls, and gadgets to make them appear more humanlike (Epley, Akalis, Waytz, & Cacioppo, 2008). It is not clear if the opportunity to alleviate the social disconnection by humanizing non-human agents may be a risk to some individuals who may prefer this easier solution over seeking connections with other human beings? Or, can it be used as a lever or a bridge to facilitate human connections following appropriate planning and training.

Summary and Conclusions

The technological environment is rapidly changing all the time. New communication technologies are continuously developed and immediately adopted by children and adolescents, including new social networking sites, new collaborative and multiplayer games, and also requiring major shifts in usages patterns. Young people have become super-communicators who are connected most of their days, using a host of new and innovative technology options for connecting with family, friends, and people that they meet online. This continuous evolution poses ongoing conceptual challenges to the traditional meanings of friends, privacy, self-identity, and intimacy. Parents, educators, health professionals, and policymakers are often confused, and by the time professionals fully understand the risks and benefits of one particular online environment, that environment may have changed so thoroughly that intervention and prevention strategies that were developed specifically for it will not be as applicable as originally designed (Mitchell & Ybarra, 2009).

Within this dynamic culture, studies attempted to understand if the adoption of different forms of communicative technologies reduced the feelings of children's loneliness by extending their options for meeting their needs for relatedness and connectivity, or perhaps just the opposite – the use of technology promoted children's loneliness. The results of several studies provided inconsistent and partial results, and repeatedly pointed out the irrelevance of the generalized approaches regarding the global impacts of online communication and relations. There is a need to move from generalized global evaluations regarding the benefits and the risks of online communication to distinguish between the rich variations of technology characteristics and usages and the differential roles of individual differences and cultural contexts (Ehrenberg, Juckes, White, & Walsh, 2008). It has also been suggested that some adolescents become so involved with certain applications of the Internet that they are no longer capable of controlling their online activity, implying that these youngsters have developed symptoms of compulsive Internet use. However, no differences were noted in this aspect between lonely and non-lonely children.

The research surveys presented in this chapter call for several conclusions: The Internet has become an integral part of the youth social environment. This environment enables youngsters to extend their current social activities, and enhance communication, relatedness to their social groups, friendships with existing companions and new acquaintances. Most youngsters play computer games not only by themselves, but also with others, at least some of the time, and gaming has become a social activity, and a key component of their overall social experiences. They mostly play games with friends and people they know, and the extended playing time extends their companionship relations. However, sometimes they play with individuals that they meet online regularly, or only few times. In contrast, lonely children tend to develop social connections and play with individuals that they meet on the net, and several of them continue to play computer games alone. The research on children's behavior online should be treated as an inseparable part of their overall behavior and development in order to achieve more consistent and meaningful answers to their social exclusion (online and offline).

Technology created and will continue to generate innovative options for connecting with people, for experimenting self-identity, for enhancing social skills and socializing patterns, for receiving and providing social support, and for enabling self-disclosure. The identity experimentation included the development of the existing identities and experimenting with various alternatives using pretence within anonymous environments. These social benefits were acquired effortlessly and applied successfully by socially competent children. They were less available to several lonely children whose limited interpersonal competence requested suitable training. In fact, these developments may make loneliness even more pronounced when children realize the enjoyable connectivity of their classmates and feel envious while facing difficulties to participate in this culture. For example, lonely children have specific difficulties in chatting and texting (writing texts) due to the inherent needs to react quickly and spontaneously during these activities. Instead, they tend to adopt the usages of unpopular connectivity options such as e-mails that will contribute to their social exclusion.

Research has already documented the empowerment and social supporting functions of forums and discussion boards. Participating in online games also provided a meaningful answer to the needs for relatedness, closeness, and companionship embedded in their competitions. Yet the same games may isolate lonely children who also lack collaborating skills both online and offline. Thus, complex interactions were identified between Internet connections, personality differences, and loneliness. The Internet relations have different meanings and functions for different children and adolescents, focusing attention on their abilities to use the varied technology options. Unique personal characteristics of individuals such as loneliness and social avoidance interacted with the technological characteristics, and affected children's life quality and wellbeing. In cultures that encourage and appreciate social connections, and in times when youngsters are socially connected most of their time after school and leisure time, the loneliness experience is more explicit and can be considered a greater risk factor.

The studies may be used to sensitize professionals to the risks of lonely children. Without detailed planning of intervention, training, support, and supervision, the Internet may not provide a venue of beneficial social interactions for lonely children and adolescents whose distress reflects their alienation to the current youth culture, and their inability to benefit from its options. It is not enough to provide them with time online. It is more important to explore what they do versus what they can and wish to do; that which they interact with and the nature of relationships that they wish to develop with their online partners. This knowledge can be used by significant adults to support and structure the children's social competence, development, and wellbeing (Subrahmanyam & Lin, 2007). The coping and social support chapters will detail children's and parents' coping options, offline and online. The Internet extends the possibilities especially for children with social difficulties and disabilities, extending the boundaries of time and space, presenting options for freeing individuals from the constraints of geography, and possibly of the isolation brought on by disability or poor social skills during typical face-to-face interactions. The Internet may enable children and adolescents to join groups on the basis of common interests without dependence on the accurate expression and interpretation of the social cues required during face-to-face relations (Kraut et al., 1998). Yet, training and support are requested in order to guarantee their benefit from the new possibilities. In order to help lonely children with the use of technological-supported solutions, there is a need for awareness to the constantly changing nature of the Internet, and to move from generic global considerations to more specified and differentiated approaches that will attempt to identify relations between the multiple options and usages of the Internet adapted to different youth cultures, and the complexity of individual differences in different cultures among users.

There is a need to reconsider the research approaches. Researchers have argued that the Internet is not one generic space. Instead of considerations of the Internet as a whole entity with a generalized impact, we should focus our attempts to explore differentiations based on a variety of the Internet's options and individual differences of the users and their modes of interactions with partners. We probably keep asking the wrong questions, and in order to identify meaningful solutions and effective intervention approaches, there is a need for an in-depth understanding of the coping strategies adopted by lonely youngsters.

References

Ando, R., & Sakamoto, A. (2008). The effect of cyber-friends on loneliness and social anxiety: Differences between high and low self-evaluated physical attractiveness groups. *Instructional Support for Enhancing Students' Information Problem Solving Ability, 24*(3), 993–1009.

Baker, J. R., & Moore, S. M. (2008). Blogging as a social tool: A psychosocial examination of the effects of bogging. *CyberPsychology & Behavior, 11*(6), 1–3.

Bargh, J. A., McKenna, K. Y. A., & Fitzsimons, G. M. (2002). Can you see the real me? Activation and expression of the "True Self" on the Internet. *Journal of Social Issues, 58*(1), 33–48.

Barker, V. (2009). Older adolescents' motivations for social network site use: The influence of gender, group identity, and collective self-esteem. *CyberPsychology & Behavior, 12*(2), 209–213.

Barlett, C. P., Anderson, C. A., & Swing, E. L. (2009). Video game effects – Confirmed, suspected, and speculative: A Review of the evidence. *Simulation & Gaming, 40*(3), 377–403.

Baumeister, R., & Leary, M. R. (1995). The need to belong: Desire for interpersonal attachments as a fundamental human motivation. *Psychological Bulletin, 117*(3), 497–529.

Baym, N. K., Zhang, Y. B., & Lin, M. C. (2004). Social interactions across media: Interpersonal communication on the Internet, telephone and face-to-face. *New Media Society, 6*(3), 299–318.

Bortee, D. S. (2005). Presentation of self on the Web: An ethnographic study of teenage girls. *Education, Communication & Information, 5*(1), 25–39.

Caplan, S. E. (2003). Preference for online social interaction: A theory of problematic Internet use and psychosocial well-being. *Communication Research, 30*(6), 625–648.

Caplan, S. E. (2005). A social skill account of problematic Internet use. *Journal of Communication, 55*(4), 721–736.

Caplan, S. E., & Turner, J. S. (2007). Bringing theory to research on computer-mediated comforting communication. *Computers in Human Behavior, 23*(2), 985–998.

Ceyhan, A. A., & Ceyhan, E. (2008). Loneliness, depression, and computer self-efficacy as predictors of problematic internet use. *CyberPsychology & Behavior, 11*(6), 699–701.

Chou, C., & Peng, H. (2007). Net-friends: Adolescents' attitudes and experiences vs. teachers' concerns. *Computers in Human Behavior, 23*(5), 2394–2413.

Deresiewicz, W. (2009). The end of solitude. *The Chronicle of Higher Education: Chronicle Review, 55,* B6.

Derlega, V., Metts, S., & Sandra, P. (1993). *Self-disclosure.* Thousand Oaks, CA: Sage.

Diener, E., Lucas, R. E., & Oishi, S. (2002). Subjective well-being: The science of happiness and life satisfaction. In. C. R. Snyder & S. J. Lopez (Eds.), *Handbook of positive psychology* (pp. 63–73). New York: Oxford University Press.

Ehrenberg, A., Juckes, S., White, K. M., & Walsh, S. P. (2008). Personality and self-esteem as predictors of young people's technology use. *CyberPsychology & Behavior, 11*(6), 739–741.

Eijnden, R. J. J. M. V. D., Meerkerk, G. J., Vermulst, A. A., Spijkerman, R., & Engels, R. (2008). Online communication, compulsive Internet use, and psychosocial well-being among adolescents: A longitudinal study. *Developmental Psychology, 44*(3), 655–665.

Eldeleklioglu, J. (2008). Gender, romantic relationships, Internet use, perceived social support and social skills as the predictors of loneliness. *Egitim Arastirmalari-Eurasian Journal of Educational Research, 8*(33), 127–140.

Engelberg, E., & Sjoberg, L. (2004). Internet use, social skills, and adjustment. *CyberPsychology & Behavior, 7*(1), 41–47.

Epley, N., Akalis, S., Waytz, A., & Cacioppo, J. T. (2008). Creating social connection through inferential reproduction: Loneliness and perceived agency in gadgets, gods, and greyhounds. *Psychological Science, 19*(2), 114–120.

Fox, A. B., Rosen, J., & Crawford, M. (2009). Distractions, distractions: Does instant messaging affect college students' performance on a concurrent reading comprehension task? *CyberPsychology & Behavior, 12*(1), 51–53.

Frostling-Henningsson, M. (2009). First-person shooter games as a way of connecting to people: "Brothers in blood". *CyberPsychology & Behavior, 12*(5), 557–562.

Gentile, D., & Gentile, J. (2008). Violent video games as exemplary teachers: A conceptual analysis. *Journal of Youth and Adolescence, 37*(2), 127–141.

Gross, E. F. (2004). Adolescent Internet use: What we expect, what teens report. *Journal of Applied Developmental Psychology, 25*(6), 633–649.

Gross, E. F., Juvonen, J., & Gable, S. (2002). Internet use and well-being in adolescence. *Journal of Social Issues, 58*(1), 75–90.

Guadagno, R. E., Okdie, B. M., & Eno, C. A. (2008). Who blogs? Personality predictors of blogging. *Instructional Support for Enhancing Students' Information Problem Solving Ability, 24*(5), 1993–2004.

Ha, J. H., Chin, B., Park, D. H., Ryu, S. H., & Yu, J. (2008). Characteristics of excessive cellular phone use in Korean adolescents. *CyberPsychology & Behavior, 11*(6), 783–784.

Hamburger, Y. A., & Ben-Artzi, E. (2000). The relationship between extraversion and neuroticism and the different uses of the Internet. *Computers in Human Behavior, 16*(4), 441–449.

Harman, J. P., Hansen, C. E., Cochran, M. E., & Lindsey, C. R. (2005). Liar, Liar: Internet faking but not frequency of use affects social skills, self-esteem, social anxiety, and aggression. *CyberPsychology & Behavior, 8*(1), 1–6.

Hart, G. M., Johnson, B., Stamm, B., Angers, N., Robinson, A., Lally, T., et al. (2009). Effects of video games on adolescents and adults. *CyberPsychology & Behavior, 12*(1), 63–65.

Heim, J., Brandtzaeg, P. B., Kaare, B. H., Endestad, T., & Torgersen, L. (2007). Children's usage of media technologies and psychosocial factors. *New Media Society, 9*(3), 425–454.

Hu, M. (2009). Will online chat help alleviate mood loneliness? *CyberPsychology & Behavior, 12*(2), 219–223.

Huffaker, D. A., & Calvert, S. L. (2005). Gender, identity, and language use in teenage blogs. *Journal of Computer-Mediated Communication, 10*(2), Article 1. Retrieved from http://jcmc.indiana.edu/vol10/issue2/huffaker.html

Jackson, L. A., Fitzgerald, H. E., Zhao, Y., Kolenic, A., Von Eye, A., & Harold, R. (2008). Information Technology (IT) use and children's psychological well-being. *CyberPsychology & Behavior, 11*(6), 755–757.

Jackson, L. A., Zhao, Y., Witt, E. A., Fitzgerald, H. E., von Eye, A., & Harold, R. (2009). Self-concept, self-esteem, gender, race, and Information Technology use. *CyberPsychology & Behavior, 12*(4), 437–440.

Joinson, A. N. (2001). Self-disclosure in computer-mediated communication: The role of self-awareness and visual anonymity. *European Journal of Social Psychology, 31*(2), 177–192.

Joinson, A. N. (2007). Disinhibition and the Internet. In J. Gackenbach (Ed.), *Psychology and the Internet* (pp. 75–92). New York: Elsevier Inc.

Jones, S. (2009). Generations online in 2009. *Pew internet & American life project*. Retrieved from http://www.pewinternet.org/~/media//Files/Reports/2009/PIP_Generations_2009.pdf

Kim, J., LaRose, R., & Peng, W. (2009). Loneliness as the cause and the effect of problematic Internet use: The relationship between Internet use and psychological well-being. *CyberPsychology & Behavior, 12*(4), 451–455.

Klimmt, C., Rizzo, A., Vorderer, P., Koch, J., & Fischer, T. (2009). Experimental evidence for suspense as determinant of Video game enjoyment. *CyberPsychology & Behavior, 12*(1), 29–31.

Klimmt, C., Schmid, H., & Orthmann, J. (2009). Exploring the enjoyment of playing browser games. *CyberPsychology & Behavior, 12*(2), 231–234.

Ko, H. C., & Kuo, F. Y. (2009). Can Blogging enhance subjective well-being through self-disclosure? *CyberPsychology & Behavior, 12*(1), 75–79.

Kraut, R. E., Kiesler, S., Boneva, B., Cummings, J., Helgeson, V., & Crawford, A. (2002). Internet paradox revisited. *Journal of Social Issues, 58*(1), 49–74.

Kraut, R., Patterson, M., Lundmark, V., Kiesler, S., Mukopadhyay, T., & Scherlis, W. (1998). Internet paradox: A social technology that reduces social involvement and psychological well-being? *American Psychologist, 53*(9), 1017–1031.

LaRose, R., Eastin, M. S., & Gregg, J. (2001). Reformulating the Internet paradox: Social cognitive explanations of Internet use and depression. *Journal of Online Behavior, 1*(2). Retrieved from http://www.behavior.net/JOB/v1n2/paradox.html

Lenhart, A. (2009). Adults and social network websites. *Pew internet & American life project*. Retrieved from http://www.pewinternet.org/pdfs/PIP_Adult_social_networking_data_memo_FINAL.pdf

Lenhart, A., Kahne, J., Middaugh E., Macgill, A. R., Evans, C., & Vitak, J. (2008). Teens' gaming experiences are diverse and include significant social interaction and civic engagement. *Pew internet & American life project*. Retrieved from http://www.pewinternet.org/pdfs/PIP_Teens_Games_and_Civics_Report_FINAL.pdf

Lenhart, A., & Madden, M. (2007). How teens manage their online identities and personal information in the age of MySpace. *Pew Internet & American Life Project*. Retrieved from http://www.pewinternet.org

Lenhart, A., Rainie, L., & Lewis, O. (2001). *Teenage life online: The rise of the instant-message generation and the internet impact on friendship and family relations*. Washington, DC: Pew Internet & American Life Project, from http//www.pewinternet.org.

Lim, S., & Lee, J. E. R. (2009). When playing together feels different: Effects of task types and social contexts on physiological arousal in multiplayer online gaming contexts. *CyberPsychology & Behavior, 12*(1), 59–61.

Margalit, M. (1990). *Effective technology integration for disabled children*. New York: Springer.

Margalit, M. (2006). Loneliness, the Salutogenic paradigm and LD: Current research, future directions and interventional implications. *Thalamus, 24*(1), 38–48.

Margalit, M., & Raskind, M. (2009). Mothers of children with LD and ADHD: Empowerment through online communication. *Journal of Special Education Technology, 24*(1), 39–50.

Matei, S., & Ball-Rokeach, S. J. (2001). Real and virtual social ties. *American Behavioral Scientist, 45*(3), 550–564.

Mitchell, K. J., & Ybarra, M. (2009). Social networking sites finding a balance between their risks and benefits. *Archives of Pediatrics & Adolescent Medicine, 163*(1), 87–89.

Morahan-Martin, J., & Schumacher, P. (2003). Loneliness and social uses of the Internet. *Computers in Human Behavior, 19*(6), 659–671.

Pennebaker, J. W., & Beall, S. K. (1986). Confronting a traumatic event: Toward an understanding of inhibition and disease. *Journal of Abnormal Psychology, 95*(3), 274–281.

Peter, J., & Valkenburg, P. M. (2006). Research note: Individual differences in perceptions of Internet communication. *European Journal of Communication, 21*(2), 213–226.

Peter, J., Valkenburg, P. M., & Schouten, A. P. (2005). Developing a model of adolescent friendship formation on the Internet. *CyberPsychology & Behavior, 8*(5), 423–430.

Pornsakulvanich, V., Haridakis, P., & Rubin, A. M. (2008). The influence of dispositions and Internet motivation on online communication satisfaction and relationship closeness. *Computers in Human Behavior, 24*(5), 2292–2310.

Punamaki, R. L., Wallenius, M., Holtto, H., Nygard, C. H., & Rimpela, A. (2009). The associations between information and communication technology (ICT) and peer and parent-relations in early adolescence. *International Journal of Behavioral Development, 33*(6), 556–564.

Radcliffe, A. M., Lumley, M. A., Kendall, J., Stevenson, J. K., & Beltran, J. (2007). Written emotional disclosure: Testing whether social disclosure matters. *Journal of Social & Clinical Psychology, 26*(3), 362–384.

Ramirez, A., Jr, & Broneck, K. (2009). 'IM me': Instant messaging as relational mainte-nance and everyday communication. *Journal of Social and Personal Relationships, 26*(2–3), 291–314.

Raskind, M. H., Margalit, M., & Higgins, E. L. (2006). "My LD": Children's voices on the Internet. *Learning Disabilities Quarterly, 29*(4), 253–268.

Rideout, V., & Hamel, E. (2006). *The media family: Electronic media in the lives of infants, toddlers, preschoolers and their parents.* Available from http://www.kff.org/entmedia/upload/7500.pdf

Roberts, D. F., Foehr, U. G., & Rideout, V. (2005). *Generation M: Media in the lives of 8–18 year-olds.* Available from http://www.kff.org/entmedia/upload/Generation-M-Media-in-the-Lives-of-8-18-Year-olds-Report.pdf

Sanchez-Martinez, M., & Otero, A. (2009). Factors associated with cell phone use in adolescents in the community of Madrid (Spain). *CyberPsychology & Behavior, 12*(2), 131–137.

Seepersad, S. (2004). Coping with loneliness: Adolescent online and offline behavior. *CyberPsychology & Behavior, 7*(1), 35–39.

Seepersad, S., Choi, M. K., & Shin, N. (2008). How does culture influence the degree of romantic loneliness and closeness? *Journal of Psychology, 142*(2), 209–220.

Stern, S. R. (2004). Expressions of identity online: Prominent features and gender differences in adolescents' World Wide Web home pages. *Journal of Broadcasting & Electronic Media, 48*(2), 218–243.

Subrahmanyam, K., & Lin, G. (2007). Adolescents on the Net: Internet use and well-being. *Adolescence, 42*(168), 659–677.

Subrahmanyam, K., Smahel, D., & Greenfield, P. (2006). Connecting developmental construc-tions to the Internet: Identity presentation and sexual exploration in online teen chat rooms. *Developmental Psychology, 42*(3), 395–406.

Swenson, L., & Rose, A. (2009). Friends' knowledge of youth internalizing and externalizing adjustment: Accuracy, bias, and the influences of gender, grade, positive friendship quality, and self-disclosure. *Journal of Abnormal Child Psychology, 37*(6), 887–901.

Tanis, M., & Postmes, T. (2008). Cues to identity in online dyads: Effects of interpersonal ver-sus intragroup perceptions on performance. *Group Dynamics: Theory, Research, and Practice, 12*(2), 96–111.

Tidwell, L. C., & Walther, J. B. (2002). Computer-mediated communication effects on disclosure, impressions, and interpersonal evaluations: Getting to know one another a bit at a time. *Human Communication Research, 28*(3), 317–348.

Turkle, S. (1995). *Life on the screen: Identity in the age of the internet.* New York: Simon & Schuster.

Valkenburg, P. M., & Peter, J. (2007). Preadolescents' and adolescents' online communication and their closeness to friends. *Developmental Psychology, 43*(2), 267–277.

Valkenburg, P. M., & Peter, J. (2008). Adolescents' identity experiments on the Internet: Consequences for social competence and self-concept unity. *Communication Research, 35*(2), 208–231.

Valkenburg, P. M., Schouten, A. P., & Peter, J. (2005). Adolescents' identity experiments on the Internet. *New Media and Society, 7*, 383–402.

Varnhagen, C. K. (2007). Children and the Internet. In J. Gackenbach (Ed.), *Psychology and the internet (Second Edition): Intrapersonal, interpersonal, and transpersonal implications* (pp. 37–54). New York: Elsevier Inc.

Vergeer, M., & Pelzer, B. (2009). Consequences of media and Internet use for offline and online network capital and well-being. A causal model approach. *Journal of Computer-Mediated Communication, 15*(1), 189–210.

Whitty, M. T., & McLaughlin, D. (2007). Online recreation: The relationship between loneliness, Internet self-efficacy and the use of the Internet for entertainment purposes. *Computers in Human Behavior, 23*(3), 1435–1446.

Wilkins, J. S. (2008). The roles, reasons and restrictions of science blogs. *Forum: Trends in Ecology and Evolution,23*(8), 411–413.

Wolak, J., Mitchell, K. J., & Finkelhor, D. (2003). Escaping or connecting? Characteristics of youth who form close online relationships. *Journal of Adolescence, 26*(1), 105–119.

Ybarra, M. L., Alexander, C., & Mitchell, K. J. (2005). Depressive symptomatology, youth Internet use, and online interactions: A national survey. *Journal of Adolescent Health, 36*(1), 9–18.

Zhao, S. (2009). Teen adoption of MySpace and IM: Inner-city versus suburban differences. *CyberPsychology & Behavior, 12*(1), 55–58.

Zhao, S., Grasmucka, S., & Martin, J. (2008). Identity construction on Facebook: Digital empowerment in anchored relationships. *Computers in Human Behavior, 24*(5), 1816–1836.

Chapter 7
Children's and Parents' Coping

Adam, a 9-year-old boy, sat at home feeling very sad and alone. He kept thinking about the group of boys who had decided to go together to the football game during the weekend. He stood in the school yard next to them, listening to their exciting planning. He had hoped that they would ask him to join them, and was distressed that they had completely ignored him. He had felt lonely, gone away, and could not stop asking himself again and again why they had not asked him to come with them, and why he had not been able to tell them how much he wanted to come.

Anna hated the school lunch. Often she sat there alone, eating her meal quickly and feeling lonely. When her teacher introduced a new student to the class, she immediately volunteered to help her, proposing to go together to lunch. She promised to show her around, and stayed with her during the school day. During dinner she told her mother: "I know what it means to be the new student at school. She probably felt alone. I stayed with her, and it was a great day for both of us."

Many children experience loneliness from time to time during short periods. However, some of them are more often lonely than others. The critical question that we have to ask ourselves is not only related to the sources of this distress, but even more importantly, what children and adolescents do when they experience alienation. Indeed loneliness is a source of their distress, and a cause for anxiety and apprehension for their parents and teachers. The study of children's coping is focused on the children's reactions (their emotional, cognitive, and behavioral responses) to loneliness in real-life contexts. Understanding the coping processes is essential to clarify the impact of stress on children and adolescents because it portrays not only how individuals deal with the social adversity, but also how these ongoing and accumulative encounters shape their future development. In addition, this understanding has a functional value, since it may provide significant indications for intervention planning. Coping research focused attention on the attempts to ameliorate the anguish and emotional pain of social alienation. In the first part of this chapter, the general coping construct is clarified, followed in the second part by the typical coping behaviors performed by children and youth when they experience loneliness. The role of family, peers, and additional sources of social support will be presented.

M. Margalit, *Lonely Children and Adolescents*, DOI 10.1007/978-1-4419-6284-3_7,
© Springer Science+Business Media, LLC 2010

Successful adaptation to various life stresses, such as the experience of loneliness, includes many coping behaviors that individuals perform in order to manage their emotions, think constructively, regulate and direct their behavior, control their autonomic arousal, and act to alter or decrease sources of stress. Coping has been defined as "cognitive and behavioral efforts to manage specific external and/or internal demands that are appraised as taxing or exceeding the resources of the person" (Lazarus & Folkman, 1984, p. 141). The goals of these efforts are to manage, master, tolerate, reduce, or minimize the demands of a stressful environment.

Skinner and Zimmer-Gembeck (2007), in her comprehensive developmental survey, defined coping as action regulation under stress, clarifying how individuals mobilize, manage, energize, and direct their attention, cognitions, emotions, and behavior under stressful conditions. Coping with loneliness consists of complex multidimensional processes that are sensitive (a) to environmental conditions; (b) to personality dispositions that influence the appraisal of the stressors; and (c) to the appraisal of the individual's available resources. When children experience loneliness and appraise it as a threat to their self-esteem and a risk to their wellbeing, the goals of their coping activities focus on decreasing this distress. The outcomes of their coping effort may affect their current efficacy beliefs, which in turn affect their future coping efforts and hopes. Children who fail in decreasing their social exclusion and feelings of alienation will probably be more frustrated and will attempt avoiding future encounters. Before further exploring the different coping strategies with loneliness, the general coping models will be illuminated.

Dual-Process Models of Coping

Early models of coping classifications proposed the adoption of several dual-process models (Cole, Martin, & Dennis, 2004). Four approaches will be presented separately to clarify their nature, in spite of their overlapping aspects:

- *Approach versus avoidance coping.* Approach (or active) coping refers to coping strategies that propose to reduce, eliminate, or manage the internal or external demands of a stressor. The coping efforts are intended to achieve some degree of personal control over the stressful aspects of the environment and one's emotions, and to decrease their impact. For example, the preschool child who was not accepted by the group of boys who played on the swings, attempted to join another group of boys and girls who were playing with a ball. Avoidance (or passive) coping, on the other hand, refers to disengagement, in which the goal is to ignore, avoid, or withdraw from the stressor or its emotional consequences (Ebata & Moos, 1991). For example, the girl who was not included in the group that planned to go together to the mall, stayed at home feeling frustrated, but did not try to call any friend.
- *Problem-focused coping versus emotion-focused coping.* Problem-focused coping seeks to change the situation or to eliminate the stressor itself (to "solve

the problem"), whereas emotion-focused coping involves seeking to reduce or manage the emotional consequences associated with the stressor (to change the perception of and emotional relation to the distressful situation), through cognitive methods of reframing (i.e., a girl that was not invited to the party told herself that she did not like dancing and hated parties), acceptance (i.e., she told herself "indeed nobody wanted to spend time with an ugly girl like myself"), or distraction through adopting alternative positive thoughts or activities (i.e., she decided to read an interesting book and not to think of the party) (Compas, Connor-Smith, Saltzman, Thomsen, & Wadsworth, 2001; Lazarus & Folkman, 1984).

- *Voluntary (controlled) versus involuntary (automatic) coping.* Voluntary coping responses to stress reflect volition and conscious effort by the individual to change the distressful circumstances whereas responses that are automatized and not under conscious control are considered involuntary coping (Compas et al., 2001).
- *Future-oriented coping (proactive) versus past-oriented coping (reactive coping).* Proactive coping is directed at an upcoming stressor, trying to prevent its occurrence or to reduce its impact, while reactive coping is directed at an ongoing stressor (Sohl & Moyer, 2009).

Approach/Avoidance Coping

Early research of coping examined the approach versus avoidance coping, and also the problem-focused coping versus emotion-focused coping. Moos (2002b), for example, proposed that coping skills could be characterized along two main dimensions: with respect to their focus (approach or avoidance), and to their method (cognitive or behavioral). When these two approaches are combined, coping skills may be categorized into the following four domains. Logical analysis and positive reappraisal of the problem reflect *cognitive approach coping*; seeking social support reflects *behavioral approach coping*. Cognitive avoidance and affective resignation exemplify *cognitive avoidance coping*, and seeking alternative rewards and emotional discharge exemplify *behavioral avoidance coping* (Moos, 2002a). In general, adolescents with an approach coping style are more likely to resolve their stressors, as well as to experience more self-confidence and less depression and dysfunction. Individuals who depend more on avoidance coping, tend to experience maladjustment and continued difficulties (Moos, 2002a). The two types of coping strategies were mutually related and individuals who perceived their situation as amendable to change reported engaging in more active coping. In contrast, individuals, whose situation was appraised as uncontrollable and unchangeable, tended to adopt higher levels of denial and disengagement from activity. Active coping was related in research to adaptation and wellbeing, whereas avoidant coping was often related to psychological distress and dissatisfaction (Holahan & Moos, 1985). Two additional models extended the insight to the complicated characteristics of the coping behavior:

Controlled/Automatic Coping

The coping reactions in several situations, especially of young children, are instantaneous and uncontrolled reactions to the stress (such as crying, or running away). In other circumstances, the reactions reveal calculated (problem solving) and planned activities (i.e., children asking themselves what can be done to find a friend). Automatic reactions to external stimuli and events (i.e., crying or running away) are initiated sometimes without prior self-awareness or knowledge and they are distinguished from processes that are consciously or intentionally put into operation. Our behavior is affected by others, their characteristic features, the groups they belong to, the social roles they fill, and whether or not we have a close relationship with them. They may automatically trigger psychological and behavioral processes. In addition, standard situations, which become automatically associated with general social norms and rules of conduct as well as with personal goals, may also trigger automatic coping reactions (Bargh & Williams, 2006). Theories of controlled coping and goal pursuit called attention to the role of conscious thought in goals' adoption. Goals have been defined as mental representations of future states that individuals wish to attain, and believe that they know how to attain (Hassin, Bargh, & Zimerman, 2009). Thus, the process of identifying personal goals is frequently assumed to involve deliberation, weighing of pros/cons, and assessing how they fit other important goals, norms, and values.

Goal pursuit is an effortful process that requires considerable amounts of flexibility. Automatic processes in general and automatic goal pursuit in particular, are usually conceived of as the opposite of controlled processes: they are unintentional, relatively effortless, and with a quick pace, without conscious direction or guidance. Their main advantage lies in freeing the limited-capacity consciousness, but the impulsive and immediate reactions may not lead to effective coping with the stress. In addition, the main drawbacks of automatic processes are their rigidity or inflexibility. However, recent laboratory experiments have validated assumptions that automatic processes of coping can react to environmental changes in a flexible manner (Hassin et al., 2009), focusing attention on the complexity of interactions and the continuation between varying levels of automated/controlled coping strategies. Children's conscience coping may become automatic reactions after many repetitions, but may also regain flexibility if they are aware of major changes in environmental conditions. The therapeutic implications of these outcomes focused attention on the needs of children to develop a wide repertoire of coping strategies in order to enable a flexible move between the different levels of conscience awareness to the coping behaviors and automatic reactions. Within the attempts of promoting children's effective coping with loneliness, there is a need to help them at the first stage to develop conscious and controlled strategies. However, effective interventions have to be extended, adopting effective training approaches until the children will reach automatic levels of coping reactions and utilize the acquired strategies without a voluntary effort. Specific explanations and examples are provided in Chapter 8.

Proactive/Reactive Coping

Proactive coping (future-oriented coping) consists of efforts undertaken in advance directed at a potentially stressful event in order to prevent it or to modify its form before it occurs, while reactive coping consists of efforts directed at current or past stressful events (Aspinwall & Taylor, 1997; Sohl & Moyer, 2009). The effective proactive coping requests appreciation of the accumulation of personal resources, such as time, money, organizational and planning skills, a social network of family and friends, and the detection of a potential stressor. Sometimes this task involves the interpretation of warning signs that come from the environment. In addition, information about potential stressors may come from one's internal processes of reflection (Gan, Yang, Zhou, & Zhang, 2007).

Proactive coping has several important benefits. It may minimize the degree of stress experienced during a stressful encounter. When a stressful event is a possibility rather than an actuality, its full impact may be lessened or averted by proactive efforts. Fewer coping resources will be requested when the stressor is tackled in its early stages rather than in its full-blown state. Specifically, an incipient stressor is likely to be modest, and because resources have not yet been expended to address it, coping resources are likely to be greater. In addition, when a stressful event is expected, a wider range of options are available to manage it, and the impact of chronic stress carried by an individual is likely to be relatively small. Because many stressful events are of long-term duration and add to the cumulative burden of obligations in an individual's daily life, proactive efforts that avoid or offset stressful events may keep chronic stress at a low level (Aspinwall & Taylor, 1997). However, there are also several potential disadvantages of proactive coping that cannot be ignored. The proactive coping may result in unnecessary plans and activities if the stressful event does not happen, and in addition, the inherent ambiguity of potential stressors may result in investing coping efforts and resources in a problem that is different from the one initially envisioned. As a possible result, coping resources may be drained at precisely the moments they are most needed for the accruing challenge.

At diverse ages, within various contextual conditions, children use different strategies to obtain the same coping goals. For example, young children who are not accepted by their group may use behavioral strategies to distract themselves in times of distress (like playing alone with something that they consider to instigate fun, or asking for a sweet), whereas older children may use cognitive strategies (like thinking about something pleasant, listening to preferred music, and also eating a chocolate). Strategies of attention redeployment can also be performed by the child or the adult who want to distract the distressed child. Overall, different coping activities are considered the building blocks in the understanding of people's actual behavioral, emotional, and cognitive responses to stress. Skinner's comprehensive survey identified the 12 coping strategies that children often used (listed here in order of the prevalence of use): support-seeking (sometimes encompassing information-seeking or help-seeking); escape (cognitive and/or behavioral reactions); distraction (cognitive and/or behavioral strategies); problem-solving (and instrumental action); accommodation; opposition and denial; self-reliance; aggression; social isolation; negotiation; helplessness; and positive cognitive reappraisal (Skinner & Zimmer-Gembeck, 2007). It is apparent that children and youth often adapt the following four coping strategies – support-seeking, problem-solving (and instrumental action), escape, and, when escape is not possible, distraction.

Among these coping types, support-seeking was the most common reaction, yet requests for help and support are complex, multidimensional activities. They are dependent on age, source of support (i.e., parents, peers, teachers), domain (i.e., medical, academic), kind of support sought (i.e., contact, comfort, guidance, instrumental aid), and means of seeking support (i.e., expressions of distress, bids and appeals, social referencing, proximity-seeking, verbal requests). Reasons for support-seeking, such as comfort, instrumental assistance with a problem, advice, or simply talking about a problem, would also change with age, family style, and individual characteristics. Parenting approaches and parents' behavior were also interrelated with children's coping styles.

Appraisal

Not every hassle or demanding situation creates stress and initiates coping reactions for each and every child. Only events that are evaluated and appraised as taxing to a person's wellbeing are most likely to generate stress (Lazarus, 1991). To cognitively appraise an event means to determine if it is personally relevant, and to interpret its meaning and value. Appraisal is commonly thought to be the first step in coping with a situation (Lazarus & Folkman, 1984). Often it consists of multiple simultaneous processes that can be considered adaptive or maladaptive. The awareness of a potential stressor often starts with initial appraisal that includes the definition of the problem and the regulation of emotional and physiological arousal. The appraisals of the stress, as well as the appraisal of the availability of social support, are critical in determining the appropriate emotional reactions. Individual differences in appraisal are powerful predictors of children's responses to a range of potentially stressful events such as those associated with social exclusion or parental conflicts (Shelton & Harold, 2008). Children faced with a potentially stressful event may try to understand and interpret cues received from their environment. Often, they try to compare a current potentially stressful event to a similar past event. Their expectations may influence their decisions regarding how to act. Appraisals can be the result of a conscious process, yet often it tends to be automatic. Appraisal may also be viewed as a style, revealing a consistent pattern of evaluating the environment. Often, children relate current potentially stressful events to their memories of comparable past events, determining their importance and evaluating how they may affect their wellbeing. Appraisals are formed and shaped by daily encounters within the family, and parents influence their children's appraisal style as well as serve as their role models and expectancy socializes. Children gradually develop their own mature appraisal style, revealing moderate consistency across situations (Hood, Power, & Hill, 2009).

Profiles of Coping Responses

In order to achieve an in-depth understanding of children's behavior, there is a need to move from understanding unique single-coping behaviors to the appreciation of specific profiles and coping families that combine several behaviors and reflect individual differences along the proposed dimensions.

The varied coping responses of children who experience social rejection by their peers demonstrate the importance of clarifying the multidimensional aspects of their reactions' style. In line with Compas et al. (2001) conceptualization, children's responses to the social stresses were distinguished along two broad dimensions: (a) voluntary/controlled coping (i.e., going to tell their teacher) versus involuntary coping (i.e., crying); and (b) engagement/approach coping (i.e., talking with a friend in order to join him and participate in the groups' activities) versus disengagement/avoidance coping (i.e., leaving the playground, starting a solitary activity). Both voluntary and involuntary responses can be further distinguished as (1) engaging with a stressor or one's responses to the stressor; or (2) disengaging from the stressor and one's responses. The roots of the engagement–disengagement (approach/avoidance) dimensions can be found in the classic human reactions to threat. Individuals react to dangers either by a tendency to participate in a fight (the engagement reaction) or by preferring a fight reaction (the disengagement reaction). Voluntary responses (coping) that involve engagement are further distinguished by their goals. Coping can be viewed as efforts to enact or mobilize competence or personal resources, and resilience can be viewed as the successful outcome of these actions (Compas et al., 2001). Volitional and involuntary responses to stress may be viewed as distinct reactions, yet involuntary responses to stress may influence volitional responses, and voluntary responses may affect involuntary reactions. For example, the release of emotions can occur through an involuntary ventilation of emotions (crying) or through a controlled process such as writing a dairy about emotional distress (Compas et al., 2001).

Compas and colleagues (2001, p. 89) distinguish between involuntary stress responses, which describe immediate and automatic reactions to stressful situations, and coping, which refers to "regulatory efforts that are volitionally and intentionally enacted specifically in response to stress."

In an attempt to clarify the complexity of coping strategies among children, a multi-factors model was identified in a study of 437 Dutch children, grades 4–6 (Boo & Wicherts, 2009). The following coping behaviors were reported:

- *Problem-focused strategies* (consisting of controlled cognitive decision-making, direct problem-solving and seeking understanding of the situation)
- *Positive restructuring* (reframing the emotional meaning of the stress including positivity, control, and optimism)
- *Distraction and avoidance strategies* (doing something else, and including physical release of emotions such as crying or shouting, distracting activities, repression, and wishful thinking)
- *Support and help-seeking strategies* (support for actions and support for feelings)

Active voluntary coping strategies, such as engagement and problem-focused coping, have been consistently associated with better adjustment. They include problem solving, cognitive restructuring, and positive reappraisal of stressors. Since these coping strategies are characterized by a careful conscience analysis of the stressful situation, they often focus attention on the positive aspects of the situation and generate alternative positive and hopeful thoughts. In contrast, attempts of avoidance coping (emotional, cognitive, and behavioral avoidance), social withdrawal, emotional ventilation or discharge, wishful thinking, and self-blame are often associated with poor adjustment, more symptoms, and lower competence. The focus is on the disengagement with the stressor or one's emotions, on negative cognitions about the self and the situation, and on unregulated release or ventilation of emotions. These responses may reflect inadequate skills in modulating and regulating the experience and expressions of negative emotions.

However, in reality, the situation is more complex, and studies showed the interactive nature of coping reactions that required a more flexible appreciation of the reciprocity of personal and environmental factors. For example, disengagement and avoidance were sometimes related to better adjustment in coping with relatively uncontrollable stressors. When children could not change the stress, their effective solution would change their emotional perceptions of and reactions to the stress. For example, avoidance strategies in reaction to conflicts with peers were associated with less risk for victimized and bullied children. Reactions of disengagement even provided some protective benefits, and coping responses were most efficacious if they matched the controllability of the stressor (Compas et al., 2001). Thus, in different situations, distraction and avoidance coping may be considered either as an expression of adjustment or of maladjustment (Boo & Wicherts, 2009; Kliewer & Sandler, 1993). In line with the salutogenic conceptualization (Antonovsky, 1979), a more generalized understanding of effective coping has been proposed, stipulating the advantage of a wide repertoire of coping approaches and the importance of personal flexibility as the predictive factors of adjustment and resilience.

In our studies (Margalit, 1994), children's observations and parents' interviewing disclosed that many children reacted to stress by individualized combined coping reactions. Their immediate reactions sometimes expressed uncontrolled anger, emotional outbursts, or attempts to distance themselves, preferring solitary activities. Yet, after a short while, several children were able to pursue effective cognitive problem-solving or to ask for help and social support, while others would continue to express their distressed and sad emotions. Thus, the impact of avoidance and approach strategies depended on their mutual interrelations and combinations. A wide repertoire of coping and a flexibility to adopt sequential coping approaches were valuable in securing resilience and effective dealing with stress. This awareness to the complex multi-stages' reactions provides clarifications to the inconsistent research results that use simplistic single-step understanding. Children tend to develop a "coping style," using several categories of coping strategy more often than others (Shiota, 2006).

It can be concluded that the wide range of coping strategies and the flexibility in children's choices were extremely important in predicting effective coping. Sociable children were noted in their wide range of coping strategies as well as in their flexible use of them. Thus, coping strategies can not be evaluated as good or bad without sufficient information on the context, the nature of the stressor, and the characteristics of the coping individual. Children's reactions to stress are a complex combination of cognitive and behavioral multi-stages of coping activities. It is usually expected that older children will be able to use more cognitive and complex strategies and emotion-regulation strategies than younger children. However, research results have not been consistent (Boo & Wicherts, 2009). The comparison of a younger group of children (9–14 year olds) with an older group (15–18 year olds) confirmed that older children used a broader range of coping strategies and made less use of distraction (Donaldson, Prinstein, Danovsky, & Spirito, 2000), Yet, no significant age differences were found in additional studies (Boo & Wicherts, 2009). Similarly, inconsistent gender differences were reported regarding the differences between boys and girls in the use of problem solving, the usages of distracting actions, wishful thinking, and the requests for social support (Boo & Wicherts, 2009; Hampel & Petermann, 2005). The results of the research demonstrated the need to acknowledge the complexity and heterogeneity of the coping behavior of children as reflecting varied individual differences within different contextual conditions.

Coping with Loneliness

In line with coping models that were presented earlier, studies that examined coping with loneliness revealed similar tendencies. The following major coping profiles were identified by studies from different cultures and age groups (Margalit, 1994; Rokach & Brock, 1998; Rokach, 1999; Van Buskirk & Duke, 1991):

Reflection, acceptance of the loneliness, and "sad passivity." These children were aware of their loneliness, but their appraisal processes (Compas et al., 2001) confirmed that they could not change it. Their activities ranged from recognition of their problem to avoidant coping behaviors, including involuntary expressions of distress such as crying, oversleeping, sitting and thinking, overeating, spending time watching television, and using the Internet. Surprisingly, the coping style of "sad passivity" did not distinguish between lonely and non-lonely adolescents. This finding emphasized the uniqueness of the non-lonely reactions even within this category. These adolescents used this coping approach only temporarily and in preparation for a more active coping style. Thus, avoidance and disengagement for some children were considered positive reactions, providing time for reflection, energizing and facilitating approach, and problem-solving coping. Non-lonely youngsters used the coping strategies of a "sad-passive" mode to provide themselves with a relief time for overcoming their frustrations toward a more active reaction. In contrast, lonely individuals remained in the sad-passive mode for much longer periods (Van-Buskirk & Duke, 1991). When asked, *"What can you do when you feel lonely?"* a lonely pre-adolescent child remarked quietly but emphatically, *"There's nothing you can do, just to be sad."* Similar behavior patterns were reported for lonely children and youth in different environmental contexts, such as the Internet. Youth who avoided dealing with their loneliness problems offline, also tended to avoid dealing with them online. Respondents who coped with loneliness, using rumination, reflection, or passive avoidant coping, also used the Internet in a similar manner (Seepersad, 2004).

Active search for social contacts and friends. This coping style referred to active attempts to change the social situation. Children's efforts were focused on creating new social contacts and extending the existing ones through the use of approach and active behaviors. Children tried to change their peers' attitude toward them by adding instrumental benefits to connections such as *"bringing a skateboard or a ball," "inviting a child to play with you new (and exciting) computer games."* Children's activities were directed at forming new relationships with children. They also tended to use the existing network more fully. This type of coping involved the initiation of activities through behaviors such as calling (or texting) a peer, suggesting help to a child who was struggling with a task, visiting someone, trying to meet new children at the local community center, and participating in youth clubs. These efforts revealed the children's willingness to compromise by seeking less desirable companionship (especially younger children), in order to play with somebody. These efforts were sometimes successful, fostering the achievement of the desired goals. Children were invited and welcomed to the group. Yet others described frustrations, disappointments, peer rejection, and feeling used and even abused when friends took advantage of their games, and afterward rejected them.

Social Support and asking for help from peers and adults. In order to avoid the loneliness experience, some children requested help from peers or adults. Children approached peers or adults asking assistance, and acknowledging the sad reality that they had not been successful in changing their social situation by themselves. The definitions of social support can be broadly described in terms of three perspectives (Vangelisti, 2009). The first is a sociological perspective reflecting the degree to which individuals are integrated into a social group and based on the number and/or the levels of interconnectedness with people's social relationships. The second is a psychological perspective that describes the perceived availability of support, assessing the type or amount of support that individuals get from their social network (*received support*) or the type or amount of support they believe is available to them (*perceived support*). The third is a communication perspective, with a focus on the interactions that occur between the providers and recipients of support, evaluating the verbal and nonverbal behaviors that individuals engage in when they are trying to provide someone with help (*enacted support*).

The psychological benefit of having reliable, dependable access to one or more supportive figures in times of need supports the effective management of distress and restoration of emotional balance. Even anticipated support and thoughts of available and supportive others has positive effects on mood and mental health (Mikulincer & Shaver, 2009). Repeated experiences of support contribute to an extensive network of positive mental representations, which play an important part in maintaining emotional stability, an optimistic and hopeful attitude toward challenges, and an inoculation against loneliness. In addition, interactions with supportive and caring others may reduce worries about being rejected, criticized, or abused. Such interactions indicate that a supportive other is unlikely to betray one's trust, react coldly or abusively to expressions of need, or respond unfavorably to bids for closeness and support. Positive self-concept and feelings of competence are often promoted by feelings of support.

Individual differences were revealed in the distinct aspects of social support such as anticipating support, perceived and experienced support, support seeking, and support provision. In addition, the beneficial aspects of the community support were also included in a wider appreciation of social support, including institutionalized support. Police and fire departments, hospitals, schools and libraries, recreation centers, and social agencies may also play supportive roles in children's lives. A welcoming teacher in the first day of high school will be considered a supportive experience even to a skeptic anxious adolescent. Receiving the first library card from a smiling librarian can be a very supportive event for an anxious child, not only with regard to the librarian as an individual, but also to the library as a welcoming institution (Sarason & Sarason, 2009).

However, research on the impact of social support has not been consistently positive, and has, in fact, provided mixed results. Indeed supportive help can have positive or negative effects, depending on several factors, including the needs of the recipient and the sensitivity of the provider. Discussing negative events with sympathetic and emphatic others can enhance feelings of competence, trust, and control. On the other hand, there is increasing evidence that discussing difficulties (including academic difficulties and loneliness) with others contributes to negative outcomes (Altermatt, 2007). This coping behavior may hurt children's self-competence when they need to recognize and to detail their social failure. For example, telling a friend about social frustration may lead to positive adjustment, if the friend emphatically provides advice and express support. Yet, if the friend criticizes or teases the child or the adolescent about the failure, regarding the distress as a true reflection of inabilities, or expresses hurting judgment, it will cause disappointment and frustrations. Several children who used social support as a coping method asked classmates to call them when they went to local youth activities. Others approached adults such as teachers, counselors, and parents, sharing with them how lonely they felt, and expecting them to help or support their efforts to find playmates. This request for help may be manifested either as a direct-approach activity, where the child expresses an expectation that the help-provider will offer assistance in finding a friend, and more often as a less-direct approach activity, where consultation or advice is sought in terms of "How can I. . .?" Sometimes the lonely child feels confident and discloses that he or she is lonely. Yet, many times the major focus of complaint may be boredom, expressed as "I have nothing to do and no friends to play with."

The responses of others play a key role in determining the consequences of social interactions. Seeking and receiving help and advice from significant others can lead to better adjustment if family members and peers respond in helpful ways. When children share and disclosed failures, expecting to get informational or emotional support, these interactions may not yield the desired effects. Personal characteristics and appraisal of the stress may promote only a little hope to get sufficient social support and help in dealing with those events, and the anxious preoccupation may decrease the adolescents' seeking for help, and contribute to feelings of loneliness (Larose, Guay, & Boivin, 2002). Social support from parents, peers, and teachers interact, and may even compensate distressful situations. Higher peer stress and less companionship support from peers were associated with lower social self-concept and experiences of social isolation. However, emotional support from the family had a buffering effect on the influence of peer stress on feelings of depression (Wenz-Gross, Siperstein, Untch, & Widaman, 1997).

Social support played a more important role for girls than for boys (Altermatt, 2007). The stronger gender differences in social support seeking were reported in the interactions of younger students with friends. Girls more than boys viewed intimate disclosure with friends as an important friendship feature at younger ages. Girls were more likely to report talking about difficulties they were having in school, expecting to receive informational and emotional support, and indeed they received the support they desired. Yet, sharing academic difficulties with friends was associated with higher levels of worry for both boys and girls. Maybe high levels of sharing reflected a continued preoccupation with the failure experience and concern with how one's friends might evaluate oneself in light of the failure. In conclusion, social support is one of the most popular and preferred modes of coping with loneliness (Sarason & Sarason, 2009). It is widely accepted that expanding social networks and establishing close relationships are among the most effective ways of coping with loneliness.

Distancing, denial, and increased solitude activities. Distancing and denial-depicted behaviors such as exaggerated consumption of food, medication, alcohol and drug abuse, self-induced isolation, and an overall denial of the experience of loneliness. Distancing is a form of coping in which the individual recognizes the problem but deliberately makes efforts to put it out of his or her mind (Folkman & Moskowitz, 2004). A denial coping style entails attempts to deny feelings of loneliness or minimize their distressful impact. Several children told us that when they heard that they were not invited to the party, they decided not to think about it. Sometimes they felt very tired and went to sleep. Others watched television, and/or went to the fridge and ate ice cream. Children described occasions when they were rejected by peers, yet they did not feel lonely, or they did not mind, yet they continuously reported overeating and minor physical complains (such as tummy aches and headaches). Sometimes they reported distancing coping, and explained that their friendships were sources of pain and distress, and they preferred loneliness than confronting with children's bullying. Distancing is considered adaptive when nothing can be done or when active alternatives may increase stress, for example, socializing with aggressive and victimizing children to avoid loneliness.

Increased leisure and extracurricular activities can be considered as part of the distancing coping category, yet it is often treated as a separate subcategory. It includes active solitary performance such as participating in leisure and sport as well as taking on extracurricular hobbies to make one's solitary time more pleasant, productive, and meaningful. It addresses the active pursuit of daily activities, including a wide range of obligations, responsibilities as well as leisure involvements. Several individuals prefer active solitary activities, while others participate more in group activities, and thus maximize their opportunities for social contacts. Being active, involved in the community and participating in activities that may open the door to new social relations and friendships are predictors of wellbeing. Being active also enables increased satisfying that has been considered beneficial regardless of age or gender (Rokach, 2001). This subcategory includes a wide variety of activities such as exercising, studying, working; reading and writing; listening to music, playing computer games, walking and running, swimming; spending time on a hobby; and going to a movie. These activities represent active efforts to change the individual's social needs or desires, through a widening of the repertoire of tasks and activities that are undertaken and considered enjoyable and satisfying, yet can be performed alone. This subcategory has an additional importance, considering research findings that pointed at the relations between loneliness and reduced physical activities. This activating strategy may buffer these tendencies and contribute to health (Hawkley, Thisted, & Cacioppo, 2009).

The disadvantage of this coping approach is that although it may reduce the inner experience of loneliness, it may not change the children's actual isolated social status. However, rather than staying immersed in self-pity, emotional pain, helplessness, and sadness, individuals who actively pursue not only their daily responsibilities, but extended leisure and fun activities, may produce new opportunities for social relations and decrease their loneliness (Rokach, 2001) In addition, since decreased social activity and increased active engagement in solitary activities were found to be two independent dimensions and not on a continuum (Csikszentmihalyi & Larson, 1984), children could be very active in both social-interpersonal and solitary activities, whereas others might remain inactive in both and complain of boredom. Thus, widening the repertoire of rewarding activities may be useful to the lonely children, decreasing their dependence on others for experiencing satisfaction, and increasing their positive mood and personal control, and yet not reducing or competing with their opportunities to identify effective ways to cope with their loneliness.

Aggressive, disruptive behaviors. Several children reported that they acted out their anger, annoyance, and frustration through expressions of overt aggression and disruptiveness when they experienced rejection by peers and loneliness (Margalit, 1994). These children and adolescents shared with us their angry and painful feelings that had lead to their disruptive and uncontrolled aggression. At times, they considered their disruptive behavior toward peers and teachers whose behavior was viewed as an intentional insult leading to their feelings of hopelessness, as justified activities. They did not attempt to control their anger, since their hopelessness triggered feelings of despair, wishes for revenge, and desperate thoughts regarding "having nothing to lose."

Self-Development and understanding. This category refers to increased understanding of one's self. It may result from newly acquired friends or following effective individualized counseling and/or participation in focused group therapy. Only few adolescents reported using this coping approach (Rokach, 2001).

Independent individuals who showed more autonomy were more engaged in individual pursuits and cognitive reframing. The more dependent individuals relied more on external sources of support and tended to participate in physical activities and ask for help. Chronic loneliness and additional personal difficulties (such as learning disabilities) also contributed to the differences, and students who had a low loneliness level used self-confident, optimistic, and social-support-seeking coping styles, while students who had high loneliness levels used hopeless and submissive coping styles (Cecen, 2008).

Interviews of children with learning disabilities (80 students aged 8–14 years) (Margalit, 1994) illustrated the impact of their disabilities on their coping activities, disclosing their acceptance of their social distresses. These students were engaged in two major coping activities: avoidance coping and alternative-solitary activities (approach coping with a focus on activities that can be performed alone, and activation of internal processing). Many students acknowledged their difficulties in developing satisfying social interrelations, and either accepted this fact trying to develop enjoyable activities to fill their free time and to replace their social needs, or stayed alone and felt self-pity. Only a few students attempted to directly change their social situation, either through active performance (searching for a friend and being ready to compromise by playing with younger students) or by asking for the help of a peer or an adult. According to students' self-reports, only a small number of children were engaged in aggressive or disruptive activities following their loneliness experience, usually when they felt very angry and hurt.

Coping with loneliness at different developmental stages is a highly neglected research issue. A recent study (Besevegis & Galanaki, in press) further examined children's ways of coping with loneliness during early, middle, and late childhood. The analysis of interviews of 180 children, fourth and sixth graders from Athens and Greece, identified several families of coping:

1. Problem solving – instrumental action (Children attempted to make new friends, seek advice usually from adults, as well as seek professional help).
2. Problem solving – self-improvement such as acquiring social skills and restoring relations.
3. Cognitive problem solving such as searching for causes and possible solutions.
4. Helplessness, passivity, or doing nothing.

5. Escape – wishful thinking, with children who expressed wishes for friends or fantasizing different social realities.
6. Self-reliance – emotion regulation (active attempts to regulate stressful thinking).
7. Self-reliance – behavior regulation (attempts to change behavior).
8. Self-reliance – emotional expression and discharge.
9. Contact-seeking with parents, siblings, peers/friends, grandparents, teachers.
10. Support-seeking, expecting to get varied types of support such as material and emotional support.
11. Accommodation – behavioral distraction and keeping busy.
12. Accommodation – cognitive restructuring, using intentional forgetting techniques, and thinking about other topics.
13. Negotiation and trying to convince their peers to include them in the desired activity.
14. Submission (rumination and catastrophizing).
15. Opposition (and expressions of aggression and anger).

Within these groups of behaviors, age-related differences for coping with loneliness were identified, and increased emphasize was noticed from early to late childhood in the following types: behavioral distraction, cognitive restructuring, and behavior regulation. Older children, who had more autonomy, knowledge, and experience, seemed to have more opportunities to engage in alternative pleasurable activities and thus were more able to regulate their behavior than younger children, yet helplessness was unique, since it did not reveal age differences. Overall, the number and variety of coping strategies increased with development and preadolescents reported significantly more ways of coping than younger children.

Although coping research has flourished during recent years, not many studies to date have examined expressions of cultural influences on coping styles. In an attempt to identify how adolescents from four European countries – Germany, U.K., France, and Italy – ($N = 3,000$, aged 12–18 years) experienced feelings of loneliness and to compare how they were able to cope with these stressors (Haid et al., 2009) adolescents' perceptions of emotional stress (i.e., feelings of loneliness and dejection) were examined. The comparisons revealed differences among the countries with respect to perceptions of loneliness. Adolescents from Italy and France reported high levels of stress related to loneliness, and German and British adolescents seemed to suffer less from feeling lonely. Perceptions of stress were slightly influenced by gender, with female adolescents experiencing more stress than their male age mates. In contrast to the differences in stress perceptions, suggesting a strict division between Northern countries and Romanic countries, similarities in coping behaviors were clearly demonstrated. In all four countries, nearly equal proportions of proactive coping strategies (i.e., discussing the problem with parents or friends, reflecting about the problem) as well as withdrawal coping strategies were reported.

An additional perspective in exploring coping is the focus on loneliness as a reaction to lack of pleasurable engagement (Joiner, Lewinsohn, & Seeley, 2002) in addition to the more conventional conceptualization of painful disconnection. To further study the conceptualization that lack of pleasurable engagement may represent the core of loneliness, there has been a need to distinguish between two aspects of the pleasure experience: anticipatory pleasure and consummatory pleasure. Anticipatory social pleasures often emerge from past experiences and memories of consummatory pleasures. Thus, many lonely children with memories of social frustrations will not anticipate pleasure from future social encounters, and these emotional anticipations will reduce their active coping efforts to join the group.

This differentiation between aspects of pleasure was further examined in studies of resilience (the ability to bounce back from negative events by using positive emotions to cope), in attempts to find out how resilient individuals "bounce back" from stressful experiences quickly and effectively. It was found that focusing attention on positive emotional granularity (the tendency to represent experiences of positive emotion with precision and specificity rather than globally) extended the clarification to the impacts of different positive emotions (Tugade, Fredrickson, & Feldman Barrett, 2004). Individual differences in the propensity to label positive emotional experiences (anticipated as well as experienced) with precision were associated with coping styles' effectiveness. Individuals who reported their emotional experience in differentiated terms with discrete emotion labels (happy, content, sad, angry, etc.), in an attempt to capture their distinctiveness, used larger repertoires of emotion-regulation strategies. They were less likely to use self-distraction during stressful times, and were more engaged in the coping process, were less automatic in their responses, and were more likely to examine their behavioral options before acting. Their reported coping seemed "proactive" and future-oriented (Tugade et al., 2004).

Entry Behavior of Young Lonely Children

In order to exemplify the complexity and interdependence of the strategies' meaning within the context of the social environment even of very young children, research on "entry behavior" among preschool and elementary school children will be provided. One of the most difficult and complex tasks that children face from the early stages of socialization development, is to join a group of children (i.e., a playing group) and to become involved in peer activities. Mothers and teachers reported that lonely and isolated children often met rejection when they tried to join their playing classmates. Many times when the teacher approached children asking why they were standing alone in the courtyard, they may have provided answers such as "nobody played with me" or "they (the group of children) told me to go away." Shy and anxious children, as well as children with attention and externalizing difficulties, encounter more barriers in joining groups of children. Their unsuccessful attempts further the development of an avoidance coping style. The coping strategies that they develop during these early unsuccessful attempts to join the group may be generalized and internalized into a coping style of lonely youngsters. Thus, researchers were motivated to explore how young children approach and enter ongoing activities of their peers (Wilson, 2006), and to find out whether lonely children adopt different coping approaches.

Successful initiation of entry into the peer play group is a prerequisite for further social interactions, whereas unsuccessful entry performance may lead to feelings of rejection and loneliness. This behavior can be considered a major, complicated task that children already face at the preschool stage (Putallaz & Wasserman, 1990). It is tempting to assume that one of the typical characteristics of socially rejected and lonely children is their failure in entry behavior, and that their coping strategies are basically different. However, research found that about 50% of initial attempts of all young children to enter a group resulted in rejection or ignorance by peers. Evidence suggested the existence of a core behavioral pattern that children exhibited with different partners and in different contexts (Guralnick, Neville, Hammond, & Connor, 2007). Those children who succeeded in joining a group gradually developed a repertoire of strategies and skills and were able to select the ones that would help them in persuading their companions to let them participate in the group's activities. Several basic skills enabled the successful entry into an ongoing group activity:

> *Understanding the group activity.* Cognitive difficulties may cause children to misjudge the group behavior and to use mistaken behaviors as a key to seeking entry.
> *Controlling impulsive behavior.* Self-control is essential to enable children to observe and listen before attempting to enter the group in order to suggest relevant activities and contents. They need self-regulation to prevent disruptive behavior that may provoke rejection.
> *Persistence.* Every child is rejected from time to time. To overcome social rejection, children have to persist in their varied attempts to enter the group.
> *Alternative activities.* Children must be able and ready to propose alternative activities should they face initial failure and rejection.

Studies of shy children further illustrated the multidimensional nature of the difficulties that children encountered in their attempts to join a group and provided in-depth insight to the developing aspects of their coping approaches (Findlay, Coplan, & Bowker, 2009). Research reported that shy children experienced difficulties in initiating social relations. In consequence, they were inclined to retreat to solitary activities and tended to stay alone, using avoidance coping more often. They obtained less social support and were reluctant to ask for help. They may have blamed themselves for being too emotional and worrying about what they were going to do. Shy children relied on more internalizing (emotion-focused) coping rather than problem-focused coping due to their wariness or anxiety. They often selected strategies which required minimal assertiveness or social involvement, or which drew minimal attention to themselves. Their internalizing coping styles may have partially accounted for some of the negative outcomes associated with shyness.

These anxious children have lower expectations for experiencing pleasurable social activities, and may be more apt to using "maladaptive" coping strategies, which lead to increased loneliness and further anxiety. By selecting internalizing strategies and avoiding stressful contacts, shy children are indeed able to delay the immediate stressor in the short term, but at the same time may feel worse for not being able to directly address the problem/stressor. In addition, in the long run, they will not learn how to manage their social anxiety nor learn and experience age-appropriate social skills – and thus exacerbate their social isolation. Sometimes, youngsters who identified themselves as victimized by peers blamed themselves for their peer-relationship problems. Self-blame and avoidant coping can lead to a variety of negative outcomes of an internalizing nature in addition to loneliness, such as depression, low self-esteem, and increased withdrawal, and seriously treated as a self-reinforcing cycle of negative socio-emotional and social-cognitive functioning for socially withdrawn children (Reijntjes, Stegge, & Terwogt, 2006; Rubin, Coplan, & Bowker, 2009). Studies of leisure activities present the wide range of coping solutions for the lonely children in their distress struggles.

Leisure Activities

Leisure may be associated with a number of risk and protective factors that enhance children and adults' resiliency when confronted with negative life experiences, or enhance their experience of social isolation (Caldwell, 2005). Specific aspects of leisure activities may act as protective factors by being personally meaningful, intrinsically interesting and/or challenging; offering social support and friendships; contributing to a sense of competence and/or self-efficacy; offering a sense of personal control, choice, and self-determination; being relaxing, and/or distracting the individual from negative life events. Yet, their value to mental health differs. Active leisure activities such as sport were widely considered beneficial. However, inconsistent results were reported regarding passive leisure activities (Holder, Coleman, & Sehn, 2009; Joudrey & Wallace, 2009). Television watching, computer involvement, and media watching were reported as the most popular activities for lonely children, yet the value seemed to vary. The usages of media as a coping strategy varied – and for some children it may be considered as a passive escapism and a way to avoid thinking about stress, while for others it was an active coping strategy. Media users may apply (a) problem-focused approach coping in aiming to find guidance from the media to solve their problems or (b) emotion-focused approach coping in seeing that others have similar problems and how they deal with them (Knobloch-Westerwick, Hastall, & Rossmann, 2009). Moore and Schultz (1983) pointed attention to the relations between loneliness and watching television. Students who reported feeling more lonely watched television for longer periods of time. Yet, several children with disabilities reported not only that they spent long hours watching television, but also that they found this time to be very enjoyable. They suggested that when they had nothing else to do, this was their preferred activity. Thus, watching television for children with difficulties may be considered a solitary alternative activity, although it may also be regarded as a passive activity, requiring careful investigation of the child's interpretations of the situation and attributions.

Playing computer games has been widely depicted as one of the most preferred activities of children (lonely and not lonely alike) (Klimmt, Schmid, & Orthmann, 2009). Computer activities are considered both age-appropriate solitary activities and active efforts to expand group activities. A recent social context of game playing has shaped the psychological experiences in multiplayer online games (Lim & Lee, 2009). Computer games and simulations are attractive and challenging, and they stimulate curiosity and fantasy. Solitary computer activities are considered extremely valuable for lonely children as an independent yet pleasurable solution for "filling" unstructured leisure time. Solitary computer games may assist these youngsters in distracting themselves from self-pity and angry thoughts, and at the same time in developing an area of competence that may foster self-esteem and be used at a later stage as a basis for expanding companionship relations and participating in multiplayer virtual contexts. However, individual differences were noticed between youngsters who developed an "addiction" to solitary computer games and continued to play alone, and those youngsters who, with renewed motivation after periods of solitary activity, actively utilized their new competency as a springboard and facilitator for new social relations.

In conclusion, both computer games and television watching can be used by lonely children as solitary activities to fill up their leisure time. The children's ability to exploit these activities for enhancing peer relations depends on their level of motivation to pursue social interactions and personal energy. An examination of the motivation of lonely students highlighted contradictory trends and reflected individual differences. Sometimes children described their experience as one of paralyzing hopelessness, fatigue, and lack of strength. In our interviews, children gave responses such as

> *When you're lonely you can't do anything. You're better off just going home and closing the door of your room behind you.*

However, if stressor-related media content helps the individual to interpret his or her situation more positively, then its beneficial value as an emotion-focused coping has to be considered. Problem-focused coping occurs more often when the individual appraises the challenging circumstances as changeable, and emotion-focused coping is more likely to be adopted if the problem seems unchangeable; however, in many stressful occurrences, both approaches are combined. Media-use can serve both coping behaviors. Individuals, who face a distressful situation of feeling excluded from a desired group of peers, can turn to the media to find unrelated, absorbing contents that will provide an effective distracter that enables them to forget the stress (emotion-focused coping). However, being attracted to contents related to their problems (individuals who are struggling with social challenges) may also provide insight and information that can help address the problems (problem-focused coping). Many times, the behavior serves both types of coping (approach coping and avoidance coping), depending on the individuals' characteristics and behavior style.

To sum up, the appraisal of the stress may predict the different usages of the media and the choices of leisure. Preferences of free-time activities vary because they have to meet specific needs and they are shaped by the resources and contexts in which they unfold. For example, individuals, who experience strains that they consider changeable, will adopt a problem-solving coping and seek advice from the media and Internet forums on how to solve the issue. In contrast, when unpleasant conditions are perceived as permanent and unchangeable, these perceptions may instigate escapist avoidance of the issue (i.e., watching a thrilling science-fiction movie) or emotion-focused coping attempts to come to terms with the adversity (such as observing fictional others' emotions in similar circumstances depicted in a movie) (Knobloch-Westerwick et al., 2009). The accompanying emotions during leisure activities reflect their coping impact, but also affect the children's behavior choices.

Emotions and Coping

Understanding emotions is critical for all phases of the coping process, from the first stages of attention, detection, and appraisals of threat to action readiness and coordinating responses during stressful situations. Emotions are considered "a kind of radar and rapid response system," or "biologically endowed processes that permit extremely quick appraisals of situations and equally rapid preparedness to act to sustain favorable conditions and deal with unfavorable conditions" (Cole et al., 2004). The differentiation between positive and negative emotions is important, and both types of emotions may have significant adaptive functions. Negative emotions such as anger or loneliness may prepare the individual in facing the difficulty and also in communicating distress and needs. Thus, adaptive coping consists of flexible access to a wide range of different emotions as well as the ongoing cooperation of emotions with other components of the action system (Holodynski & Friedlmeier, 2006). Since coping refers to a subset of inner self-regulatory processes during stressful circumstances (Compas et al., 2001), the processes include the regulation of emotion and the regulation of behavior during the emotional arousal. When confronted with stress, individuals attempt not only to deal with the emotional experience, but also to coordinate motor behavior, attention, cognition, and reactions adaptable to the social and physical environments.

The experience of positive emotions is hypothesized to facilitate more adaptive responses to environments, which create greater learning opportunities and accrual of resources, further facilitating effective coping. Positive emotions are current markers of wellbeing, and also produce future adjustment. The study of affect and coping at two assessment periods indicated that positive affect predicted improved coping, that predicted increased positive affect. In other words, positive emotions create upward spirals toward effective coping and wellbeing (Fredrickson & Joiner,

2002). In contrast, frequent negative emotions are believed to narrow thoughts and behaviors, reducing learning and adaptation resources. Yet, positive and negative emotions may each be adaptive, depending on the circumstances. In life-threatening situations, narrowed thought action patterns that emerge due to negative emotions facilitate swift and focused actions with immediate benefits to the individual, such as survival. Positive emotions, however, are adaptive in circumstances that are not dangerous, enriching personal resources, promoting broadening global thinking, growth in coping resources, and contributing to psychological resiliency (Fredrickson, 2001). Negative emotions are part of life, but since the proportions of positivity and negativity (positivity about three times more than the negativity) were associated with human flourishing (Fredrickson & Losada, 2005), there is a need to explore children's loneliness within the wider perspective of hope, positive affect, and coping. Children's positive emotions in school were considered protective factors that were related to effective coping strategies, including problem-solving coping as well as social-support-seeking coping, and promoted school engagement (Reschly, Huebner, Appleton, & Antaramian, 2008). Positive affect was also associated with interpersonal trust. Low trust in others and their social support were predictive of increased current and future negative affect (Burns et al., 2008).

Children's loneliness cannot be treated in isolation, and it has been a source of distress not only to the children but also to their parents. Stressful events can shape family life through the different coping responses that family members adopt. The conceptualization of the family as a system and recognizing the reciprocal ongoing impacts of the family members require awareness of family coping styles.

Stress and Coping in the Family

Parents cope with family stresses, and react to children's requests for help. In addition, children's coping reactions are influenced by parental approaches and reactions to stress in general and to social distress in particular. Furthermore, parental stresses are not exclusively originated at home. They also reflect stresses initiated and occurring outside the home such as at work and with friends. Yet, the overall parental coping with their children's requests for support and help cannot be treated as isolated from their children's experiences, or from their coping and experiences at work. Within the systemic conceptualizations of the family, stressors experienced outside the home affect the emotional reactions and cognitions of all the family members. The term "spillover" has often been used to describe states such as negative mood or physiological arousal that are experienced and expressed within the family, even though the original precipitating conditions occurred outside the family setting, at school or at work. There is evidence of a straightforward carryover of physiology and mood from one context to the next (Repetti, Wang, & Saxbe, 2009). Negative mood generated outside the home may not only influence subsequent social behavior and coping of family members, but may also color the social perceptions within the family. Stresses experienced outside the family may increase the vulnerability to additional stresses, expressed both in children's appraisals as well as in their actual behavior. Thus, the understanding of appraisal processes is decisive for in-depth consideration of children's coping choices.

In addition, the expression "crossover" was also used to describe how stressors experienced by one family member affect another family member, such as a spouse or child. Crossover may occur through emotion-transmission processes, short-term links between one family member's momentary mood and another member's concurrent or subsequent emotional experience. Studies indicate (Repetti et al., 2009) that, like a row of falling dominos, the mood of one family member may be affected by the experiences encountered by another family member hours earlier and in a different setting (such as at school or at work). Parents also play a central role in determining the stressors, both chronic and acute, to which children are exposed and their appraisals. Of course, parents and children are not passive participants in emotion transmission, appraisals, and co-regulation processes. The understandings of these reciprocal processes whereby family members shape one another's unfolding coping responses to stressful days have preventive and intervention importance.

These reciprocal interactions play an important role in structuring parental coping reactions. Parents cannot avoid reacting to their children's distress and expressions of suffering. A mother told us that seeing her child excluded from the group's enjoyable activities "broke her heart." Parents' problems outside the home and conflicts between the parents can become additional stressors for children. Parents' characteristics, their strengths and challenges also contribute to the development of children's coping resources, such as their self-efficacy or social skills. Parents act as models for their children's coping through their own behavior, their interpretations of events, and accompanying emotions. Parents can also help children understand and learn from good and bad social experiences, including planning proactive coping to prevent their reoccurrence. Sometimes, when parents consider their children vulnerable and consistently distressed, parents may develop an over protective style, attempting to shield their children from stress. Yet, they may also prevent their children from developing effective age-appropriate coping strategies (Fox, Henderson, Marshall, Nichols, & Ghera, 2005). Thus, parents have to develop skills to appraise children's abilities and vulnerabilities, to adapt children's exposure to stress to their strengths, while providing sufficient support so that their children can learn to manage the stress well (Skinner & Zimmer-Gembeck, 2007). This challenge is especially difficult for parents of children with atypical development, who face increased overall general stress (Margalit & Raskind, 2009).

Parents use different coping approaches to meet the varied needs of stressful situations. Many parents of children with difficulties and disabilities adopted the avoidance coping style as an expression of their stressful reactions to their children's chronic difficulties (Margalit & Ankonina, 1991). This increased use of avoidance coping in families with and without disabled children predicted higher levels of negative and distressed parental affect, pinpointing attention to the crucial maladaptive role played by parents' attempts to deny a stressful reality. Additionally, many parents used active coping expressed through requesting and allocating help and support outside the family, including a search for relevant information in the Internet and active participation in parents' forums and discussion boards. Research focusing on the availability of social and community support has emphasized its importance for the growth and wellbeing of the family members.

The important role of families during different developmental stages in promoting children's academic achievement was widely reported in several studies, yet their contribution to children's social competence or loneliness was less examined. Academic socialization as an important part of parenting style had the strongest positive relation with children's achievements at school. Academic socialization included parents' communication of their expectations for achievement and value for education, fostering educational and occupational aspirations in their adolescents, discussing learning strategies with children, and making preparations and plans for the future, including linking ideas discussed in school with students' interests and goals (Hill & Tyson, 2009). We expected that parental social socialization would have a similar impact on children's social success and loneliness. Our current study (Idan, Sade & Margalit, 2009) consisted of 1,309 adolescents (679 boys and 630 girls) divided into two age groups (453 junior high students and 856 senior high students). Among these adolescents, 471 students were diagnosed as students with learning disabilities. A specific coping strategy was the focus of our concerns – the children's investment of effort. We wanted to identify the role of loneliness and hope in the children's coping, and to consider personal and familial characteristics.

Effort investment as children's coping style with their academic challenges was predicted by personal and systemic factors such as family cohesion (the closeness that family members feel toward one another), sense of coherence (self-perception), hope expectations, and the loneliness experience. Earlier research reported that adolescents with positive and close family relationships used more active coping both at home and at school. Positive relationships with teachers also predicted active-coping behaviors, especially at school (Zimmer-Gembeck & Locke, 2007). In our study, as presented in Fig. 7.1, children's loneliness and their sense of coherence did not predict the readiness to invest effort in their academic roles, but was mediated by the impact of hope. Lonely children who had hopeful coping styles were ready to invest more effort in different age-appropriate tasks and obligations. Family climate, the closeness that family members felt toward each other, the flexibility of their adaptation to change, and their sense of coherence predicted the children's loneliness as well as their hopeful thinking. Children from cohesive and flexible families and children with a stronger sense of coherence were more hopeful and less lonely. Family cohesiveness also predicted the children's effort. Interestingly, loneliness did not directly predict children's investment of effort (even though the correlations between effort and loneliness were significant and negative), but rather indirectly, through the levels of hope (that were negatively related to loneliness).

The examination of the students with learning disabilities revealed similar results with two major differences. Loneliness predicted effort both directly (more loneliness predicted lower levels of effort), but also indirectly through hope, enabling hope to jointly impact effort. In addition, family cohesion predicted not only loneliness but also hope. However, it did not predict effort investment directly. The results of the study emphasized the importance of loneliness, relating the

a. Children with typical development

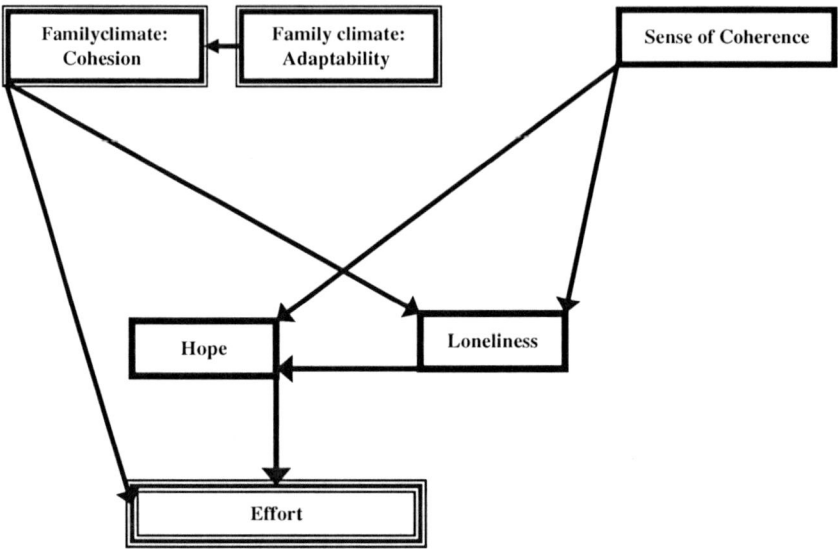

b. Children with learning disabilities

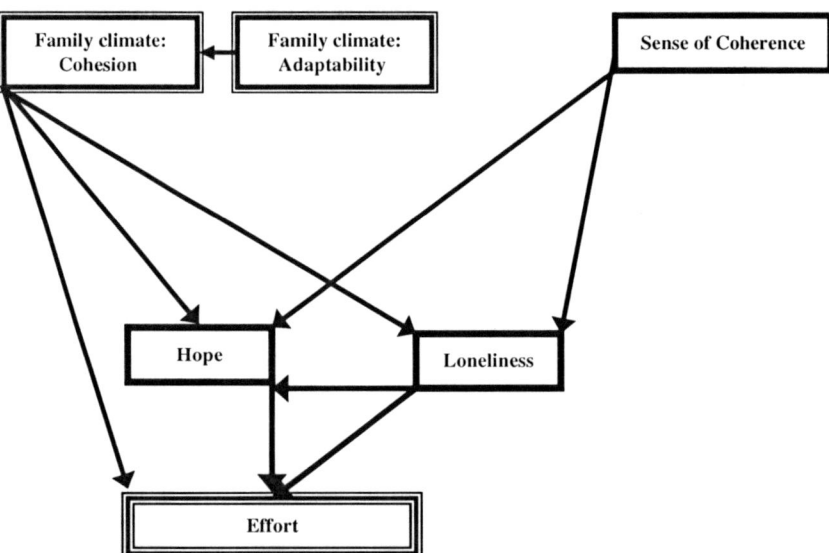

Fig. 7.1 Personal and familial predictors of children's effort: (**a**) children with typical development and (**b**) children with learning disabilities

significance of the social distress for explaining children's coping with academic challenges. Additionally, hopeful thinking had an important buffering role regarding risk factors. Thus the significant value of the search for hope, and the adaptation of hopeful thinking were established in this study. In addition to hope as a personal strength, additional studies proposed the importance of social support for empowering children and families when the individual strengths were not sufficient.

Parental Access to Social Support

Social support was theoretically considered a major resource for meeting family challenges, and fulfilling different parental needs (Adler & Fagley, 2005). Asking for help was considered an important coping strategy, yet research provided inconsistent results regarding the value of the social support for the parents' wellbeing. The social support construct consists of the people who are important in a parent's life, including a spouse or significant other, relatives, friends, and neighbors. Support may serve different needs such as requests for information, advice, and counseling. It may also provide important resources such as providing/sharing time to care for children, emotional support, and material support. Social support can be provided in different ways including formal help by professionals (i.e., psychologists, teachers) and informal support by nonprofessionals (i.e., extended family members, friends, and other parents) (Kossek, Pichler, Meece, & Barratt, 2008). Social support can improve parenting satisfaction, affecting the availability of mothers to their infants as well as the quality of mother–infant interactions (Bradley, Whiteside Mansell, Brisby, & Caldwell, 1997). Well-supported mothers were less restrictive and punitive with their infants than were less well-supported mothers, and frequency of contacts with sources of support improved the quality of parent–infant relationships (Crnic, Greenberg, Robinson, & Ragozin, 1984) as well as the parents' sense of their own effectiveness and competence (Bornstein, 2002).

Mothers often reported that community and friendship support were beneficial, but they insisted that the intimate support from spouses provided the most general positive consequences for maternal competence (Crnic et al., 1984). Emotional and practical support from extended family members and friends also enhanced maternal behavior and fostered positive parent–child relationships. Mothers with higher levels of social support were more nurturing and consistent in their parenting and less likely to use punitive strategies such as scolding and ridiculing. In addition, being a father or a mother may instigate feelings of loneliness especially during stressful periods, while the social support can reduce this distress by providing closeness and companionship (Cohen & Wills, 1985). Companionship and emotional support refer to feeling mutually close, expressing appreciation, and regarding the person as valued.

Material support is related to the provision of resources and actual assistance, whereas informational support involves advice and counseling. Often both types of supports were considered beneficial to families, yet contextual conditions and specific characteristics of the support providers and recipients interacted with their process. For example, in poorer, high crime neighborhoods, the positive influence of social support in bolstering parental nurturance and reducing punitiveness was diminished. In addition, receipt of social support was not always a positive process because, at times, the providers of support may have also served as sources of distress, dominating or criticizing the parent and causing him/her to feel incompetent (Ceballo & McLoyd, 2002). Thus, there is a need for in-depth examination of different forms of social support.

Most social support research has investigated the type and style of the different supports and support providers. Many mothers and fathers face difficulties in balancing their obligations to their working career and familial expectations. In order to take advantage of available support possibilities within the extended family and community, the parent must be able to ask for help and to accept it, in addition to maintaining interpersonal relations. Many studies deal with social support needs and provisions to families of children with disabilities. It is surprising that the needs of parents who struggle with day-to-day conventional demands and especially their needs for social support were not the focus of research, and were often neglected.

Parents of lonely children often felt the need for advice and support. Their distress was escalated when their children's agony awoke their own childhood memories of sad social disappointments. A mother shared with our research team that her daughter's loneliness left her completely helpless. She told us that when her daughter had difficulties in mathematics – she sat with her and taught her. She was not trying to avoid her responsibilities, and she was ready to provide help to her lonely child. Yet, she did not know what to do. When she tried to share her distress with friends, she felt threatened regarding the need to maintain her child's reputation as a "successful child." In addition, she did not have the confidence that she would get meaningful help. She was exploring different possibilities of consulting a professional such as the school's psychologist, but in addition she was eager to hear if other parents experienced similar problems, and what they were able to do. Thus she started looking for parental discussion groups.

The following messages were taken (with age and gender changes to protect anonymity) from several parents' discussion groups, illustrating the distress that parents experienced when their children shared their loneliness. Boys and girls of different ages struggled with social exclusion, loneliness experiences, bullying, and staying alone in the morning at school and during afternoons at home, and their mothers and fathers were looking for social support and advice in forums and discussion boards.

A mother wrote

> My first-grade daughter felt left out in the playground today. She told me that there were three girls playing together during recess time. She wanted to join them, but they ran away when she talked to them. So she felt bad today. What should I do? I told her that she didn't have to play with specific kids. She could play with any girl that she liked. But she said that she felt lonely. She was not a shy-type of girl and she was doing well in school and happy before this had happened.

The mother got a supportive answer from another mother:

"My heart goes out to you; it's very upsetting when you see your child upset." She got several advices from parents who shared similar experiences and reported how they dealt with the problem (encouraging the child, inviting children to their home, etc.).

A father of a 5-year-old boy wrote

My son has a tough time making friends. He is well liked in school, has several "friends," but no one seems to want to come over to play. He spends most of his time at home on the computer . . .because he says he has many virtual friends.

He got an answer from a mother:

When my son was in Kindergarten he did not take his first "I don't want to play with you" well either. You are not alone in your boat. I felt so bad for my "baby" when he cried over those boys.

Another mother wrote

My eight-year-old daughter is lonely. She loves to play with everyone. Now all the kids have grouped and she feels left out. She hangs out with the recess teacher a lot. This breaks my heart. She comes home sad and. . .doesn't want to go to school.

Bullying was raised by several parents as a cause for their children's loneliness:

My son is a victim of bullying. He is in middle school, and although he is very intelligent and a very good student, he is completely excluded now. It started off with a few boys and girls starting rumors presenting him as annoying/irritating, etc, and now he feels completely lonely. He often cries when he thinks that nobody is watching, and screaming at us and at his brother and sister.

These few typical examples bring the voices of concerned parents (in ways that protect their anonymity) to exemplify parental emotions and reactions when they are confronted with their children's loneliness. In today's "Internet World," virtual social connections challenge the classical conceptualization of social supports as resources, in terms of style and proximity. Parents feel that the anonymity together with the virtual companionship provides meaningful solutions. The immediate reactions of many mothers, their different proposals and expressions of understanding and empathy energize them. Extended discussion on virtual social support can be found in Chapter 6.

Raising a child with difficulties involves balancing a number of challenges, including seeking and gaining support (Canary, 2008). Thus, many studies explored the social-support possibilities available to parents with children from different medical and intellectual challenges. Parents, whose infants and young children with established disabilities have significant problems in cognitive, social-emotional, motor, or sensory domains of development, faced various challenges and difficulties in parenting (Guralnick, 2006). These challenges in turn created a set of stressors related to parents' increased needs not only to obtain information, but also to identify services for their child, to cope with issues related to family support and interpersonal relationships, and in addition to instill a sense of confidence in their ability to parent their child (Guralnick, 2001), but to provide support.

In addition to the function of the Web as a rich resource for information regarding special topics concerning children's disabilities, the Web also contains many electronic groups, chat rooms, and bulletin boards whose main purpose is to enable communication between parents with similar interests. Virtual support communities have been defined as a group of people with similar concerns who communicate via information technology (Zaidman-Zait & Jamieson, 2007). The goals of on-line support groups include collaboration between participants, information sharing, social and emotional support, and personal empowerment. The interaction with other parents whose children face similar challenges has been reported to provide support, reduce the parental sense of isolation, and suggest models and strategies for coping.

Many parents have benefited from these groups, and their dynamic formation reflected many needs from practical information to emotional support (Zaidman-Zait & Jamieson, 2007). Parents living in rural areas, who do not have close or regular contact with other parents of children with similar disabilities, may find on-line parent groups to be virtually the only regular means of parent-to-parent support. Those parents who have little or no time to spend outside the home, due to work obligations, children's challenging conditions or limited resources, benefit from this option. In addition, parents whose children have a low-incidence condition, such as rare syndromes, may locate other parents of similar children only through the worldwide community accessing the Internet. The analysis of the communication occurring in the Down Syndrome Discussion Group for a period of 6 months (Jones & Lewis, 2000) revealed that the group exchanged information on issues such as medical matters, new treatments, services, policies, and personal life stressors. In addition, there was a sense of shared identity and support. The content analysis of the on-line interactions indicated that the discussion group served as a support system for distressed parents, including exchanging information, expressing personal opinions, sharing experiences, obtaining advice, and receiving mutual support.

Summary and Conclusions

Studies of coping with loneliness emerged from the recognition of the significance of children's social distress as well as the appreciation of its importance for predicting parents' and teachers' anxiety and apprehension. This chapter explained how children and adolescents deal with the social adversity, calling for awareness of their ongoing and accumulative encounters that may shape their future development. Coping research focused attention on the attempts to ameliorate the anguish and emotional pain of social alienation. Indeed the study of children's coping has been focused on their emotional, cognitive, and behavioral responses to loneliness in real-life contexts. The in-depth understanding of the coping processes extends the understanding of the meaning of loneliness because it not only portrays how children deal with social adversities, but also how these ongoing and accumulative distresses shape their future development. Several coping-behavior categories are used to manage children's disturbing emotions, to help them think constructively, regulate and direct their behavior, control their autonomic arousal, and act to alter or decrease sources of stress. In this chapter the coping categories were first presented separately for methodological purposes. In reality, the interactive nature of coping reactions requires a more flexible appreciation to the reciprocity of personal and environmental factors. In this chapter the complexity of the construct was discussed focusing on the multidimensional processes that reflected (a) the choices of coping possibilities; (b) the personality dispositions that influenced the appraisal of the stressors to environmental conditions; (c) the appraisal of the individual's available resources; and (d) the contextual condition that enhanced or buffered the distressful experience. To exemplify the complexity of the different coping strategies and their impact, parental social support and children's entry behavior were presented.

There is a need to move from the conceptualization of differentiated typologies of coping, including dual-process models to families of coping, and further more to the understanding of individualized coping styles that dynamically reflect the interactions of individuals and contextual conditions. The dual-processes proposed several points of view based on psychological theories and theoretical emphasizes, and there was a noticeable correspondence between them. The approach/avoidance coping proposed the direction of the mental activities. The problem-focused/emotion-focused coping processes (cognitive/affective) described the nature of the mental processes. The voluntary/involuntary (controlled/automatic) coping processes provided information on the controllability and flexibility of the behavior and the reactive/proactive coping processes (past/future oriented coping) introduced the time element, and the ability to prepare, reduce, or even prevent stress. These coping strategies were combined into families of strategies and to more individualized profiles in which their impact was related and clearly understood only within the contextual and cultural background. Children's individual differences interacted with stressful reactions in different contextual conditions, and their evaluation was dependent on these complex connections.

For example, the commonly accepted views regarding the negative impact of avoidance approaches to children's wellbeing were challenged by circumstances in which the best solution was avoidance coping (i.e., distraction and alternative solitude activities were beneficial in unsolvable social threats). In addition, the behavior could be considered not only along a complex of similar coping strategies (families) but also as related to hierarchical multi-step solutions (for example, starting with avoidance passive reaction and after emotional ventilation moving to a more active problem solving). In order to achieve in-depth understanding of children's behavior, there is a need to move from examining unique single-coping behaviors to the appreciation of specific individualized profiles and coping families that combine several behaviors and reflect personal differences along the contextual dimensions. It can be concluded that the wide range of coping strategies and the flexibility in children's moving among them are extremely important in predicting effective coping. Sociable children were noted in their wide range of coping strategies as well as in their flexible use of them. Thus, coping strategies can not be evaluated as good or bad without sufficient information on the context, the nature of the stressor, and the characteristics of the coping individual. Children's reactions to stress are a complex combination of cognitive and behavioral multi-stages of coping activities. Usually it is expected that older children will be able to use more cognitive, complex, and emotion-regulation strategies than younger children, but individualized differences between children-necessitated dynamic approaches.

Examples were provided to clarify the complex and multidimensional interacting coping behavior: the children's entry behavior, leisure activities, and parental support seeking, including online social support. Overall, the number and variety of coping strategies increased with development and older children reported significantly more ways of coping than younger children. Older children, who had more autonomy, knowledge, and experience, seemed to have more opportunities to engage in alternative pleasurable activities and thus were more able to regulate their behavior than younger children, yet helplessness was unique, since it did not reveal age differences. In addition, since loneliness was often a reaction to lack of pleasurable engagements, the differentiation between anticipatory pleasure and consummatory pleasure provided a unique perspective (Gard, Gard, Kring, & John, 2006). Children, who did not anticipate that their social relations would be enjoyable, tended to cope with avoidance. A more detailed examination revealed individual differences in the propensity to label positive emotional experiences (anticipated as well as experienced) with precision, associated with coping styles' effectiveness. Individuals, who reported their emotional experience in more differentiated terms using discrete emotional labels (happy, content, sad, angry, etc.) and attempting to capture their distinctiveness, tended to use a more extended repertoire of emotion-regulation coping strategies. Sociable children were noted in their wide range of coping strategies as well as in their flexible use of them.

Thus, coping strategies can not be evaluated as good or bad without sufficient information on the context, the nature of the stressor, and the characteristics of the coping individual. Children's reactions to stress are a complex combination of cognitive and behavioral multi-stages of coping activities.

In conclusion, lonely children were caught in a vicious circle. Inadequate social behavior led to stress in social relationships, which was not countered by adequate repertoire of coping. This resulted in more rejection and more stress. The therapeutic implications of the coping research focused attention on the needs of children to develop a wide repertoire of coping strategies in order to enable a flexible move between the different levels of conscience awareness to the coping behaviors and automatic reactions. Chapter 8 will explore therapeutic and intervention implications.

References

Adler, M. G., & Fagley, N. S. (2005). Appreciation: Individual differences in finding value and meaning as a unique predictor of subjective well-being. *Journal of Personality, 73*(1), 79–114.
Altermatt, E. R. (2007). Coping with academic failure: Gender differences in students' self-reported interactions with family members and friends. *The Journal of Early Adolescence, 27*(4), 479–508.
Antonovsky, A. (1979). *Health, stress and coping.* San Francisco: Jossey-Bass.

Aspinwall, L. G., & Taylor, S. E. (1997). A stitch in time: Self-regulation and proactive coping. *Psychological Bulletin, 121*(3), 417–436.

Bargh, J. A., & Williams, E. L. (2006). The automaticity of social life. *Current Directions in Psychological Science, 15*(1), 1–4.

Besevegis, E., & Galanaki, E. P. (in press). Coping with loneliness in childhood. *European Journal of Developmental Psychology.*

Boo, G., & Wicherts, J. (2009). Assessing cognitive and behavioral coping strategies in children. *Cognitive Therapy & Research, 33*(1), 1–20.

Bornstein, M. H. (Ed.). (2002). *Handbook of parenting* (2nd ed.). Mahwah, NJ: Lawrence Erlbaum Associates.

Bradley, R. H., Whiteside Mansell, L., Brisby, J. A., & Caldwell, B. M. (1997). Parents' socioemotional investment in children. *Journal of Marriage and the Family, 59*(1), 77–90.

Burns, A. B., Brown, J. S., Sachs-Ericsson, N., Plant, E. A., Curtis, J. T., Fredrickson, B. L., et al. (2008). Upward spirals of positive emotion and coping: Replication, extension, and. initial exploration of neurochemical substrates. *Personality and Individual Differences, 44*(2), 360–370.

Caldwell, L. L. (2005). Leisure and health: Why is leisure therapeutic? *British Journal of Guidance and Counselling, 33*(1), 7–26.

Canary, H. E. (2008). Creating supportive connections: A decade of research on support for families of children with disabilities. *Health Communication, 23*(5), 413–426.

Ceballo, R., & McLoyd, V. C. (2002). Social support and parenting in poor, dangerous neighborhoods. *Child Development, 73*(4), 1310–1321.

Cecen, A. R. (2008). The effects of gender and loneliness levels on ways of coping among university students. *College Student Journal, 42*(2), 510–516.

Cohen, D. S., & Wills, T. A. (1985). Stress, social support, and the buffering hypothesis. *Psychological Bulletin, 98*(2), 310–357.

Cole, P. M., Martin, S. E., & Dennis, T. A. (2004). Emotion regulation as a scientific construct: Methodological challenges and directions for child development research. *Child Development, 75*(2), 317–333.

Compas, B. E., Connor-Smith, J. K., Saltzman, H., Thomsen, A. H., & Wadsworth, M. E. (2001). Coping with stress during childhood and adolescence: Problems, progress, and potential in theory. *Psychological Bulletin, 127*(1), 87–127.

Crnic, K. A., Greenberg, M. T., Robinson, N. M., & Ragozin, A. S. (1984). Maternal stress and social support – Effects on mother–infant relationship from birth to 18 months. *American Journal of Orthopsychiatry, 54*(2), 224–235.

Csikszentmihalyi, M., & Larson, R. (1984). *Being adolescent: Conflict and growth in the teenage years.* New York, NY: Basic Books.

Donaldson, D., Prinstein, M. J., Danovsky, M., & Spirito, A. (2000). Patterns of children's coping with life stress: Implications for clinicians. *American Journal of Orthopsychiatry, 70*(3), 351–359.

Ebata, A., & Moos, R. H. (1991). Coping and adjustment in distressed and healthy adolescents. *Journal of Applied Developmental Psychology, 12*(1), 35–54.

Findlay, L. C., Coplan, R. J., & Bowker, A. (2009). Keeping it all inside: Shyness, internalizing coping strategies and socio-emotional adjustment in middle childhood. *International Journal of Behavioral Development, 33*(1), 47–54.

Folkman, S., & Moskowitz, J. T. (2004). Coping: Pitfalls and promise. *Annual Review in Psychology, 55*, 745–774.

Fox, N. A., Henderson, H. A., Marshall, P. J., Nichols, K. E., & Ghera, M. M. (2005). Behavioral inhibition: Linking biology and behavior within a developmental framework. *Annual Review in Psychology, 56*, 235–262.

Fredrickson, B. L. (2001). The role of positive emotions in positive psychology. The broaden-and-build theory of positive emotions. *American Psychologist, 56*(3), 218–226.

Fredrickson, B. L., & Joiner, T. (2002). Positive emotions trigger upward spirals toward emotional well-being. *Psychological Science, 13*(2), 172–175.

Fredrickson, B. L., & Losada, M. F. (2005). Positive affect and the complex dynamics of human flourishing. *American Psychologist*, *60*(7), 678–686.

Gan, Y., Yang, M., Zhou, Y., & Zhang, Y. (2007). The two-factor structure of future-oriented coping and its mediating role in student engagement. *Personality & Individual Differences*, *43*(4), 851–863.

Gard, D. E., Gard, M. G., Kring, A. M., & John, O. P. (2006). Anticipatory and consummatory components of the experience of pleasure: A scale development study. *Journal of Research in Personality*, *40*(6), 1086–1102.

Guralnick, M. J. (2001). A developmental systems model for early intervention. *Infants and Young children*, *14*(2), 1–18.

Guralnick, M. J. (2006). The system of early intervention for children with developmental disabilities. In J. W. Jacobson, J. A. Mulick, & J. Rojahn (Eds.), *Handbook of mental retardation and developmental disabilities* (pp. 465–480). New York: Plenum.

Guralnick, M. J., Neville, B., Hammond, M. A., & Connor, R. T. (2007). Linkages between delayed children's social interactions with mothers and peers. *Child Development*, *78*(2), 459–473.

Haid, M. L., Seiffge-Krenke, I., Hoareau, E., Menna, A., Bergsland, C., & Howson, L. (2009, August). *Coping with loneliness in adolescence across four European countries (Germany, U.K., France, Italy)*. Paper presented at The XIVth ESDP European Society Conference on Developmental Psychology Vilnius, Lithuania.

Hampel, P., & Petermann, F. (2005). Age and gender effects on coping in children and adolescents. *Journal of Youth and Adolescence*, *34*(2), 73–83.

Hassin, R. R., Bargh, J. A., & Zimerman, S. (2009). Automatic and flexible: The case of nonconscious goal pursuit. *Social Cognition*, *27*(1), 20–36.

Hawkley, L. C., Thisted, R. A., & Cacioppo, J. T. (2009). Loneliness predicts reduced physical activity: Cross-sectional & longitudinal analyses. *Health Psychology*, *28*(3), 354–363.

Hill, N. E., & Tyson, D. F. (2009). Parental involvement in middle school: A meta-analytic assessment of the strategies that promote achievement. *Developmental Psychology*, *45*(3), 740–763.

Holahan, C. J., & Moos, R. H. (1985). Life stress and health: Personality, coping, and family support in stress resistance. *Journal of Personality and Social Psychology*, *47*(3), 739–747.

Holder, M. D., Coleman, B., & Sehn, Z. L. (2009). The contribution of active and passive leisure to children's well-being. *Journal of Health Psychology*, *14*(3), 378–386.

Holodynski, M., & Friedlmeier, W. (2006). *Development of emotions and emotion regulation*. New York: Springer.

Hood, B., Power, T., & Hill, L. (2009). Children's appraisal of moderately stressful situations. *International Journal of Behavioral Development*, *33*(2), 167–177.

Idan, O., Sade, S., & Margalit, M. (2009, August). *Loneliness and hope: Risk and protective factors for predicting adolescent students' academic effort*. Paper presented at the XIV European Conference on Developmental Psychology, Vilnius, Lithuania

Joiner, T. E., Lewinsohn, P. M., & Seeley, J. R. (2002). The core of loneliness: Lack of pleasurable engagement – More so than painful disconnection predicts social impairment, depression onset, and recovery from depressive disorders among adolescents. *Journal of Personality Assessment*, *79*(3), 472–491.

Jones, R. S. P., & Lewis, H. (2000). Debunking the pathological model: The functions of an Internet discussion group. *Down Syndrome Research and Practice*, *6*(3), 126–131.

Joudrey, A. D., & Wallace, J. E. (2009). Leisure as a coping resource: A test of the job demand-control-support model. *Human Relations*, *62*(2), 195–217.

Kliewer, W., & Sandler, I. N. (1993). Social competence and coping among children of divorce. *American Journal of Orthopsychiatry*, *63*(3), 432–439.

Klimmt, C., Schmid, H., & Orthmann, J. (2009). Exploring the enjoyment of playing browser games. *CyberPsychology & Behavior*, *12*(2), 231–234.

Knobloch-Westerwick, S., Hastall, M. R., & Rossmann, M. (2009). Coping or escaping? Effects of life dissatisfaction on selective exposure. *Communication Research*, *36*(2), 207–228.

Kossek, E. E., Pichler, S. M., Meece, D., & Barratt, M. E. (2008). Family, friend, and neighbour child care providers and maternal well-being in low-income systems: An ecological social perspective. *Journal of Occupational & Organizational Psychology, 81*(3), 369–391.

Larose, S., Guay, F., & Boivin, M. (2002). Attachment, social support, and loneliness in young adulthood: A test of two models. *Personality and Social Psychology Bulletin, 28*(5), 684–693.

Lazarus, R. S. (1991). *Emotion and adaptation.* Oxford: Oxford University Press.

Lazarus, R. S., & Folkman, S. (1984). *Stress, appraisal and coping.* New York: Springer.

Lim, S., & Lee, J. E. R. (2009). When playing together feels different: Effects of task types and social contexts on physiological arousal in multiplayer online gaming contexts. *CyberPsychology & Behavior, 12*(1), 59–61.

Margalit, M. (1994). *Loneliness among children with special needs: Theory, research, coping and intervention.* New York: Springer.

Margalit, M., & Ankonina, D. B. (1991). Positive and negative affect in parenting disabled children. *Counselling Psychology Quarterly, 4*(4), 289–299.

Margalit, M., & Raskind, M. (2009). Mothers of children with LD and ADHD: Empowerment through online communication. *Journal of Special Education Technology, 24*(1), 39–50.

Mikulincer, M., & Shaver, P. R. (2009). An attachment and behavioral systems perspective on social support. *Journal of Social and Personal Relationships, 26*(1), 7–19.

Moore, D., & Schultz, N. R. (1983). Loneliness at adolescence: Correlates, attributions and coping. *Journal of Youth and Adolescence, 12*, 95–100.

Moos, R. H. (2002a). Life stressors, social resources, and coping skills in youth: Applications to adolescents with chronic disorders. *Journal of Adolescent Health, 30*(4, Suppl. 1), 22–29.

Moos, R. H. (2002b). The mystery of human context and coping: An unraveling of clues. *American Journal of Community Psychology, 30*(1), 67–88.

Putallaz, M., & Wasserman, A. (1990). Children's entry behavior. In S. R. Asher & J. D. Coie (Eds.), *Peer rejection in childhood* (pp. 60–89). Cambridge: University Press.

Reijntjes, A., Stegge, H., & Terwogt, M. M. (2006). Children's coping with peer rejection: The role of depressive symptoms, social competence, and gender. *Infant and Child Development, 15*(1), 89–107.

Repetti, R., Wang, S. W., & Saxbe, D. (2009). Bringing it all Back home: How outside stressors shape families' everyday lives. *Current Directions in Psychological Science, 18*(2), 106–111.

Reschly, A. L., Huebner, E. S., Appleton, J. J., & Antaramian, S. (2008). Engagement as flourishing: The contribution of positive emotions and coping to adolescents' engagement at school and with learning. *Psychology in the Schools, 45*(5), 419–431.

Rokach, A. (1999). Cultural background and coping with loneliness. *The Journal of Psychology, 133*(2), 217–218.

Rokach, A. (2001). Strategies of coping with loneliness throughout the lifespan. *Current Psychology, 20*(1), 3–18.

Rokach, A., & Brock, H. (1998). Coping with loneliness. *Journal of Psychology, 132*(1), 107.

Rubin, K. H., Coplan, R. J., & Bowker, J. C. (2009). Social withdrawal in childhood. *Annual Review of Psychology, 60*, 1–31.

Sarason, I. G., & Sarason, B. R. (2009). Social support: Mapping the construct. *Journal of Social and Personal Relationships, 26*(1), 113–120.

Seepersad, S. (2004). Coping with loneliness: Adolescent online and offline behavior. *CyberPsychology & Behavior, 7*(1), 35–39.

Shelton, K. H., & Harold, G. T. (2008). Pathways between interparental conflict and adolescent psychological adjustment: Bridging links through children's cognitive appraisals and coping strategies. *The Journal of Early Adolescence, 28*(4), 555–582.

Shiota, M. N. (2006). Silver linings and candles in the dark: Differences among positive coping strategies in predicting subjective well-being. *Emotion, 6*(2), 335–339.

Skinner, E. A., & Zimmer-Gembeck, M. J. (2007). The development of coping. *Annual Review of Psychology, 58*, 119–144.

Sohl, S. J., & Moyer, A. (2009). Refining the conceptualization of a future-oriented self-regulatory behavior: Proactive coping. *Personality and Individual Differences, 47*(2), 139–144.

Tugade, M. M., Fredrickson, B. L., & Feldman Barrett, L. (2004). Psychological resilience and positive emotional granularity: Examining the benefits of positive emotions on coping and health. *Journal of Personality, 72*(6), 1161–1190.

Van Buskirk, A. M., & Duke, M. P. (1991). The relationship between coping style and loneliness in adolescents: Can 'sad passivity' be adaptive. *Journal of Genetic Psychology, 152*(2), 145–157.

Vangelisti, A. L. (2009). Challenges in conceptualizing social support. *Journal of Social and Personal Relationships, 26*(1), 39–51.

Wenz-Gross, M., Siperstein, G. N., Untch, A. S., & Widaman, K. F. (1997). Stress, social support, and adjustment of adolescents in middle school. *The Journal of Early Adolescence, 17*(2), 129–151.

Wilson, B. J. (2006). The entry behavior of aggressive/rejected children: The contributions of status and temperament. *Social Development, 15*(3), 463–479.

Zaidman-Zait, A., & Jamieson, J. R. (2007). Providing web-based support for families of infants and young children with established disabilities. *Infants & Young Children, 20*(1), 11–25.

Zimmer-Gembeck, M. J., & Locke, E. M. (2007). The socialization of adolescent coping behaviours: Relationships with families and teachers. *Journal of Adolescence, 30*(1), 1–16.

Chapter 8
Prevention and Intervention Approaches

Loneliness is a threat to the positive development of children's adaptation and reflects several cumulative risk and protective factors. The continuous professional efforts to support positive development and resilience require multifaceted strategies and strategic, sequential timing plans (Masten, Herbers, Cutuli, & Lafavor, 2008). In order to prevent and buffer the cumulative risks of social isolation, and to empower children in their developmental struggles, specific attention to multiple components and processes is requested at multiple levels to promote resilience. Resilience has been broadly defined as the skills, attributes, and abilities that enable individuals to adapt to hardships, difficulties, and challenges. Although some of these attributes are biologically determined, research showed that resilience skills could be strengthened as well as learned and trained (Alvord & Grados, 2005). Prevention programs strive to reduce, avoid, and prevent children's distress of loneliness and/or its impact. Intervention programs are requested when the prevention efforts have limited results. The goals of intervention planning are to "treat" lonely children, to reduce their pain, and to help them manage or cope with their loneliness. Since these two concepts have several overlapping segments, it is important in the beginning of this chapter to define what each one of these two terms mean, as well as what they comprise. In the first part of this chapter the definitions of prevention in general will be provided, and different aspects of loneliness prevention will be proposed, including empowerment of self-perception and self-presentation, examination of social and solitude competencies, and cultivation of the hopeful approach. In the second part of this chapter, the focus will be on different intervention approaches. Following the general definition of the intervention and therapeutic constructs, several intervention approaches will be presented including suggestions to families and proposals of virtual solutions.

The Meaning of Prevention

In line with Caplan (1964) general definition, prevention consists of three groups of goals:

(a) Stopping a problem from ever occurring.

M. Margalit, *Lonely Children and Adolescents*, DOI 10.1007/978-1-4419-6284-3_8,   235
© Springer Science+Business Media, LLC 2010

(b) Delaying the onset of a problem, when it cannot be avoided or stopped.
(c) Reducing, limiting, and capsulating the impact of a problem, when it is unavoidable.

   In an attempt to emphasize the importance of personal strengths and competences, as well as to convey the significance of contextual-based comprehensive approaches, Romano and Hage (2000) proposed the following two extensions to this early prevention model:

(d) Strengthening knowledge, attitudes, and behaviors that promote emotional and physical wellbeing as an inoculation approach.
(e) Promoting institutional, community, and government policies that foster physical, social, and emotional wellbeing.

Hence, prevention in this chapter includes two major focuses: a salutogenic, strength-based approach and a "risk-reduction" approach (Antonovsky, 1987). A key idea is that prevention programs will focus on developing assets, personal strengths and resources for children and adolescents who may be at risk for developing loneliness instead of the more traditional approach of focusing on risk amelioration. In line with contemporary theory and research, prevention programs are considered most effective when they are not limited to a single factor, but address comprehensive and multiple factors across several contextual domains, including the neighborhood, school, community, and social–political contexts. In line with studies that assumed that children's difficulties were often not isolated, and several developmental challenges tended to appear together (Yates & Masten, 2004), comprehensive approaches that addressed a wide range of problems and behaviors, and that strived to coordinate a varied range of services and activities across multiple contexts, such as the family, school, and community, were considered more advantageous than a series of isolated and uncoordinated programs that focused on a single problem from time to time (Hage et al., 2007). Our goals in proposing preventive procedures aiming at children's loneliness were to provide meaningful answers and suggestions to concerned parents and to committed teachers.

It is widely recognized that contemporary prevention initiatives warrant attention to both individual and contextual factors. Research conclusions have clarified individual and interpersonal characteristics within different contextual conditions – at home, at school, and in the neighborhood. The goals of the current chapter are to explore the implications of these studies for preventive effort. Developmental theories and research highlighted the important role of protective factors as well as risk factors as determinants of personal adjustment and resiliency. The study that examined the impact of cumulative risk factors in early and middle childhood on child behavior outcomes in adolescence, supported the cumulative risk hypothesis that considered the number of risks in early childhood as a critical index in predicting adjustment in adolescence (Appleyard, Egeland, Van Dulmen, & Sroufe, 2005). In line with this approach, more risks during developmental stages predicted a poorer quality of children's outcomes. Moreover, the presence of multiple risks in early childhood continued to explain variations in predicting adolescent behavior outcomes. The results supported the need for early awareness of children's lone-liness, and to comprehensive prevention efforts with high-risk children. It seemed that every risk factor that could be reduced or avoided was significant to adjusted development. Yet, the group of resilient children who flourish, regardless of their cumulative risks, necessitated a more in-depth examination of contextual conditions.

In conjunction with the growing body of research examining the role of risk factors in development, research has also focused attention on the identification of individual and contextual factors that contribute to positive development out-comes despite exposure to significant adversity or trauma (Luthar & Zelazo, 2003; Luthar, Cicchetti, & Becker, 2000). The construct of resilience referred to the processes or causal mechanisms that explain positive adaptation at a given point in time, despite the presence of considerable risks (Cicchetti & Rogosch, 2009; Masten & Obradovic, 2008). Resilience described positive patterns of adaptation in the context of past or present adversity, or in other words, positive outcomes from high-risk contexts, recovery from trauma, overcoming adversity to succeed in life, and unexpected positive development. The study of resilience stimulated interest in positive development because of its emphasis on promoting competence throughout development (Yates & Masten, 2004). The focus on positive develop-ment stemmed from the awareness to the roles of protective factors in reducing the likelihood of maladaptive outcomes (Catalano, Hawkins, Berglund, Pollard, & Arthur, 2002). Whereas the concept of protective factors retained a focus on reduc-ing risk, positive youth development theory acknowledged the roles of strengths and assets for a successful life. By definition, protective factors operated only under conditions of risk, whereas assets and capacities contributed to positive developmen-tal outcomes as an inoculation, independent of the level of risk (Yates & Masten, 2004). The development of competencies thus served the dual functions of offer-ing protective factors that decreased problem behaviors and at the same time also built foundations for healthy development across the life span (Greenberg, 2006; Greenberg et al., 2003).

Resilience constructs concentrated discussions on dynamic processes. They examined transactional interactions between individuals and the environment and proposed developmental processes that were not static over time. Resilience did not deal with individual characteristics nor did it imply a sense of individual responsibility and personal blame for poor developmental outcomes (Luthar et al., 2000). Just as developmental research revealed that risk factors were often interre-lated, research also demonstrated an interrelationship among competencies (Yates & Masten, 2004). Promoting social competence and habits of age-appropriate activ-ities, for example, could have a positive preventive impact on academic failure and would contribute to achievement and vice versa. Academic success might enhance success in self-perception and adjustment. Based on protective factors and resilience conceptualization, prevention programs were designed to increase protec-tive factors that might decrease the contextual probabilities of the risks' emergence, delimit their powers, or empower individuals to effectively cope when the risk factors would appear. Thus, prevention was most effective when direct attempts to enhance health and competence were combined with efforts to reduce risks

surfacing (Peck, Roeser, Zarrett, & Eccles, 2008). Focusing only on building competencies or only on preventing problems might not be as effective as addressing both
together (Catalano et al., 2002). An emphasis on simultaneously reducing risks and
developing competencies was consistent, furthermore, with research concerning the
foundations of positive youth development (Catalano, Berglund, Ryan, Lonczak, &
Hawkins, 2004). Durlak and Wells's (1997, 1998) meta-analysis revealed that primary prevention programs developed for children and adolescents were effective in
building competencies, such as communication skills and self-confidence, and in
reducing emotional and behavioral problems, which were done with demonstrated
effectiveness.

Suggestions to Parents

Thus the concept of resilience and its associated evidence suggested several implications for loneliness prevention planning. A resilience approach emphasized the
promotion of personal assets as well as increasing family or educational resources
as an effective support. The internal resources that were critical for the prevention of loneliness included the promotion of positive self-perceptions and academic
competence, the enhancing of age-appropriate social skills to enable satisfactory
peers' relations, self-efficacy for age-appropriate leisure activities, and participation in extracurricular and community activities. The planning of prevention efforts
involved both the family and the school environments. Several preventive programs
were directed at schools, and the family was neglected. Concerned parents who anxiously observed their children struggling often asked what they needed to know and
how they could help.

During international lectures, following theoretical presentations, I was often
asked what could be done, or more specifically, if parents could prevent or decrease
their children's risks for developing chronic loneliness. We have to bear in mind that
it is not realistic to prevent children's loneliness altogether. Everybody experiences
loneliness from time to time. Controlled preventive studies are scarce. However,
based on theory and research, several conclusions can be reached and used to advise
parents on how they may reduce and limit the emergence of social distress and
alienation. The following recommendations demand different levels of awareness
and knowledge, with focused timing, self-awareness, and empowering approaches
in effective parenting:

1. *Start early.* The most important recommendation appreciates the strong impacts
   of early intervention, and proposes to develop awareness and adopt socialization strategies at an early developmental stage, when parents start to be aware
   of their children's social risks. The results from the large-scale, longitudinal
   sample of the NICHD SECC provided a complex and intriguing picture of the
   associations between early childcare-based peer experiences and later social
   competence at school, in the world of peers (Brownell et al., 2008).

Even in playgroups, several infants and young children already disclosed their difficulties while trying to form interpersonal relations. These difficulties predicted future social and behavior problems, emphasizing the significant roles of the family and child characteristics. Early positive relations with peers predicted social competence in the third grade, while early social difficulties predicted the continuation of social isolation. In another study (Burchinal et al., 2008), early intervention supported the development of social competence and social skills, in addition to academic achievements. Responsive and stimulating interactions with teachers and the instructional quality aspects of the pre kindergarten classroom predicted the acquisition of language, pre-academic and social skills by the end of the kindergarten year.

Shyness was also considered a risk factor, although sometimes it was less pronounced than children's reluctance, aggression, and/or indifference to other children. At this young age, parents may have been able to intervene more effectively before the loneliness became a dominant interpersonal style and a habit. Since loneliness is first of all an expression of unsatisfactory self-perception and presentation, empowering young children's capacities, helping them to develop awareness of their abilities and supporting their experimentations in positive but realistic self-presentation may be the building blocks of their emerging self-confidence to initiate future interrelations with other children. Even when parents have to set boundaries regarding their children's behavior, they can do it in an encouraging fashion that recognizes and appreciates strengths.

2. *Interpersonal modeling.* Parents provide vital models of behavior in general and especially social behavior for their children, even when they are not aware of it. Children listen to their conversations and self-remarks when they value (or criticize) their friendship relations, and communicate appreciation to the meaning of their social interrelations with their own acquaintances. Children start developing their insights on how friends are expected to behave by listening and observing their family members.

3. *Active instigation.* Parents may initiate meetings with families who also have young children, invite children from the playgroups, and suggest modes of social interactions, not only to create social opportunities, but also to model social initiatives. For example, a mother told us that at the beginning of the school year she watched enviously while other children invited "friends" after school, while her 5-year-old son kept complaining that nobody invited him, but did not try to invite his peers. She was distressed, remembering the agony of his father who was a loner, and viewed this behavior pattern as a risk. Consequently, she started arriving earlier to school, waiting with other mothers and initiating conversations with them (sharing difficulties among overworking mothers). She invited their children, and sometimes together with the mothers to their home. She told us that she wished she had done it earlier. She decided to ignore the disturbing fact that many times she invited children that never invited her son, and turned their house into a playground. She became friendly with mothers that she had never related to them before. Yet she decided: "My son needs this help, and gradually he will start to initiate social connections by himself." Yet,

she sighed – "it is not easy after a long working day to be friendly to strangers, and I need lots of patience."

4. *Establishing and strengthening social support connections* within the family or outside the family. Children, who experienced quality and consistent interactions with supportive individuals, with the parents and in addition to the parents, had significantly fewer internalizing and externalizing problems at school. Early social support was related to positive behavioral and emotional outcomes, and decreased loneliness (Appleyard, Egeland, & Sroufe, 2007). The quality of support comprised several aspects such as stability in relationships, extensiveness of the social network, and mutual positive regards in relationships. These aspects of support contributed to children's sense of self-worth, which then portended less anxiety and depression in future stressful situations. One mechanism through which these effects might have operated was through the child's representational models of self and others. However, not every social support had beneficial outcomes (Gleason, Iida, Shrout, & Bolger, 2008). Paradoxically, sometimes the receipt of social support from close others was associated with negative outcomes, calling attention to the quality of the support. Only responsive social support that displayed understanding, validation, and caring would be beneficial (Maisel & Gable, 2009).

   There was significant variability in the individuals' capacity to elicit and utilize social support. Children who could play an active role in seeking support, and who showed the capacity to utilize this resource, had better outcomes (Egeland, Carlson, & Sroufe, 1993). Parents can model these skills, support and promote them from early developmental stages. The critical question that fathers and mothers have to ask themselves is related to their abilities first to ask and accept help, and second to encourage their children to seek support and to reinforce their explorations for help in an appropriate communication style. The balance between the encouragement toward independence and autonomy on the one hand, and the ability to ask for and accept help and support on the other hand, require a sophisticated and sensitive parenting style.

5. *Promoting of hopeful thinking and habits of hope* from early age. The advantages of high hopes were detailed in Chapters 1 and 2. Hopes could be distinguished from general wishes and specific plans. However, unlike general wishes, hopeful thinking was recognized as requiring specific programs and plans. The introduction of hope language at home enabled the development of different and new mental pictures – the identification of new goals and strategies (Pound & Duchac, 2009). Hope theory posited that the development of an individual's hope disposition occurred during early childhood (Creamer et al., 2009), and thus prevention efforts required the parents' focusing attention on their significant role in establishing family climate and communication styles that enhanced their children's hope from the early developmental stages as an inoculation strategy to reduce social distresses. More importantly, parents who promoted hopeful thinking in themselves would be able to teach it to their children more effectively. Three stages for this learning process were suggested (Shade, 2001).

The first stage dealt with identifying specific meaningful hopes. These specific contents of hopes were closely related to current activities, but aspiring to change involvements and challenges. Parental goals at this stage were to embrace hope and to actively resist the debilitating effects of fear and despair. Parents' communication style with their children included the language of hopes, grounded in specific targets, and day-to-day occurrences. They often used sentences of specific planning and future expectations such as "I hope that tomorrow . . .," related to small practical expectations. This "hope" language was the foundation for the development of a hope communication style, and the building blocks for a more general positive approach.

The second stage was the development of hope habits. Habits of hope are the skills that structure (directly or indirectly) personal commitments, enabling persistence, resourcefulness, and courage. Habits were developed through repeated interactions with environments, providing a structure which directed energy and facilitated more complex modes of activities. Repeated engagement with the environment shapes and structures human plasticity into powerful, purposive modes of parsimonious activity – the habits. Repetitions of "hope" communication and activities develop habits that save personal energy, facilitating the performance of recurring and repeated events with ease. These habits enable the focus of personal energy on the more complicated and demanding modes of actions.

The third stage was the developing of hopefulness. Hopefulness was a general orientation of open attentive readiness to possibilities that promise future satisfaction. It differed from particular hopes since it lacked the specifiable end. It enriched life, since it was defined not only by past accomplishments, but also by expectations for future achievements that would enhance growth, satisfaction, and self-fulfillment. A series of successful experiences in particular hopes fostered the development of habits, and those habits were gradually generalized through repetitions and training to hopefulness orientation.

Prevention planning within the suggested hope model needs to capture two major aspects: first, hopes have to be age appropriate for children, practical, and grounded in real contextual conditions through which they can be realized. Second, hopes may generate new and creative ways to prevent children's social distress (Shade, 2001). In order to develop habits of hopes, persistence, resourcefulness, and imagination are required. Attention to actual conditions is thus coupled with exploration of the possibilities pregnant in those conditions. Finally, hoping calls for enhancing courage to discover and act in new ways, and to realize the means that actually bring about desired ends. Sometimes, there is also a need to postpone immediate gratifications that compete with future hopes, as well as to identify conditions that impede or make possible their realization, and generate and act on alternate possibilities.

Parents use several approaches to promote their children's hopeful thinking regardless of realistic challenges. They use stories in varied ways, such as sharing stories of personal challenges, emphasizing optimistic and persistent expectations and successful outcomes; they can propose (or read to the children) relevant literature as powerful means of inspiring hopes. Stories help cultivate hope by providing concrete illustrations of the complex steps of hoping, prompting self-reflection and understanding, and inspiring children to generate creative alternatives. These stories also offer insight into the process of hoping, generating new and alternative possibilities (Shade, 2006).

The results of a recent study (Creamer et al., 2009) called attention to the need to differentiate between the hope factors (i.e., goals, pathways, and agency), and to adapt the support accordingly. For example, research reported that childhood trauma did not affect the children's abilities to generate creative ideas about ways to achieve goals. However, they lost the belief in their ability to succeed in using these identified pathways. These results suggested that agency, a self-referential belief in the child's abilities, was more vulnerable and at a higher risk for development. Parental support, caring, and responsiveness could enhance their children's beliefs in their own abilities to reach goals and find in themselves the personal energy necessary in order to persist in trying to obtain desired goals.

6. *Enable and respect different expressions of temperament and solitude.* Research focused interest on individual differences in temperament and in the need for social relations, reflecting genetic, contextual, and cultural differences. The ability of children to stay alone and enjoy solitary activities develops along individualized paths and cultural conventions. Individuals (adults as well as children) have different needs for social relations. Several children need a small and close/intimate network of friends, while others are satisfied only with active extensive social activities during most of their day. An additional group needs time for solitude activities – time for themselves. These differences are expressed in quantity and preferences since, in fact, everybody has different social needs at different times. There are times when we wish for the intimacy of a close friend, and times we yearn and long for time alone – for ourselves. The importance of the developmental capacity to stay alone was supported by research of children, who had difficulties in staying alone, and felt lonelier when they were left on their own. Thus, respecting children's individual differences in their needs of social connections by their parents can reduce the risk for distress. In addition, parental promotion of their children's abilities to stay alone will help them to develop solitude habits. Planning periods of enjoyable activities alone from early developmental stages and consistent expressions of appreciation, not only of the children's abilities to keep friendships with peers but also of their ability to stay alone, will support the children's solitude abilities without experiencing distressed loneliness.

7. *Promoting children's self-competence.* The experience of childhood loneliness was consistently related to children's self-perceptions and their experiences of different difficulties (Coplan, Findlay, & Nelson, 2004). Early competence in various domains predicted developmental outcomes (Denham, Wyatt, Bassett, Echeverria, & Knox, 2009). Nobody can promise parents that their children will always be successful, or that they can help them in avoiding failure and difficulties. However, the children's and parents' inclination to consider

difficulties as stable characteristics, unchangeable and generalized, may contribute to children's lower self-perception and loneliness.

Parents have an important role in promoting their children's generalized feeling of competence. Their perceptions of their children's competence affect the development of children's functioning (Pomerantz & Wei, 2006). Through their perceptions of children's competence, parents may act as interpreters of reality for their children, and their attitudes further function as self-fulfilling prophecies. Thus, they will influence children's academic and affective functioning in a consistent manner with their perceptions. In addition, when parents view their children's competence as a stable characteristic, their perceptions have a stronger impact than among parents who consider the competence as relatively changeable. The keys to parental perceptions of children's competence are their belief that competence is not easily changeable (Pomerantz, Moorman, & Litwack, 2007). In order to enhance children's competence as a way to prevent loneliness, children need varied opportunities to perform well in various age-appropriate tasks and to be appreciated by responsive parents for their successful achievements and thus develop competent self-perceptions. Parents, who believe in their children's competence, are able to accept challenges since their attitudes will recognize the specific and changeable multiple aspects of competence.

8. *Responsive understanding to children's protective self-presentation.* The protective style was associated with social anxiety, reticence, conformity, and help in avoiding disapproval (Arkin, 1981). Protective self-presentations and attempts of individuals to present themselves as more positive than they are emerge from efforts to avoid undesirable rejected self-presentations. Socially anxious children may have doubts about their interpersonal competencies and capacities to create favorable impressions on others. Thus sometimes children adopted a protective self-presentation style, and their social goals were to avoid others' disapproval. Tendencies to view interpersonal encounters as threats, others as rejecting and the self as less socially skilled maintained or even increased social anxiety and/or avoidance of social interactions. This pattern resulted in reduced social contacts and increased loneliness. High-school students who were particularly concerned with others' disapproval were more lonelier than their peers (Jackson, 2007). These children who valued social approval but lacked confidence in their own abilities to discern or enact desired impressions, often protected themselves from losses of approval by avoiding undesired, contestable, or even noticeable impressions.

If longing for interpersonal contacts was a hallmark of loneliness, somewhat paradoxically, lonely students were more concerned about others' disapproval. Parents have to develop awareness of and insight to their children's modes of self-presentation from early developmental stages. Prevention planning has to promote and enable opportunities for building children's competence as well as enhancing their positive and realistic self-presentation. Parents have to develop awareness of their children's protective self-presentation as an indicator of risk factor. Yet, they have to treat it with sensitivity and caution considering the research which indicated that the protective self-presentation of children with disorders was an effective coping strategy, adaptive and protective of children's self-esteem and positive affect (Heath & Glen, 2005).

9. *Parental communication for modeling affect's expressions, and empowering emotion regulation.* Children at risk for developing loneliness tend to use a limited communication style reflecting vague and over generalized positive and negative emotions. It is important for children to learn and use the concepts of universal versus specific as well as permanence versus temporary in relation to their emotional reactions, and to practice them in different events. When interpreting negative events, and in line with Taylor's (2006) suggestions, permanence is considered as a rigid, pessimistic style that defines the timing of events in terms of "always" or "never." For example, "I was always lonely," or "I never had a true friend." Individuals with a temporary interpretation of negative events consider negative events as occurring "sometimes" and "lately." Similarly, the interpretations of events as either universal or specific are also related to emotion regulation. According to this approach, parents are encouraged to model their children's communication and encourage the adoption of universal and permanent attributions to positive events (i.e., "I am always a good friend") and specific and temporary attributions to negative events (i.e., "Yesterday at the sport competition, I was not invited to join the group"). Instead of saying "you *always* make me angry," it is better to say, "I did not like it this morning when you did not prepare your notebooks in the satchel." Parents can encourage their child to be specific and say "Yesterday (or sometimes) I was so sad and lonely" instead of "I am always lonely and sad."

10. *Encouraged experiencing of anticipatory pleasures from social interactions.* Often research on pleasure experiences revealed that the anticipation for a pleasure was as pleasurable as, or even more than, the pleasure experiences. Let us consider our own enjoyments. We often enjoy visualizing our future vacation, planning a trip, and looking forward to a meeting with a good friend. Our expectations and anticipations from enjoyable experiences are sometimes better and stronger than the true experiences. Anticipatory pleasure is thought to involve the pleasure experienced in anticipation and the ability to imagine it. Research identified the differences between anticipatory pleasures, consummatory pleasures (one's ability to enjoy something at the moment of occurrence), and memories of pleasurable times in the past (Gard, Kring, Gard, Horan, & Green, 2007; Joiner, Lewinsohn, & Seeley, 2002). This differentiation may facilitate the engagement of motivational processes and self-preparation. Children who have difficulties in anticipating an enjoyable future social interaction due to painful memories will lose interest in pursuing social relationships. Anticipatory pleasures are often related to social encounters. We repeatedly and continually plan what to say and expect to hear friendly responses. Anticipation has been closely linked to motivation and goal-directed behavior, leading one to wish more of the positive experience (Gard, Gard, Kring, & John, 2006).

In other words, it may be that anticipatory pleasure (or wanting, planning, and imagining the event) is the factor that activates motivational processes, which subsequently encourage individuals to seek out a particular stimulus and look forward to pleasurable experiences (Gard et al., 2007). Two components were identified: (1) prediction and envision of the future experience of pleasure; and (2) the concurrent experience of pleasure in knowing that a future enjoyable activity is going to occur. In addition, anticipatory pleasure is linked to motivational processes that promote goal-directed efforts and behaviors aimed at achieving the desired rewards from the activity. Lonely children did not expect that their social encounters would be enjoyable and, as a result of their anxiety, they avoided thinking about it and focused their attempts on evading it. This was often a self-fulfilling prophecy. Thus, in order to reduce the risks for loneliness, parents may communicate to children using modeling and sharing personal experiences and their positive anticipations of social experiences. Their responsiveness to their children's social anxiety and reluctance can be combined with their support for the children's needs and difficulties to anticipate pleasurable social experiences.

11. *Supportive planning of leisure and extracurricular activities.* The relation between children's active leisure activities and their wellbeing, including happiness, social satisfaction and self-concept were established in several studies. However, this participation in leisure activities may be the source of frustrations, peer exclusion and loneliness. Many parents believe that they don't have the time or the energy for their own leisure activities, not realizing their importance for relieving parental stress and feelings of tensions in their life. Yet, parental involvement, participation and support of leisure activities may enhance the children's participation (Holder, Coleman, & Sehn, 2009). Persistence in extracurricular activities may contribute to children's gradual development of skilled performance and satisfaction. A positive association was found between parental involvement in their children's activities and youths' persistence of participation in leisure activities over time (Denault & Poulin, 2008). In order to reduce the risks of loneliness, parents and children are encouraged to plan and to participate in different leisure activities, responsive to personal preferences and anticipated sources of enjoyment. These activities create opportunities for developing feelings of competence and social participation.

The beneficial value of the participation in extracurricular activities was demonstrated and its contribution to youth resilience. When vulnerable youth were exposed to a broad variety of extracurricular activity settings that afforded them constructive, developmentally appropriate opportunities (i.e., to make friends, develop competencies and skills, exercise some autonomy, and develop long-term mentoring relationships), their opportunities of becoming resilient were enhanced (Peck et al., 2008).

12. *Forecasting and preventive preparation of specific risk periods.* Lonely children are not lonely all the time. Weekly loneliness refers to all the temporary, short-term periods that children experience loneliness regularly, such as weekends, a specific time at school (i.e., lunch time), or during a special hour in the afternoon. In order to reduce the risks of chronic loneliness, it is important to

identify these periods and be prepared to avoid the risks by proposing alternative actions. Parents can plan enjoyable activities and/or social contacts for these periods. They can also sensitize the children to identify distressful periods and to increase their awareness of challenges of emotional regulation.

Overall, successful prevention programs may alter the balance between risks and assets and mobilize powerful systems toward adaptive human development. They will include individualized profiles composed of the proposed above different segments that will target effective parenting skills as well as their communicative abilities related to supporting and affirming children's strengths and competence, their self-perceptions as well as their self-presentations, hopeful orientation in general, and specifically focusing at satisfactory interpersonal relations and anticipations for relations. Parenting roles include developing and maintaining social-support networks and maintaining interpersonal relationships with others, including family members, such as enhancing siblings' connectedness in order to create an environment that prevents/decreases children's social isolation, as well as modeling satisfactory interrelations and companionships. Indeed creating preventive approaches is not simple. Teaching and coaching parents how to enhance their support, relationships, and connectedness with their children, in order to help them in developing appropriate empowering and monitoring interpersonal activities, that will include adapted cultural elements, requires comprehensive learning opportunities for parents (Fergus & Zimmerman, 2005).

Preventive Effort at School

The mentioned above prevention approaches for parents were presented as an example. In fact the participation of additional significant adults such as teachers and leisure time instructors in these preventive planned efforts is important and beneficial. The participation of teachers, for example, in these prevention efforts can make a difference in children's development if they structure the classes' and schools' climate as environments that support and appreciate collaborations and cooperation as well as children's individual differences, strengths, and basic needs for autonomous and relatedness, embedded with hopeful thinking within the school curriculum. Teachers can blend hope in the curriculum. As they face their own challenges in the classroom, teachers are in a prime position to serve as role-models of hopeful behavior. By designing cooperative activities among students, and creating cooperative opportunities they extend agency processes and foster trust and interpersonal connection. Through this process, the classroom will become a community of hope and companionship that will reinforce hope's habits and nurture the hopes of its members (Shade, 2006).

Social changes are slow and difficult processes, and meaningful answers to individual factors still continue to warrant extensive consideration. Yet at the same time, prevention efforts are also needed to address the contextual factors. Since preventive interventions will target the empowerment of individuals in coping adaptively with environmental conditions, school-based interventions are requested to support individual processes.

We started experimenting with structured workshops for teachers and school counselors, targeting increased hopeful thinking for both the adults and the students. Several pilot interventions were performed as case studies. They documented a wide range of outcomes, reflecting individual differences. Future research is needed to refine and evaluate these approaches that target changing the school climate and teachers support to include sensitization to children's interpersonal needs. Yet, it is unrealistic to expect that even these preventive comprehensive approaches will provide inclusive solutions to the challenging social distress – children's loneliness. Intervention approaches that focus on those children who experience chronic loneliness may complement the prevention programs.

Intervention Programs and Therapeutic Approaches

Intervention programs consist of planned activities that treat and modify the distressful social experience of loneliness. In this chapter various types of interventions and therapies are included. Similar to preventive approaches, effective intervention programs nowadays propose two interrelated focuses, those that are based on deficit models and attempt to cure or reduce the negative symptoms, and those that are focused on empowering models, promoting personal strengths, and enhancing positive emotions and emotional regulation (Seligman, Rashid, & Parks, 2006). Psychological therapy is a common way of treating loneliness. Different psychotherapeutic approaches can provide relief from chronic loneliness especially when the distress is accompanied by several additional psychological problems, but their specifics are beyond the scope of this book. Their goal is to clarify the causes of the problem; reversing the negative thoughts, feelings, and attitudes resulting from the problem; and exploring ways to cure the patient. In a psychodynamic model of therapy, the therapists become a presence in the children's life, by communicating their awareness of the distressed experiences that the child shares and thereby decreasing the experience of loneliness and social isolation associated with internal conflict or crisis. In this respect, the therapeutic aim is to "be with the patient" (Viederman, 2008).

Sometimes, the group therapy has been recommended as a channel to connect with other individuals who suffer from loneliness, and in order to establish a support system. For example, in cognitive–behavioral group therapy (that concentrates on thinking processes and their interrelations with emotions), the therapist asks the lonely individuals to record their pessimistic, self-critical, and globally negative thoughts and then helps them to identify how such thinking causes and maintains their social isolation and sad affect. In positive therapy the therapist asks the individuals to introduce themselves through telling each other a real-life story that shows them at their best. This is followed by their identifying signature strengths and the therapist coaching them to find practical ways of using and expressing these strengths more often. Individuals are asked to set goals and to enhance their strengths through real-life exercises. Substantial time is spent in coaching them to focus on what is good and positive in their lives, with the goal of providing them with a more balanced context to their problems. Although some problem-solving and discussion of troubles does take place in both approaches, the goals of the positive approaches are to "teach" behaviors that bring positive feedback from others, and to strengthen already existing positive aspects, rather than clarification and reinterpretation of negative aspects (Seligman et al., 2006).

The described above approaches are not unique to children or to loneliness. They are applied by child therapists for dealing with various emotional difficulties. Intervention research that directly focused on loneliness' alleviation of children is scarce. Loneliness has been considered a symptom among various children's difficulties. However, many studies have already explored the children's social difficulties, peer rejection, and maladaptive behavior manifestations at different developmental stages, including children with typical development as well as those with different difficulties and disabling conditions such as behavior difficulties, learning disabilities, and developmental disabilities. Comprehensive surveys of research revealed different levels of positive impact, yet inconsistent results were reported by various intervention approaches. In order to promote intervention significance, crucial issues were identified, and especially the limited value of simplistic models. The following section presents major intervention approaches within the deficit and empowerment approaches that were applied to children's loneliness beside the traditional psychodynamic approaches.

Social Skills Training

Social skills' deficits are many times among the roots of chronic loneliness. Many programs for social skills assessment and training have been developed. Social skill intervention approaches such as social skills' training consider the delay or deficit in critical social skills as the cause for social distress. There is growing evidence that peer relations and the experience of loneliness may emerge in consequence of the children's behavior or their lack of or delayed age-appropriate social skills with peers resulting in poor social interrelations and lower social competence (Asher & Paquette, 2003). In order to act in a socially skilled manner, children must (a) possess social knowledge how to initiate social interactions and how to maintain satisfactory social connections and friendships; (b) be able to translate the knowledge into skilled performance; (c) continuously monitor and evaluate their environmental contextual conditions and their impact on socially accepted behaviors; and (d) regulate emotional arousal and behavior in order to adapt them to environmental expectations and norms (Gresham, 1986). Within this conceptualization, children's difficulties may stem from deficient cognitive processing and understanding of the complex environmental interactions, from performance difficulties, and/or from faulty emotional self-monitoring.

Since deficits in social skills and social competence played a significant role in the development and maintenance of social distress, social skills' training aimed at increasing the children's ability to perform key social behaviors that were considered important in achieving success during social situations (Elliott, Malecki, & Demaray, 2001). For example, some children felt uneasy when other children became very close to them. Yet, they could learn to regulate the permissible degree of contact and closeness and still felt comfortable. They could learn whether to look at other children and adults and how long to keep the eye contact. They could learn to plan whether to talk to another child and what to say. Once they realized that they could regulate the amount of interpersonal contacts, they had to experiment their new skills in order to reach competent performance. Examining intervention models revealed that most social skills' programs were comprehensive, including instructions and teaching how to perform the social activities, modeling competent age-appropriate behavior by teachers or parents, emphasizing the significance of behavior rehearsals after the child acquired the desired skills until reaching fluency and automaticity in performance and providing consistent feedback and reinforcement to appropriate performance of the acquired skills (Lane, Menzies, Barton-Arwood, Doukas, & Munton, 2005).

Many social skills were targeted, reflecting the theoretical conceptualization of interpersonal problem-solving and social perception skills training, such as participation in group activities, cooperation with dyads and small groups, and communication skills (Nangle, Erdley, Carpenter, & Newman, 2002). Several additional programs trained conversation skills such as asking questions in a friendly manner as a means for initiating and maintaining social contacts. In addition, effective changes in social behavior required interventions that would reduce inhibiting and competing behaviors, such as cognitive restructuring, self- and emotional-regulation methods, and contingency management. Comprehensive reviews of empirically rigorous studies provided support to the effectiveness of social skills' training in varied tasks such as performing social skills and improving social relations and emotional adjustment of children and youth with a wide range of problematic behaviors and psychopathology (Harrell, Mercer, & DeRosier, 2009). Meta-analytic studies suggested that social skills' training interventions that combined behavioral modeling with direct instruction in social perception and performance skills, emotional self-regulation techniques, and social problem-solving skills might produce the most positive and consistent treatment effects (Spence, 2003). In addition, results showed that teaching children a wider range of strategies to use during peer interactions supports their abilities to employ the most appropriate strategy and to change it should the outcomes not validate their choice (Mize & Cox, 1990). Several children also need specific learning and experimenting of flexible strategies' utilization within the wide repertoire of behaviors. There is a need to move from general social learning programs to individualized peer-interaction interventions adapted to different needs/deficits and contexts (Brown, Odom, & Conroy, 2001). For example, an evaluation of comprehensive social skills' interventions focused on aggressive children clarified the critical value of the training intensity for ensuring successful outcomes (Lochman et al., 2009). Systemic interventions in various childhood difficulties, and the participation of the family in the therapeutic process, may also support the effective and stable-desired changes (Carr, 2009).

Several social skills' programs applied approaches that were developed within the cognitive–behavioral therapy paradigm. Cognitive behavior therapy (CUT) is a structured, collaborative psychotherapy, which emphasizes the link between thoughts, feelings, and behavior in maintaining psychological disorders (Goldfried, 2003; Vickers, 2002). The study of children's coping strategies revealed their strengths and weaknesses in their cognitive and behavioral repertoire when they dealt with loneliness. Problem-solving skills aim to extend the child's response repertoire in difficult situations. Cognitive restructuring interventions aim to alter the children's interpretations of threatening events into less-problematic thoughts, enabling changes in emotions and behavior. An additional goal is to support the child's self-confidence, which may be reflected by a more active coping approach and by positive cognitive restructuring. An important part of the therapeutic effort with children is to influence their social context by teaching their parents and teachers how to apply supportive and positive reinforcing attitudes and behavior. Therefore, it can be expected that children may also need to acquire support-seeking strategies adapted to their age.

Most programs did not directly target children's reports of loneliness. Often they included similar segments and reported positive short-term results and inconsistent long-term efficacy outcomes. It was not surprising, since contextual conditions and the severity of children's social problems were related to the outcomes, presenting heterogenic needs and environments. At Tel-Aviv University we developed and assessed the programs "I found a solution." These were social learning programs for children with special needs from kindergarten to high schools, working in the first stage directly with the children, and in the second stage, we trained teachers and parents. These teachers worked in inclusive classes and in special schools in order to promote companionship and cooperation in their classes. Many children with special needs experienced loneliness and social rejection due to their social-skills' deficits. Within the empowering models, our goals were first to empower the children by sensitizing them to their capacities and strengths. Second, the instruction of social problem-solving skills and collaboration strategies provided children with abilities to deal with social challenges. They learnt and were reinforced to develop companionship in dyads and afterward in small groups. In our programs we utilized active learning approaches and provided many opportunities for experimentation of the new skills. We taught the children self-instruction and instructed them how to devise and monitor their solution plans. Gradually they developed self-guidance through practice with self-directed commands, suggestions, and rewards.

Our program (based on cognitive–behavioral models) consisted of the following activities:

- Explaining the strategy, detailing each step within the strategy;
- Pointing out and discussing with the children the advantages of applying the strategy;
- Modeling of the strategy by the teacher, followed by peer tutoring;
- Verbal and behavioral rehearsal of the strategy by the children;

- Comprehensive training, using a wide variety of materials (such as stories, role playing, games, and computer games) presented by a variety of agents (i.e., different teachers, peers, family members) in a variety of settings (i.e., classrooms, school yards) with varied conditions (Margalit, 1995, 1998).

Our conclusions confirmed the significance of the decisions to start early with preschool children. The impact of the programs was larger for this age group. However, it was clear that the preschool environments were more flexible and supportive of companionship, and the teachers were more prepared to embed the programs in their curriculums and to instruct social networking. We avoided simplistic approaches and applied comprehensive programs that combined strategy learning, teachers' training, and parents' involvement, emphasizing motives of children's empowering and establishing a wide repertoire of social-coping strategies. All these factors contributed to the global program's impacts. However, these factors were interrelated, and since this was a school-based intervention, we were not able to differentiate between the various factors. Our studies confirmed that reducing loneliness was a long process. It takes time to change children's loneliness, and repeated assessment revealed that there was not a quick fix. It was quicker for the preschool children, but required a longer intensive intervention for the older children.

School transitions were added risks to the return of the difficulties. In addition to the realization that it was more difficult to change the chronic-established loneliness of adolescents, special attention had to be focused on the children's coping style with loneliness. When the training did not include a specific segment of awareness of children's loneliness and their choices of individualized coping strategies, only partial results were obtained. Even when positive general outcomes were reached, such as a decrease in peer rejection, wider social networks, even fewer behavior difficulties (although this achievement was a side effect and was not the target of the program), no changes in the loneliness levels were found. Only when we added a special and focused training unit that dealt directly with the children's understanding of their loneliness (their feelings in terms of consistencies and severity, the causes for the distress, the ability to predict risk periods for experiencing the distress and the coping outcomes), a change in the level of loneliness was achieved. We trained the children in self-monitoring procedures and encouraged them to experiment different coping procedures, to identify their personal priorities and trained them to use the preferred modes effectively. The children and significant adults (parents and teachers) reported significant lower levels of social alienation and loneliness following these comprehensive procedures.

Future-Oriented Coping Interventions

Most intervention programs focused attention on past experiences and present challenges. Two intervention approaches concentrated on the anticipation of the future: hope intervention and proactive coping intervention.

Hope-Based Interventions

The hope intervention was developed within the cognitive–behavioral group therapies (Cheavens, Feldman, Gum, Michael, & Snyder, 2006), and based on the hope
theory. As opposed to more problem-oriented therapies that direct effort with past
and present challenges, hope interventions direct attention to future expectations,
framing goals as positive outcomes that have to be actively pursued rather than
focusing on ways to avoid problems or remove symptoms. Hope has been defined
as a cognitive process through which individuals pursue their goals. It is a gradual process of regaining inner strength and building self-confidence to make sense
of current and future situations. This therapeutic approach offers instruction and
training of planning skills, including group processes' components. In several locations this approached was developed, with similar outcomes. As an example, the
following description is provided.

Group participants first were introduced to the theoretical principles of the hope
theory and thereafter discussed how to apply these principles to their own lives. In
doing so, participants learned how to

- Set meaningful, achievable, and measurable goals
- Develop multiple pathways to work toward those goals
- Identify sources of motivation and counteract any drains on motivation
- Monitor progress toward goals
- Modify goals and pathways as needed

This intervention was conducted in a group setting to enable transactional processes between participants. During the treatment procedures (Cheavens et al.,
2006), participants were taught hope-related skills within three categories – goals,
pathways, and agency. They discussed ways of applying these skills to the participants' lives. At the outset of the meeting, each participant was asked to select a
specific goal to "work" on during the intervention period, as well as to learn to
apply each session's specific skill to that goal. Written narratives were applied, and
the participants examined the level of hope expressed in their personal narratives
and were invited to generate more hopeful narratives, when appropriate. Therapists
also used storytelling as a way to model children's optimism and striving toward
goals in promoting hope (Gillham & Reivich, 2004).

Participation in the 8-week treatment program using the Hope approach resulted
in increased agency thinking (a component of hopeful thinking), life meaning, and
self-esteem as well as decreases in anxiety and depressive symptoms, when compared to a wait-list control group (Cheavens et al., 2006). Additionally, results
indicated that changes in Hope Scale scores were associated with reductions in
post-treatment anxiety and depression scores.

Along this line, a pilot study was performed in several high schools in Israel in
order to develop with teachers a protocol for enhancing adolescents' at-risk hopeful-
thinking style using the format of 1-h group sessions every week during the whole
school year. The follow-up revealed that teachers and school counselors acquired

successfully the hope theory conceptualization. They were able to develop effective interventions with their middle-school students in order to enhance their abilities to identify personal goals. These workshops enabled the youngsters to develop personalized goals according to their needs and concerns. They used group discussions, written descriptions, and self-monitoring. These workshops did not focus on children's loneliness, but they may be applied as a prototype of developing interventions that will target promoting satisfactory social relations and challenging loneliness experiences among adolescents. Individual differences between groups' effectiveness were disclosed, reflecting not only the differences between children but also between teachers. In several studies we established the negative relations between loneliness and hope (Lackaye & Margalit, 2008), but only future longitudinal controlled studies will be able to evaluate the impact of the hope intervention on children's loneliness.

Proactive Coping Interventions

Proactive coping was defined as the strategies that people apply to prevent future stressors or to minimize their effects (Bode, de Ridder, Kuijer, & Bensing, 2007). This approach is different from the hope intervention since it has a clear focus on potential stresses, and the hope theory targets positive goals in addition to avoiding challenging stresses. Proactive coping is a psychological process which was divided into five stages (Ouwehand, de Ridder, & Bensing, 2007). The first requirement for engaging in proactive coping was related to personal resources which may be accumulated during life (stage 1), in order to build up resistance and to be prepared as much as possible (Aspinwall & Taylor, 1997). The environment was screened for dangers to identify a potential stressor (stage 2), and cues indicating a potential stressor were recognized and appraised as a threat that required actions (stage 3). Individuals who experienced a threat (such as loneliness) directed their attention to potential stressors and became motivated and engaged in proactive coping. Initial coping efforts (stage 4) included both behavioral actions, such as seeking more information about the stressor, and cognitive strategies, such as planning, aimed at preventing or minimizing the stressor. This approach proposed that proactive coping efforts were active rather than avoidant, because avoidance of thinking about the stressor did not contribute to controlling the problem. Feedback (stage 5) was a necessary final stage in proactive coping, since it provided information about the development of the potential stressor and the results of one's coping efforts. Proactive coping included skills such as planning, regulation of negative emotions invoked by thinking about the stressor, and mental simulation.

Proactive coping included the promotion of desired future outcomes and the prevention of undesired changes (Bode et al., 2007). A brief educational intervention was developed using a group format. The program aimed at adults and trained them in proactive coping competencies, supporting future-oriented behavior. In the first session, trainers helped participants to identify the advantages of preparing oneself for the future. Homework assignments were used, and participants were asked to write down warning signals of challenges. The assignments required them to anticipate topics or write narratives about risks that they would regret in the future should they not work on them in the present. In the next sessions, the participants learnt to identify and handle early warning signals of worry, and to specify strategies to meet their personal goal. Strategy training was followed by feedback and evaluation of attempts to reach the individual goal. In addition, they discussed the productive use of feedback, and the increased knowledge about their own potential, the supportive or hindering function of their environment, and the attainability of their future goals and plans.

The results demonstrated that brief interventions (4 weekly sessions) can substantially improve competencies with regard to future-related behavior. Yet, only the concrete formulation of the individual goal facilitated improvement of proactive competencies. This therapeutic approach was mentioned in this chapter, although it was not used with children because of its resemblance to the hope theory intervention approach. However, the hope theory emphasized positive and negative goals, while the proactive coping approach dealt mostly with worries and negative expectations for future stresses. However, its emphasis on feedback and self-monitoring, the suggestions regarding the effectiveness of concrete personal goals and the advantages of exploring and securing environmental help and support are valuable for future interventions' planning.

Overall, several approaches were developed, but controlled research did not provide confirming results. Maybe the complexity of individuals, contexts, and interrelations prevented simplistic answers. However, several conclusions were consistently demonstrated. It was also important to recognize the debilitating impact of helplessness that often accompanied loneliness. The motivation to avoid threatening feedback about the self might at times be stronger than the motivation to establish social relationships (Solomon, 2000). Two additional contextual agents have to be presented: social-support interventions and animal-assisted interventions. Since the core of loneliness is rooted in the difficulties to establish meaningful interpersonal close relations, the potential of planned supported relations with others, such as social-support intervention and animal-assisted intervention have to be considered.

Social-Support Interventions

Several intervention programs assumed that since loneliness reflected feelings of social distancing and isolation, the planned presence of social support – characterized by close and supportive human relations – could facilitate the development of meaningful and close relations that would reduce loneliness. Varied intervention approaches were proposed by different programs, including training and counseling of family members, peers and recently the emergence of virtual connections by forums and discussion groups. A comprehensive survey of social-support interventions, mostly with adults, including different samples and a wide range of therapeutic approaches (Hogan, Linden, & Najarian, 2002) reported inconsistent results. Naively it was expected that the optimal answer to social connections' deficit would be to provide structured companionship and supportive relations. However, the conclusions of several studies accentuated a differentiated understanding of the critical roles of the types and contents of social support, as well as of the individuals who provided the support, without ignoring the effect of contextual issues. They all jointly determined whether the support was beneficial and empowering or harmful and distressing. Thus, detailed examination why the children feel lonely and what they mean when they complain about lack of social support may provide important clues as to how their support needs are best met.

The emerging virtual support provided through the participation in forums and discussion boards created a bridge between coping and intervention, and sensitized intervention planning to the paradox between the anonymity and distance proposed by Internet sites and the feelings of closeness. One of my graduate students at Tel Aviv University, in a research seminar, decided to explore a parents' forum (Swablearning, July, 2006) and sent a message to mothers of children with learning difficulties. She wrote "I was wondering if you could share with me what this board means to you." She got 20 answers such as … "this board means knowledge, support, and friendship to me. It is funny, but I trust most of the members here regarding my feelings before my other colleagues and some family…" "I can tell these people anything and have told them things that I haven't told anyone else." "It helps knowing you are not alone…" "This group is a lifeline to sanity. Because of the anonymity, what would be a stupid question to someone that knows us well is answered with an unbiased reply from someone that understands why we need the answer." Another mother advised my student: "read the fun posts, read the heartbreakers – read the triumphs and then I think it will be very clear to you how we support each other." It is clear from the answers that the forum provided mothers with the kind of social support that was not available in any other form. They emphasized the developing culture of the group, including socializing, joking and sharing various narratives. They shared sorrows, and celebrations.

In another study that analyzed children's messages (Raskind, Margalit, & Higgins, 2006), children with learning disabilities and ADHD presented their identities and appreciated the provided help. In some instances, it appeared that they did not feel trusting enough to ask for help from friends, family members, teachers, or other adults, but expressed trust and closeness to other children on the website, and seemed more than willing to share their difficulties and seek the advice of those with whom they identified (i.e., "some people don't understand me and I hope you do"). In another study (Margalit & Raskind, 2009), mothers' messages were analyzed. Mothers described the supportive value of the forum not only as a provider of valid information, but especially as a source of encouragement and help, providing emotional assistance, empathy, companionship, and prevention of loneliness. They appreciated the immediate responsiveness and help of the participants in this virtual community, the reassurance of privacy and safety. They appreciated the lack of judgment by others. Not only people provide support. Animals may also provide close relations and facilitate the intervention processes.

Animal-Assisted Therapy

Animal-assisted therapy differs from common interaction with companion animals. This is an intentional and distinct healing modality involving a patient, a trained animal as therapist, and the human owner or handler having a goal of facilitating the patient's success in achieving therapeutic goals. Such goals can include improvement in physical, social, emotional, and cognitive functioning, and decreasing loneliness. Animal therapists are most commonly dogs or cats but can also include birds, guinea pigs, fish, horses, dolphins, and others. The aim is to match the patient's needs with the animal best suited to meet that need. The animals are trained, the meetings have a clear therapeutic goal and the relationship terminates when the therapy is complete (Braun, Stangler, Narveson, & Pettingell, 2009). The interest in animal-assisted therapy has been fueled by studies supporting the many health benefits related to pet participation in therapy. A survey (Braun et al., 2009) of animal-assisted therapies demonstrated their beneficial contribution in a wide variety of settings, interventions approaches, goals, children's and adults' characteristics, and their needs, such as reductions in anxiety and fear. Patients reported reduced pain, decreased negative mood and an increase in perceived energy level, decreased tension/anxiety and fatigue, and improved overall mood (Coakley & Mahoney, 2009). In children research (Braun et al., 2009), animal-assisted therapy that included dogs in the intervention reported reduced pain experiences during painful medical procedures, promoted calmness in a child with post-traumatic stress disorder, and increased attention and positive behaviors in children with pervasive developmental disorders.

The efficacy of Equine (horses)-Assisted Counseling during 12 weekly counseling sessions was presented by comparing it to the impact of classroom-based counseling. It had increased positive impact on children's adaptive behavior and decreased negative behaviors. The 164 children who participated in this study were identified as being at high risk for academic and/or social failure (Trotter, Chandler, Goodwin-Bond, & Casey, 2008). Results also provided a physiological explanation to these positive outcomes, indicating that higher levels of the neurochemicals that were found during the therapy were related with increased attention-seeking behavior during sessions. Positive interactions with companion dogs showed significant increases of the neurochemicals associated with positive affect, bonding, and affiliation (Odendaal & Meintjes, 2003). The animal-assisted therapy was used not only in individualized therapy sessions, but also within group therapy with adolescents, revealing similar beneficial impacts (Lange, Cox, Bernert, & Jenkins, 2007). In conclusion, these companion animals can be considered therapeutic agents.

A different interpretation to the process was provided by researchers of anthropomorphism, who compared the impact of pets with the impact of animal robots, assuming that animal assisted therapy was related to human needs for anthropomorphism. Anthropomorphism means attributing and perceiving humanlike characteristics in nonhuman agents. Often people say sentences such as "our dog loves us," "this cat shows envy." People also say "our computer is angry at us," and "our car is tired." When individuals attributed human emotions and cognitions to nonhuman agents, it may have compensated for desired and unfulfilled social connections with other individuals (Turkle, 2004). It also enhanced a sense of understanding and control on nonhuman agents (a jammed computer), supporting the needs for environmental control.

Children and adults need other humans in their daily life for reasons ranging from the practical to the existential, and often tend to "create" humans out of non-humans objects through a process of anthropomorphism. Research reported that participants, who felt more socially disconnected, provided higher rankings of the supportive anthropomorphic traits. Those who were chronically lonely created agents of social support by anthropomorphizing their pets to satisfy their need for social connection (Epley, Waytz, Akalis, & Cacioppo, 2008). Thus, planners of intervention programs that used pet supported therapy assumed the pet may provide the experience of relations, unconstrained love, and devotion, enhancing personal feelings of competence. However, it had to be realized that interactive robots provided similar impacts. Research that compared interactive robotic dogs to live dogs in an animal-assisted therapy program showed the effectiveness of both therapeutic agents, and both were able to reduce loneliness (Banks, Willoughby, & Banks, 2008).

In conclusion, animal-assisted therapy seems a promising intervention approach for helping lonely children. The affection and bonding provided by animals may offer meaningful answers to children's needs for closeness and bonding. However, further controlled studies are needed to explore procedures and different mediating and assisting agents including the robotic agents in order to assess its impact and to develop effective procedures for their future use. The results also further enhance the importance of the mindset of lonely individuals and not only the objective realities of social exclusion.

Summary and Conclusions for Future Interventions

Reviews of intervention and therapeutic literature provided detailed approaches that differed in their theoretical models, procedures, complexity, and intensity. There is a risk that lonely children will continue to feel isolated, socially excluded and rejected through their adolescence and into their adult life without intervention planning. The therapies described above provide a useful set of recommendations for developing future programs to deal effectively with children's loneliness:

- *Systemic and comprehensive approaches.* In order to enhance the interventions' impact, they have to involve both the home and the school. Family-intervention programs that consist of direct interactions with family members may provide all the family members with opportunities to learn, rehearse, and refine social skills and thus disrupt the intergenerational cycles of loneliness. Including families in the intervention processes provided children with opportunities to practice new skills in safe social contexts, and to develop a sense of social judgment (Solomon, 2000). Social judgment is the ability to choose the correct behavior in varied situations, to recognize when the social actions are being well received, and to decide how, when, and why to change the behavior. School-based interventions, involving active participation of teachers and peers, may provide opportunities to apply and refine the new skills in the educational environments, and to support the children's experimentation and learning. Thus, future programs will be beneficial if they are based on these two environments.

- *Focused approaches on the loneliness experience.* Loneliness was often accompanied with additional developmental challenges. Many times, following comprehensive programs the children reported improved wellbeing, higher self–esteem, and fewer behavior challenges. Yet, many times the intervention did not change significantly major goals that initiated the intervention, i.e., the loneliness experience. For example, in our loneliness prevention studies, an overall improvement was reported. Yet, the target of the intervention – the loneliness reduction – was accomplished only after we included a specific focus on the children's risks of social alienation and experiences of loneliness.

- *Promote social identity.* The goals of loneliness programs was not only to teach new skills and behaviors, but to blend these skills into a seamless social identity that children can present to their peers and family members, and consider it as part of their self-identity. School personnel, especially classroom teachers, have a valuable role in providing objective perspectives of the child's peer relations, and supporting their attempts by creating opportunities for using the new social skills and developing social relations with peers. Parents and siblings may support children's attempts to connect with others by creating empowering and enjoyable social encounters that will empower their renewed social identity. Only through repeated successful social connections will social identities be adapted to the renewed social style.

- *Loneliness conceptualization and social skills' training models.* Interventions that target loneliness must be conceptually based on loneliness theory and research. The paradigm of loneliness as a multivariate construct that jointly deals with self-perceptions and perceptions of others, reflecting individual differences that interact dynamically with environmental characteristics have to guide the programs' development. Effective interventions have to target the sources of the loneliness such as deficits and developmental challenges, but also to consider children's strengths and future hopes to promote buffering of risk factors. Since research already demonstrated that the simplistic approaches to social skills' training had limited impact, research-based and elaborated planning are required.

- *Solitude appreciation and self-awareness.* Intuitively, it seems paradoxical to promote the abilities for solitude as an important part of interventions for decreasing loneliness. However, children's difficulties to stay alone predicted increased feelings of alienation, jealousy of others who participate in enjoyable social activities, despair and loneliness. Effective interventions have to explore opportunities for enhancing enjoyable solitary activities adapted to individual needs and developmental stages and to support and train children to get involved in leisure and extracurricular solitary activities. As their abilities to stay alone develop, they will be less emotionally desperate and more adequate in their practice of the new companionship skills. The solitude activities can be enjoyable and empowering to the children's feelings of competence, if they are targeted within an intervention to support self-understanding and emotional regulation, and viewed as a satisfying part of overall activities. It is valuable to support and enable enjoyable solitary time from early developmental stages, side by side with collaboration and companionship.

- *Self-awareness to emotions.* Self-awareness to emotions played an important part in coping selection (Lambie, 2009). When parents talked with their children about emotions, and supported the development and experimenting of their conscious emotional expressions and regulation, they contributed to their adjustment. Intervention programs have to promote awareness to emotions and their expressions, and the abilities to regulate their expressions and related behavior, since self-awareness improved the ability to inhibit actions and facilitated the choice of alternative actions. Reflective emotion experiences supported self-understanding and provided information about concerns and about biases. Children's understanding and regulation of emotions was associated with general social competence across development in socially adjusted as well as maladjusted populations. Parental awareness and understanding of emotions, and the value that they attributed to the emotional socialization of their children predicted their children's wellbeing and developmental adjustment (Cunningham, Kliewer, & Garner, 2009).

    Emotions affected not only the children who experienced them, but also the behavior of their peers' who reacted to the information provided by the children's emotional expressions (Van Kleef, 2009). The instrumental account of emotion regulation highlights the benefits of promoting knowledge on the utility of emotions. If people know when particular even unpleasant emotions are useful, they may prefer and subsequently cultivate emotions that will help them attain their goals. Such knowledge should apply to pleasant and unpleasant emotions, each promoting unique sets of goals. People want to feel emotions that may be useful for attaining their goals, even when those emotions are unpleasant, such as anger, when they are preparing for a confrontation (Tamir, 2009). Intervention approach that trains children to be aware of their emotions, to understand their impact on the self and on others, can promote effective emotion regulation.

- *Emotion regulation.* For developing effective intervention programs, distinctions need to be made between regulation of emotion and regulation by emotion and between conscious and nonconscious/automatic emotion regulation (Gross, 1999). In a meta-analysis of 34 studies (Augustine & Hemenover, 2009), several coping strategies related to emotion regulation were compared, such as reappraisal (attempts to view negative experiences in a positive manner or to concentrate on any positive aspects of a negative situation) and self-distraction (removing one's self-cognitively or behaviorally from the cause of a negative affect). The purposes of these strategies were to stop thinking about the distressing event and negative emotion. Engaging in alternate activities, such as turning on the television or getting involved in pleasant/rewarding activities such as a hobby, were the most effective regulation/repair strategies.

- *Thinking and doing.* Behavioral strategies (doing) created a larger positive shift than cognitive (thinking) strategies. Whereby cognitive strategies required skilled training or level of cognitive resources for effective use, the behavioral strategies (i.e., playing basketball, walking) could be used by those with less matured affect regulation abilities such as young children or children with disabilities. Surprisingly, shorter strategies were more effective than longer ones (Augustine & Hemenover, 2009). It is commonly accepted that people want to feel pleasant and positive and avoid unpleasant emotions. Social and environmental support can alleviate loneliness experiences and enable the instruction of social skills within the context of satisfactory relations, by providing experiences of closeness, companionship, help, and reduction of stress. It can be provided by children and adults, by family members, and by professionals outside the family. It can also be mediated by animals and robots. The key to their effectives is in their abilities to meet the children's needs, and change their emotional experiences of social relations as a source of threat and distress. The focus of these processes and their guiding principle is the child's preferences and needs. Only planned and theory-based procedures of intervention will contribute to successful outcomes.
- *Future expectations and hope.* Most interventions focused their effort on the cure of the deficient social skills and the development of competent self-identity. The power enclosed in defining future goals and devising routes for achieving these goals was demonstrated through positive psychology models (Feldman, Rand, & Kahle-Wrobleski, 2009). In order to motivate youngsters to invest effort in challenging their loneliness, they have to envision enjoyable social closeness in their future, and to identify personal strength and contextual resources to change their social isolation and dissatisfaction. However, this approach showed the advantage of specific and individualized goals over generalized solutions (Feldman, Hayes, Kumar, Greeson, & Laurenceau, 2007). Effective interventions often combined strategies that promoted competence with those that reduced problems; focused effort on learning from past challenges and attempting to actualize future visions and wishes.

In conclusion, there are many developmental roads to travel and many junctions along the way. Interventions are more effective when they start early. Yet, development can follow different routes, and it is possible to change course at many points, even at an old age. For example, a study that aimed at old people in six communities and seven study sites throughout Finland targeted their loneliness and implemented comprehensive psychosocial group rehabilitation (Pitkala, Routasalo, Kautiainen, & Tilvis, 2009). The participants were trained to share their experiences with people of their own age, discuss their feelings of loneliness, receive peer support, surpass their own limits, and develop feelings of solidarity. This in turn led to the empowerment of the participants, better mastery over their own lives, and support for their self-respect. The results demonstrated not only the reduced loneliness, but also the improved health and wellbeing. The results of this study supported the beliefs in the effectiveness of loneliness interventions at different ages.

It is possible to reverse the deteriorating effects of social isolation and loneliness for adults. However, comprehensive interventions for lonely children may change interpersonal habits, facilitate processes, and avoid loneliness scars. However, the intervention of younger children was more effective. In addition, planning interventions for childhood loneliness required a multi-dimensional approach (Taylor & Stanton, 2007), since risks factors often don't appear in isolation, and cumulative risks call for cumulative protection approaches.

The survey of prevention and intervention approaches can be divided into two groups: prevention and intervention approaches that are directed toward the children and their coping processes; and interventions directed toward changing environments – in order to create alternative environmental opportunities at home and in schools that reinforce closeness, companionship, and support. Moving the field forward requires innovative complex research designs and a willingness to develop prevention and intervention models that reach beyond the current body of treatment outcomes and prevention research.

References

Alvord, M. K., & Grados, J. J. (2005). Enhancing resilience in children: A proactive approach. *Professional Psychology: Research and Practice, 36*(3), 238–245.

Antonovsky, A. (1987). *Unraveling the mystery of health.* San Francisco: Jossey-Bass.

Appleyard, K., Egeland, B., & Sroufe, L. A. (2007). Direct social support for young high risk children: Relations with behavioral and emotional outcomes across time. *Journal of Abnormal Child Psychology, 35*(3), 443–457.

Appleyard, K., Egeland, B., Van Dulmen, M. H. M., & Sroufe, L. A. (2005). When more is not better: The role of cumulative risk in child behavior outcomes. *Journal of Child Psychology & Psychiatry, 46*(3), 235–245.

Arkin, R. M. (1981). Self-presentation styles. In J. T. Tedeschi (Ed.), *Impression management theory and social psychological research* (pp. 311–333). New York: Academic Press.

Asher, S. R., & Paquette, J. A. (2003). Loneliness and peer relations in childhood. *Current Directions in Psychological Sciences, 12*(3), 75–78.

Aspinwall, L. G., & Taylor, S. E. (1997). A stitch in time: Self-regulation and proactive coping. *Psychological Bulletin, 121*(3), 417–436.

Augustine, A. A., & Hemenover, S. H. (2009). On the relative effectiveness of affect regulation strategies: A meta-analysis. *Cognition & Emotion, 23*(6), 1181–1220.

Banks, M. R., Willoughby, L. M., & Banks, W. A. (2008). Animal-assisted therapy and loneliness in nursing homes: Use of robotic versus living dogs. *Journal of the American Medical Directors Association, 9*(3), 173–177.

Bode, C., de Ridder, D. T. D., Kuijer, R. G., & Bensing, J. M. (2007). Effects of an intervention promoting proactive coping competencies in middle and late adulthood. *Gerontologist, 47*(1), 42–51.

Braun, C., Stangler, T., Narveson, J., & Pettingell, S. (2009). Animal-assisted therapy as a pain relief intervention for children. *Complementary Therapies in Clinical Practice, 15*(2), 105–109.

Brown, W. H., Odom, S. L., & Conroy, M. A. (2001). An intervention hierarchy for promoting young children's peer interactions in natural environments. *Topics in Early Childhood Special Education, 21*(3), 162–175.

Brownell, C., Belsky, J., Booth-LaForce, C., Bradley, R., Campbell, S. B., Clarke-Stewart, K. A., et al. (2008). Social competence with peers in third grade: Associations with earlier peer experiences in childcare. *Social Development, 17*(3), 419–453.

Burchinal, M. R., Howes, C., Pianta, R., Bryant, D., Early, D., Clifford, R., et al. (2008). Predicting child outcomes at the end of kindergarten from the quality of pre-kindergarten teacher–child interactions and instruction. *Applied Developmental Science, 12*(3), 140–153.

Caplan, G. (1964). *Principles of preventive psychiatry.* New York: Basic Books.

Carr, A. (2009). The effectiveness of family therapy and systemic interventions for child-focused problems. *Journal of Family Therapy, 31*(1), 3–45.

Catalano, R. F., Berglund, L. M., Ryan, J. A. M., Lonczak, H. S., & Hawkins, D. J. (2004). Positive youth development in the United States: Research findings on evaluations of positive youth development programs. *The Annals of the American Academy of Political and Social Science, 591,* 98–124.

Catalano, R. F., Hawkins, J. D., Berglund, M. L., Pollard, J. A., & Arthur, M. W. (2002). Prevention science and positive youth development: Competitive or cooperative frameworks? *Journal of Adolescent Health, 31*(6, Suppl. 1), 230–239.

Cheavens, J. S., Feldman, D. B., Gum, A., Michael, S. T., & Snyder, C. R. (2006). Hope therapy in a community sample: A pilot investigation. *Journal Social Indicators Research, 77*(1), 61–78.

Cicchetti, D., & Rogosch, F. A. (2009). Adaptive coping under conditions of extreme stress: Multilevel influences on the determinants of resilience in maltreated children. *New Directions for Child and Adolescent Development, 2009*(124), 47–59.

Coakley, A. B., & Mahoney, E. K. (2009). Creating a therapeutic and healing environment with a pet therapy program. *Complementary Therapies in Clinical Practice, 15*(3), 141–146.

Coplan, R. J., Findlay, L. C., & Nelson, L. J. (2004). Characteristics of preschoolers with lower perceived competence. *Journal of Abnormal Child Psychology, 32*(4), 399–408.

Creamer, M., O'Donnell, M. L., Carboon, I., Lewis, V., Densley, K., McFarlane, A., et al. (2009). Evaluation of the dispositional hope scale in injury survivors. *Journal of Research in Personality, 43*(4), 613–617.

Cunningham, J. N., Kliewer, W., & Garner, P. W. (2009). Emotion socialization, child emotion understanding and regulation, and adjustment in urban African American families: Differential associations across child gender. *Development and Psychopathology, 21*(1), 261–283.

Denault, A. S., & Poulin, F. (2008). Associations between interpersonal relationships in organized leisure activities and youth adjustment. *The Journal of Early Adolescence, 28*(4), 477–502.

Denham, S. A., Wyatt, T. M., Bassett, H. H., Echeverria, D., & Knox, S. S. (2009). Assessing social-emotional development in children from a longitudinal perspective. *Journal of Epidemiology and Community Health, 63*(1), 137–152.

Durlak, J. A., & Wells, A. M. (1997). Primary prevention mental health programs for children and adolescents: A meta-analytic review. *American Journal of Community Psychology, 25*(2), 115–152.

Durlak, J. A., & Wells, A. M. (1998). Evaluation of indicated preventive intervention (secondary prevention) mental health programs for children and adolescents. *American Journal of Community Psychology, 26*(5), 775–802.

Egeland, B. R., Carlson, E., & Sroufe, L. A. (1993). Resilience as process. *Development and Psychopathology, 5*(4), 517–528.

Elliott, S. N., Malecki, C. K., & Demaray, M. K. (2001). New directions in social skills assessment and intervention for elementary and middle school students. *Exceptionality, 9*(1/2), 19–32.

Epley, N., Waytz, A., Akalis, S., & Cacioppo, J. T. (2008). When we need a human: Motivational determinants of anthropomorphism. *Social Cognition, 26*(2), 143–155.

Feldman, G., Hayes, A., Kumar, S., Greeson, J., & Laurenceau, J.-P. (2007). Mindfulness and emotion regulation: The development and initial validation of the cognitive and affective mindfulness scale-revised (CAMS-R). *Journal of Psychopathology and Behavioral Assessment, 29*(3), 177–190.

Feldman, D. B., Rand, K. L., & Kahle-Wrobleski, K. (2009). Hope and goal attainment: Testing a basic prediction of hope theory. *Journal of Social & Clinical Psychology, 28*(4), 479–497.

Fergus, S., & Zimmerman, M. A. (2005). Adolescent resilience: A framework for understanding healthy development in the face of risk. *Annual Review of Public Health, 26,* 399–419.

Gard, D. E., Gard, M. G., Kring, A. M., & John, O. P. (2006). Anticipatory and consummatory components of the experience of pleasure: A scale development study. *Journal of Research in Personality, 40*(6), 1086–1102.

Gard, D. E., Kring, A. M., Gard, M. G., Horan, W. P., & Green, M. F. (2007). Anhedonia in schizophrenia: Distinctions between anticipatory and consummatory pleasure. *Schizophrenia Research, 93*(1–3), 253–260.

Gillham, J., & Reivich, K. (2004). Cultivating optimism in childhood and adolescence. *The Annals of the American Academy of Political and Social Science, 591*, 146–163.

Gleason, M. E. J., Iida, M., Shrout, P. E., & Bolger, N. (2008). Receiving support as a mixed blessing: Evidence for dual effects of support on psychological outcomes. *Journal of Personality & Social Psychology, 94*(5), 824–838.

Goldfried, M. R. (2003). Cognitive-behavior therapy: Reflections on the evolution of a therapeutic orientation. *Cognitive Therapy & Research, 27*(1), 53.

Greenberg, M. T. (2006). Promoting resilience in children and youth. *Annals of the New York Academy of Sciences, 1094*(Resilience in Children), 139–150.

Greenberg, M. T., Weissberg, R. P., O'Brien, M. U., Zins, J. E., Fredericks, L., Resnik, H., et al. (2003). Enhancing school-based prevention and youth development through coordinated social, emotional, and academic learning. *American Psychologist, 58*(6–7), 466–474.

Gresham, F. M. (1986). Conceptual and definitional issues in the assessment of children's social skills: Implications for classification and training. *Journal of Clinical Child Psychology, 15*(1), 3–15.

Gross, J. J. (1999). Emotion regulation: Past, present, future. *Cognition and emotion, 13*(5), 551–573.

Hage, S. M., Romano, J. L., Conyne, R. K., Kenny, M., Matthews, C., Schwartz, J. P., et al. (2007). Best practice guidelines on prevention practice, research, training, and social advocacy for psychologists. *The Counseling Psychologist, 35*(4), 493–566.

Harrell, A., Mercer, S., & DeRosier, M. (2009). Improving the social-behavioral adjustment of adolescents: The effectiveness of a social skills group intervention. *Journal of Child and Family Studies, 18*(4), 378–387.

Heath, N. L., & Glen, T. (2005). Positive illusory bias and the self-protective hypothesis in children with learning disabilities. *Journal of Clinical Child and adolescent Psychology, 34*(2), 272–281.

Hogan, B. E., Linden, W., & Najarian, B. (2002). Social support interventions: Do they work? *Clinical Psychology Review, 22*(3), 381–440.

Holder, M. D., Coleman, B., & Sehn, Z. L. (2009). The contribution of active and passive leisure to children's well-being. *Journal of Health Psychology,14*(3), 378–386.

Jackson, T. (2007). Protective self-presentation, sources of socialization, and loneliness among Australian adolescents and young adults. *Personality and Individual Differences, 43*(6), 1552–1562.

Joiner, T. E., Lewinsohn, P. M., & Seeley, J. R. (2002). The core of loneliness: Lack of pleasurable engagement – More so than painful disconnection predicts social impairment, depression onset, and recovery from depressive disorders among adolescents. *Journal of Personality Assessment, 79*(3), 472–491.

Lackaye, T., & Margalit, M. (2008). Self-Efficacy, loneliness, effort and hope: Developmental differences in the experiences of Students with learning disabilities and their non-LD peers at two age groups. *Learning Disabilities: A Contemporary Journal, 6*(2), 1–20.

Lambie, J. A. (2009). Emotion experience, rational action, and self-knowledge. *Emotion Review, 1*(3), 272–280.

Lane, K. L., Menzies, H. M., Barton-Arwood, S. M., Doukas, G. L., & Munton, S. M. (2005). Designing, implementing, and evaluating social skills interventions for elementary students: Step-by-step procedures based on actual school-based investigations. *Preventing School Failure, 49*(2), 18–26.

Lange, A. M., Cox, J. A., Bernert, D. J., & Jenkins, C. D. (2007). Is counseling going to the dogs? An exploratory study related to the inclusion of an animal in group counseling with adolescents. *Journal of Creativity in Mental Health, 2*(2), 17–31.

Lochman, J. E., Boxmeyer, C., Powell, N., Qu, L., Wells, K., & Windle, M. (2009). Dissemination of the coping power program: Importance of intensity of counselor training. *Journal of Consulting and Clinical Psychology, 77*(3), 397–409.

Luthar, S. S., Cicchetti, D., & Becker, B. (2000). The construct of resilience: A critical evaluation and guidelines for future work. *Child Development, 71*(3), 543–562.

Luthar, S. S., & Zelazo, L. B. (2003). Research on resilience: An integrative review. In S. S. Luthar (Ed.), *Resilience and vulnerability: Adaptation in the context of childhood adversities* (pp. 510–550). New York: Cambridge University Press.

Maisel, N. C., & Gable, S. L. (2009). The paradox of received social support: The importance of responsiveness. *Psychological Science, 20*(8), 928–932.

Margalit, M. (1995). Social skills learning for students with learning disabilities. *Educational Psychology, 15*(4), 445–457.

Margalit, M. (1998). *"I found a solution" – Report to Yad-Avi-Hyishuv.* Tel Aviv: Tel Aviv University.

Margalit, M., & Raskind, M. (2009). Mothers of children with LD and ADHD: Empowerment through online communication. *Journal of Special Education Technology, 24*(1), 39–50.

Masten, A. S., Herbers, J. E., Cutuli, J. J., & Lafavor, T. L. (2008). Promoting competence and resilience in the school context. *Professional School Counseling, 12*(2), 76–84.

Masten, A. S., & Obradovic, J. (2008). Disaster preparation and recovery: Lessons from research on resilience in human development. *Ecology and Society, 13*(1), 9–25.

Mize, J., & Cox, R. A. (1990). Social knowledge and competence: Number and qualities of strategies as predictor of peer behavior. *Journal of Genetic Psychology, 151*(1), 117–127.

Nangle, D. W., Erdley, C. A., Carpenter, E. M., & Newman, J. E. (2002). Social skills training as a treatment for aggressive children and adolescents: A developmental-clinical integration. *Aggression and Violent Behavior, 7*(2), 169–199.

Odendaal, J. S. J., & Meintjes, R. A. (2003). Neurophysiological correlates of affiliative behaviour between humans and dogs. *The Veterinary Journal, 165*(3), 296–301.

Ouwehand, C., de Ridder, D. T. D., & Bensing, J. M. (2007). A review of successful aging models: Proposing proactive coping as an important additional strategy. *Clinical Psychology Review, 27*(8), 873–884.

Peck, S. C., Roeser, R. W., Zarrett, N., & Eccles, J. S. (2008). Exploring the roles of extracurricular activity quantity and quality in the educational resilience of vulnerable adolescents: Variable- and pattern-centered approaches. *Journal of Social Issues, 64*(1), 135–155.

Pitkala, K., Routasalo, P., Kautiainen, H., & Tilvis, R. (2009). Effects of psychosocial group rehabilitation on health, use of health care services, and mortality of older persons suffering from loneliness: A randomized, controlled trial. *The Journals of Gerontology, 64A*(7), 792–800.

Pomerantz, E. M., Moorman, E. A., & Litwack, S. D. (2007). The how, whom, and why of parents' involvement in children's academic lives: More is not always better. *Review of Educational Research, 77*(3), 373–410.

Pomerantz, E. M., & Wei, D. (2006). Effects of mothers' perceptions of children's competence: The moderating role of mothers' theories of competence. *Developmental Psychology, 42*(5), 950–961.

Pound, P., & Duchac, N. (2009). Driven by goals: Choice theory and the HELP method. *International Journal of Reality Therapy, 28*(2), 36–39.

Raskind, M. H., Margalit, M., & Higgins, E. L. (2006). "My LD": Children's voices on the Internet. *Learning Disabilities Quarterly, 29*(4), 253–268.

Romano, J. L., & Hage, S. M. (2000). Prevention and counseling psychology: Revitalizing commitments for the 21st century. *The Counseling Psychologist, 28*(6), 733–763.

Seligman, M. E. P., Rashid, T., & Parks, A. C. (2006). Positive psychotherapy. *American Psychologist, 61*(8), 774–788.

Shade, P. (2001). *Habits of hope: A pragmatic theory.* Nashville, TN: Vanderbilt University Press.

Shade, P. (2006). Educating hopes. *Studies in Philosophy and Education, 25*(3), 191–225.

Solomon, S. M. (2000). Childhood loneliness: Implications and intervention considerations for family therapists. *The Family Journal, 8*(2), 161–164.

Spence, S. H. (2003). Social skills training with children and young people: Theory, evidence and practice. *Child and Adolescent Mental Health, 8*(2), 84–96.

Tamir, M. (2009). What do people want to feel and why: Pleasure and utility in emotion regulation. *Current Directions in Psychological Science, 18*(2), 101–105.

Taylor, R. R. (2006). Instilling hope in people with chronic conditions. In R. R. Taylor (Ed.), *Cognitive behavioral therapy for chronic illness and disability* (pp. 172–183). New York: Springer.

Taylor, S. E., & Stanton, A. L. (2007). Coping resources, coping processes, and mental health. *Annual Review of Clinical Psychology, 3*, 377–401

Trotter, K. S., Chandler, C. K., Goodwin-Bond, D., & Casey, J. (2008). A comparative study of the efficacy of group equine assisted counseling with at-risk children and adolescents. *Journal of Creativity in Mental Health, 3*(3), 254–284.

Turkle, S. (2004). Whither psychoanalysis on computer culture. *Psychoanalytic Psychology, 21*(1), 16–30.

Van Kleef, G. A. (2009). How emotions regulate social life: The emotions as social information (EASI) model. *Current Directions in Psychological Science, 18*(3), 184–188.

Vickers, B. (2002). Cognitive behaviour therapy for adolescents with psychological disorders: A group treatment programme. *Clinical Child Psychology & Psychiatry, 7*(2), 249–263.

Viederman, M. (2008). A model for interpretative supportive dynamic psychotherapy. *Psychiatry, 71*(4), 349–359.

Yates, T. M., & Masten, A. S. (2004). Fostering the future: Resilience theory and the practice of positive psychology. In P. A. Linley & S. Joseph (Eds.), *Positive psychology in practice* (pp. 521–539). Hoboken, NJ: Wiley.

Chapter 9
Risks, Resilience, Empowerment, and Hope: Summary and Future Directions

In our time, the constantly growing technology supported connectedness choices through communication paths such as social networking sites (i.e., Facebook) and cells' oral and written communication, in addition to face-to-face contacts, the importance of children's loneliness is accentuated, especially in the background of the extended and varied options for social interactions, and it is getting more and more difficult to stay unresponsive to their social distress. Childhood loneliness is indeed a painful experience, affecting current quality of life, and representing a developmental risk for future adjustment. It signals the existence of a failure in the valued areas of personal perception and interpersonal relationships. The formation and maintenance of positive close relationships can be characterized as one of the primary motivations for individuals. Additionally, social exclusion can threaten people at such a basic level that it impairs their sense of meaningful existence, by reducing their sense of purpose and the desire to meet objective goals and attain desired states of subjective fulfillment, reducing their perceptions of self-control and self-worth (Stillman et al., 2009). Thus the experience of loneliness and social isolation affect individuals' thinking, feelings, and development. Various aspects of children's behavior such as their learning, extracurricular activities, and even sleeping, eating, and shopping may reflect distressful experiences of social disconnections and attempts to cope with the aversive feelings, by adopting varied strategies (Kim, Kim, & Kang, 2003).

Nowadays young people keep contacts with family, friends, and classmate peers as well as "friends of friends" and total strangers. Social networking has been growing in magnitude and importance, enabling diverse routes to challenge social isolation. Yet, many children and adolescents fail to use them, and continue to feel alone even among friends and family members. Parents shared deep concerns when realizing their children's social suffering. Educators articulated their frustrations when they identified children's social exclusion, and felt unprepared to provide meaningful help. My goals in writing this book were to sensitize families and schools to the children's distress, to promote the awareness and the understanding of mental health professionals to the theoretical complexity of the construct in order to advance the realization for urgent needs to develop prevention and intervention programs.

M. Margalit, *Lonely Children and Adolescents*, DOI 10.1007/978-1-4419-6284-3_9,
© Springer Science+Business Media, LLC 2010

Children and adolescents maintain a wide variety of social contacts during their waking time, since all human beings have fundamental needs and desires to belong (Carvallo & Gabriel, 2006). Some children experience loneliness, but often they are reluctant to share it, since it is generally treated as a negative embarrassing condition (Killeen, 1998). Loneliness does not mean that they do not have social contacts. However, it means that their needs to be connected with favorite and preferred individuals are not met in a satisfactory manner, and they feel excluded and socially alienated. The objectives of this chapter are to integrate the updated research that was presented in the different chapters of this volume into a comprehensive working model that will promote in-depth understanding of children's loneliness, connectedness, and subjective social dissatisfaction as related to genetic, typical development and specific difficulties. Human needs' models, psychoanalytic theories of attachment, and social learning theories of attribution were joined together in this book within the developmental and salutogenic perspectives, trusting that any attempt to provide research-based answers to long-term difficulties request careful clarification and integration of inconsistencies. The working paradigm proposed in this book presented loneliness as a risk factor; individual and systemic resources as protective factors; and activities as effective coping strategies proposed not only to enhance theoretical understanding but in particular for promoting effective empowering approaches that will focus effort on developing children's resilience through improved competence for solitude encounters and social networking as well as friendship formation.

The description of the shrinking networks in America reflected a significant ongoing social change (McPherson, Smith-Lovin, & Brashears, 2006). This survey reported that the number of people who had someone to talk to about matters that were important to them had declined dramatically between the years 1985 and 2004, and more people feel nowadays socially isolated than before (McPherson, 2008). The decreasing social networks of people that individuals feel close to them, and confident in their support and friendship, predict increased loneliness including children's loneliness. This survey has a special meaning, considering people's attempts to keep ongoing social contacts, using cells, messages, and e-mails. The paradox between limitless connectivity due to Internet and cell communication, the blurring boundaries between private and public environments, and the distress of social isolation and alienation requested in-depth clarification. Reading adolescents' blogs and listening to children's conversations on cells or messages exposed very short messages and short reports such as "where are you and what you are doing." They spent short periods between the "Hi" and the "Bye" in their conversations. They often used instant messaging to perform a relational maintenance function (Ramirez & Broneck, 2009), signaling their struggles to avoid alienation and social disconnection.

Loneliness and Solitude

We started the book with the commonly accepted understanding that almost everybody is lonely to some degree, and even young children experience social alienation, and are able not only to express their distress in various ways, but also to communicate and elaborate their social pain, indicating individual differences in their interaction styles. Loneliness as a subjective concept is surprisingly comprehensible in different cultures. When the word loneliness is mentioned during a conversation in different countries, people understand what it means, and how a distressing ordeal it can be. Contacts with other people are valued in instrumental and socio-emotional senses and the closer and stronger our ties with someone, the broader the scope of their support for us.

The goals of the first chapter were to provide an overview of loneliness research as a basis for the developmental discussions. It was clarified that loneliness was a subjective complex set of painful experiences and feelings, reflecting a gap between existing and expected social relations and connections, and unfulfilled social needs. The complexity of loneliness as a multivariable construct was extensively considered by scholars that proposed different interrelated subtypes with different origins and characteristics. The emotional loneliness captured the distress related to the lack of close satisfying interpersonal relations, while social loneliness focused interest on the frustrations emerging from unsatisfactory network connectedness and belonging. The third type – the existential loneliness – clarified the personal painful feelings of isolation and worthless, while the fourth type – the representational loneliness – focused discussion on the conflictual awareness to personal alienation and the remoteness from others whose connectedness enhanced the personal feelings of separation and distance. Loneliness and solitude represented two distinct yet related constructs, and staying alone could be enjoyable and a source of satisfaction. Children who had difficulties in staying alone often experienced increased loneliness.

Individual Differences, Developmental Challenges, and Hope

The second chapter focused on the personal distinctiveness of lonely children, their personal abilities and difficulties. However, before detailing their uniqueness, it was important to clarify that children's reports of their loneliness could be treated as valid information, reflecting their ability to understand the construct from early developmental stages. Their needs for relatedness and social networking were identified even before entering school. They understood what loneliness meant, and were able to define it and differentiate it from solitude. In this chapter the evolutionary theory of loneliness was outlined, and primary genetic roots of loneliness were presented within a dynamic model that considered the genetic vulnerability as an increased risk within a wide range of interacting risk and protective factors. Children's temperament, their emotional style, and emotion regulation abilities continuously interacted with personal strengths and difficulties. Since loneliness is a subjective experience, special attention was devoted to varied self-perceptions and their predictive power. The differentiation between several self-perceptions and their relations with loneliness such as Sense of Coherence, social self-concept, social self-efficacy beliefs, hope expectations, and attribution styles were presented as interlocked within networks of qualities linked with gender and age.

Special attention was devoted in the second chapter to children with special needs, rejecting a simplistic approach that children whose development was marked with a personal history of failures in highly valued tasks were at an increased risk for lower self-competence, decreased social skills, and different attribution styles. Indeed their social difficulties reflected their deficient social cognition, ineffective social skills, and difficulties to adopt age-appropriate behaviors. However, individual differences in the quality and quantities of challenges during typical developmental paths, the contribution of temperament differences, and the impact of specific difficulties (i.e., ADHD, dyslexia, etc.) interacted with protective factors. Social difficulties emerged from children's deficient social cognition, ineffective social skills, and difficulties to adopt age-appropriate behaviors, but the survey also accounted for factors that predicted resilience and their characteristics for predicting hope regardless of risk factors.

Loneliness in the Family

Individual traits and contextual components jointly and dynamically contribute to human connections and relations. The impacts of ecological factors have received major research attention, in addition to studies on personal characteristics. The third chapter provided insights to the family role in the development of loneliness. The social connections of parents provided models for children's social interactions. Children learned their first social interactions and intimate relations with parents and siblings. In this chapter, the importance of the family was established and explained the connections between children's loneliness and their relations with fathers and mothers (Le Roux, 2009). The breakdown of the nuclear family, the reduced involvement on the part of several fathers, the rising divorce statistics, and the increasing mobility of modern society all contributed to increased loneliness until it reached epidemic proportions. The third chapter presented the roots of childhood loneliness in the family, with a focus on two major concepts, the attachment outcomes and the family climate, with parental styles and communication patterns as models for interpersonal relations. Children's characteristics, strengths, and difficulties were dynamically interrelated to different modes of family functioning.

The nature of parent–child interactions have been considered the roots of social competence, providing children with the confidence, knowledge, and experience that serve as the basis for later social growth and peer relations. This paradigm identified factors which may either exacerbate parental feelings of distress and children's social difficulties or may serve a stress-resistance role in buffering stressful realities and in empowering parental active coping and children's social growth. The contradictory emotions of parents who felt desperately alone in their parenting roles and responsibilities, yet they also wished for time alone to empower themselves, exemplified the dynamic complexity of parental roles as well as the human struggles between the needs to be connected and the necessity for distanced solitude times.

The current conceptualization of attachment was proposed in this chapter as a dynamic process that throughout the life cycle predicted different levels of social connections, social support, and isolation (Mikulincer & Shaver, 2009). From early developmental stages, infants needed intimacy and continuous contacts with parents. Gradually the dynamic conceptualization of attachment relations was expressed through the youngsters' negotiations for a satisfactory balance between staying close and connected to their parents and cherishing their independence and autonomy. Social role models were provided by different profiles of family climates and parental interpersonal behaviors with family members as well as with friends and work mates outside the family. Various aspects inside families, such as the cohesion and supportive relations among family members, communication styles, problem solving, siblings' conflicts, and parental social activities provided guidance for their children's social development. These behaviors were considered the joint outcomes of parental distinctiveness, children's characteristics including specific needs, and family resources. Parents' Sense of Coherence, the family's strengths and capacity for successful adjustment (Al-Yagon & Margalit, 2009), and parental beliefs, attitudes, hopes, and coping abilities, all joined together and are related to children's functioning within environments that either promoted their capacity to form meaningful companionship and intimacy or may have created risks for elevating social isolation and alienation. Children's characteristics, strengths, and disabilities interacted with these familial factors, predicting loneliness at home and at school.

School Is a Lonely Place

School was presented as a lonely environment in Chapter 4. The goals of this chapter were to provide expanded views of children's loneliness at school, as related to their wellbeing, including their success or failure and the outcomes in terms of their self-perception of academic competence and their relations with teachers. Several children and adolescents experienced loneliness at schools, sometimes regardless of their social status, their friendship networks, or their behavioral profile. A partial explanation was proposed by the transactional model of development (Sameroff & Mackenzie, 2003) that emphasized the bi-directional nature of interactions between children and schools. The ongoing interplay between children and school environment predicted outcomes in terms of teacher–child relationship quality and feelings of closeness and confidence. The ecologic and dynamic model of transition (Rimm-Kaufman & Pianta, 2000) extended the former conceptualization by focusing on children's successful transitions and considering them as multi-determined processes of development emerging from combinations of children and educational contextual characteristics. It has been commonly accepted that teachers influence children but also children influence the teachers' reactions. Gradually these reciprocal relationships became over time more patterned as participants created expectations and behaved accordingly.

The distinctiveness of students' interpersonal relations with teachers and the attachment processes were presented to clarify factors that predicted children's wellbeing (Al-Yagon & Margalit, 2006). Teachers' attitudes and perceptions of children's competence affected their beliefs, classroom climate, competitive or collaborative working style and values. In addition, children's characteristics that contributed to their vulnerability to loneliness at school such as giftedness and learning disabilities were presented to exemplify the complexity of the interacting contextual factors in the educational environments. In this chapter it was clarified how teachers could play a role in children's loneliness, and, additionally, how they could provide help to lonely children. Overall, children's school adjustment was facilitated by obtaining close relationships with teachers, whereas teacher–child conflicts predicted the children's poorer adjustment (Ewing & Taylor, 2009). These relations are complex and multidirectional, and for some children they have a tremendous impact on their wellbeing, even when teachers are not aware of their origin, characteristics, and manifestations.

Teachers were able not only to identify distressed and unhappy children, but also to empower their struggle for finding their place among peers. The teachers' perceptions of children's characteristics, including their unique areas of competence and challenges contributed to their behavior patterns in class. These modes of adults–children's relatedness support and closeness predicted children's experiences of wellbeing or loneliness at school and their relations to self-perceptions and interpersonal expectations. Children needed and longed for teachers' closeness, appreciation, and affection. The attachment conceptualization provided a theoretical background for these ongoing complex transactional relations between children and teachers.

Children's unique personal characteristics such as their giftedness, shyness, learning disabilities, and ADHD provided in-depth illuminations to these multifaceted processes. For example, shy children initiated fewer interactions with teachers at the preschool level, and these fewer child-initiated interactions predicted lower levels of closeness, and increased loneliness. Similarly, children with learning disorders, behavior problems, and attention difficulties often reported higher levels of loneliness as related to their emotional distancing by their teachers. In addition, these children also expressed lower levels of hope for changing their school situation and many felt isolated and alienated at school. These relations reflected children's struggles for identity construction during developmental stages and educational transition. School climate and academic demands extended the complexity of these relations, accentuating the importance of a dynamic conceptualization, and at the same time calling attention to the surprising relative consistency of children's loneliness distress within these multidimensional changing processes and different school environments. School climate, classroom relations, and teaching styles were important predictive factors for children's interactions, relations with peers, friendships, conflicts, and alienation. In addition, teachers' attitudes, their perceptions and interpretations of children's competence, effort, behavior, and success reflected their beliefs regarding classroom climate, competitive or collaborative working style, and classroom values, and affected peer relations, especially at younger ages.

Companionships and Peer Relations

The goals of the fifth chapter were to portray the rich variety of peer relations and their contribution to the understanding of children's loneliness. Peer relations have been considered an important challenge for boys and girls during different developmental stages. Social difficulties and problematic peer interactions can be identified already at early developmental stages. Two major categories were presented: close friendships ("best friends") and social status (such as acceptance, popularity, and rejection). In addition, special attention was devoted to the harmful impacts of conflicts among children, bullying and "identified enemies." Friendship was defined at the dyadic level as the voluntary and reciprocal relationship between two individuals. Loneliness emerged not only as a result of the lack of friends, but sometimes also as a result from problematic friendship relations. High-quality and trustful friendships relations were considered effective protective factors that fostered children's self-esteem, improved their social adjustment, protected them from loneliness, and increased their ability to cope with social alienation (Waldrip, Malcolm, & Jensen-Campbell, 2008). However, several negative qualities of friendship such as jealousy, conflicts, aggression, and victimization may extend the impact of developmental risks. Not all friendships were necessarily considered adaptive or had a positive influence on adjustment (Burgess, Wojslawowicz, Rubin, Rose-Krasnor, & Booth-LaForce, 2006). Thus the quality of interpersonal connections with friends and classmates may be treated both as an index of current and future developmental adjustment or as a contributor to difficulties.

The concept of peer status refers to the group's acceptance of a child and it is different from the concept of friendship that refers to a specific relationship between children's dyads. Research showed that children do not have to be exceptionally popular or well-liked to avoid feeling lonely, but peer rejection and social skills' difficulties clearly contributed to loneliness even among young children. Rejected children with difficulties in establishing satisfactory peer relations, and those with low social status were considered at risk for experiencing increased alienation. Children's disabilities and difficulties in establishing satisfactory social connections within different cultural contexts exemplified the complexity and multidimensional aspects of having friends and belonging to groups. Not all of the children with difficulties were lonely. The value of positive self-perceptions and hope orientation were recognized as protective factors and as predictors of resilience and effective coping with challenges. Even when the positive self-perception reflected an illusory bias, it could have been a developmental risk, but also had a protective quality.

The expressions of loneliness differed across cultures. If a given behavior was viewed by the community as acceptable or even desirable, then parents and teachers would attempt to encourage its development and enable its expressions; if the behavior was perceived as maladaptive or pathological, then they would attempt to discourage its appearance and manifestation. Children played an active role in selecting and adopting different segments of the existing culture while ignoring others. Overall, the experience of loneliness was significantly affected by cultural heritage, especially when the cultures were different economically, geographically, religiously, and socially. These differences between individualistic and group-oriented cultures were influenced not only by the existing ideologies, but also reflected the dramatic ongoing social changes that may have lead to the progress of a global youth culture. Within this acknowledgement for cultural differences, comparative research clearly demonstrated the universality of the loneliness experience. Children who were socialized under different social and cultural backgrounds experienced similarly the feelings of loneliness and social distress. These results were rather surprising, given the differences among cultural norms and values concerning social connections and personal relationships (Rubin, Coplan, & Bowker, 2009).

The conception of peer relations provided only a partial insight for the understanding of social distress. Social satisfaction and distress were often the joint impacts of companionships and peer status that dynamically interacted with subjective self-perceptions and feelings of competence. Several individuals reserved positive self-perceptions and hopeful expectations, regardless of their low social status and social distresses. However, often children and adolescents, who over time demonstrated the worst social outcomes, were those who lacked a strong sense of their own social acceptance and were also rated as rejected and unpopular by their peers.

Loneliness Online: The Virtual World

The contribution of different cultures to social adjustment and loneliness focused attention on the emerging culture of the Internet that challenged conventional concepts of environments, interpersonal relations, friendships, and social connections. Chapter 6 dealt with the impact of technology on loneliness. New technologies are continuously developed, updated, and immediately adopted by children and adolescents, especially social-networking sites, forums, and collaborative multiplayer games. Young people have become super-communicators who are motivated to stay connected most of their days, using a host of new and innovative technology options for connecting with family, friends, and people that they meet only online. Studies demonstrated the empowerment and social-supporting functions of forums and discussion boards, enabling personal disclosure and developing interpersonal trust and closeness. Complex interactions were identified between Internet connections, personality differences, and loneliness. The Internet relations had different meanings and functions for children and adolescents with different personal characteristics, focusing attention on their self-disclosure of "true selves" or their pretended self-identity.

The information and communication technologies enabled youngsters to extend their current social activities, to enhance communication, and to enrich their involvement and relatedness to their current social groups and companionship relations. Computer games can be treated as an example of these dynamic developments. Most youngsters play computer games. They often play not only by themselves, but also with others, at least some of the time, and gaming has become a social activity, and a key component of their overall social experiences. They mostly play games with friends and people they know, and the extended playing time expands their companionship relations. However, sometimes they also play and communicate with individuals that they meet online regularly, or only a few times. This generalized consideration of overall youngsters' socialization focused attention on the increased social distress experienced by lonely children, demonstrating the principle that "the rich get richer and the poor get poorer." Often lonely children were not able to benefit from the enhanced networking opportunities, they were more vulnerable to communicate and develop social connections with individuals that they met online. In addition, several of them continued to play computer games alone, while they were aware that their peers played together.

Many concerned parents, educators, and researchers asked themselves if the adoption of different forms of communicative technologies reduced the feelings of children's loneliness by extending their options for meeting their needs for relatedness and connectivity, or perhaps just the opposite – the use of technology promoted children's loneliness. The results of several studies provided inconsistent and partial results. They repeatedly pointed out the irrelevance of the generalized approaches regarding the global impacts of online communication and relations. There is a need to move from generalized global evaluations regarding the benefits and the risks of online communication and to try to distinguish between the rich variations of technology usages and the differential roles of individual differences and cultural contexts (Ehrenberg, Juckes, White, & Walsh, 2008). In order to clarify these processes, the conclusions of many studies recommended to treat children's online connectedness as an inseparable part of their overall social behavior (online and offline) in order to achieve more consistent, coherent, and meaningful answers to their social exclusion. This chapter accentuated the detrimental and harmful characteristics of loneliness that were expressed online and offline, regardless of the increased opportunities for maintaining connectedness. In order to enhance hope for changes, there is a need to develop an in-depth understanding regarding what children do to alleviate their loneliness in different environments, and how they cope with their distress. This knowledge will be employed for considering preventive and interventional approaches.

Coping and Social Support

Chapter 7 clarified how children and adolescents dealt with their social adversity. Studies of children's coping behavior explored their emotional, cognitive, and behavioral responses to loneliness in real-life contexts. Several coping categories were presented in this chapter to illuminate how children managed disturbing emotions and regulated their behavior. The coping categories were first presented separately for methodological purposes, yet, in reality, the interactive nature of coping reactions requires a more flexible appreciation of the reciprocity of personal and environmental factors. Thus, the understanding of the multidimensional coping processes called for awareness of the selection of coping possibilities, the consideration of the personality dispositions that influenced the appraisal of stressors, the availability of resources and contextual conditions that enhanced or buffered the distressful social experiences. Two examples were provided to illustrate the complexity of the coping behaviors: the entrance behavior (how children enter a group of playing children), and parental social support.

The survey of coping research demonstrated the necessity to move from differentiated typologies of dual-process models of coping to understanding individualized coping styles that were dynamically adapted to individuals and contextual conditions. Children's individual differences interacted with stressful reactions in different contextual conditions, and their evaluation was dependent on these complex connections. For example, the commonly accepted views regarding the negative impact of avoidance approaches to children's wellbeing were challenged by circumstances in which the best solution was avoidance coping (i.e., distraction and alternative solitude activities were a beneficial alternative in unsolvable and even threatening social bullying). In addition, the behavior could be considered not only along a complex group of similar coping strategies (families of coping strategies) but as related to hierarchical multi-step solutions (for example, children who reacted to a social rejection, started their coping reactions with an avoidance passive reaction, i.e., crying or leaving the playground), and after a period of emotional ventilation they were able to start a more active problem-solving as a second step.

In general, children reacted to social distress by various behaviors (i.e., by passive awareness and avoidance behavior that employed distractions; or by active searches for alternative social relations and provisions of social support). Children also used distancing coping activities, preferring solitude activities, and getting involved in increased leisure and extracurricular activities. Others reacted with anger, overt aggression, acting out, and disruptiveness. It can be concluded that the examination of the wide range of coping strategies, children's emotional reactions, emotion regulation, and the flexibility in children's moving among the distress consequence were extremely important in predicting their effective coping. When confronted with stress, individuals attempted not only to deal with the negative emotional experience, but also struggled to coordinate motor behavior, attention, cognition, and reactions adaptable to the social conventions and physical environments.

Thus, coping strategies should not be evaluated as "good" or "bad" without acquiring sufficient information regarding the contexts, the nature of the stressors, and the unique characteristics and personal resources of the children. Reactions to stress are a complex combination of cognitive and behavioral multi-stage coping activities. Older children, who had more autonomy, knowledge, and experience, were able to use more sophisticated complex strategies that applied specific cognitive and emotion regulation processes adapted to situations than younger children. They were able to stay engaged in alternative pleasurable activities and thus were more able to regulate their reactions. Overall, regardless the wide varieties of children's coping options, lonely youngsters were often caught in a vicious circle. Inadequate social behavior led them to experience more stress in social relationships, which was not countered by an adequate repertoire of coping. This resulted in increased painful rejection and more stress, emphasizing the needs to promote a wider repertoire of coping strategies to enable a flexible move between the different levels of conscience selection to the coping behaviors and development of automatic reactions.

The extended clarification of children's coping with loneliness required awareness not only of children, but also of family coping styles. Parents cannot avoid reacting to their children's social distresses. They often model the children's coping strategies. The study on a parental forum was provided in this chapter as an example of the new technology options for providing coping with stress and social support within virtual communities. This example demonstrated the accommodating importance of virtual communities, and at the same time showed the continuity and complementary between coping behavior online and offline.

The importance of the hope theory was offered to exemplify the value of moving from consideration and deliberation of painful past occurrences, to dynamically exploring future perspectives. By adopting hopes (i.e., future goals) the motivation of individuals to get involved in active coping efforts and energy investment was enhanced. Hopeful thinking and expectations seemed to boost effort investment in social and academic challenges not only for typical developing children, but also for those children and adolescents with learning disabilities whose academic learning had been their main source of stress and frustrations (Lackaye & Margalit, 2008). Their difficulties required focused coping involvement, labor investment, extended struggling, and personal commitment. Children applied effective and non-effective coping behavior following their experiences in social isolation. The challenges to prevent or reduce the impact of loneliness resulted in developing prevention and intervention programs.

Hope and Resilience: Prevention and Intervention

In order to clarify approaches for supporting children's hope and resilience, Chapter 8 explored prevention approaches in addition to therapeutic and intervention implications of the models and studies that were presented throughout this book. Resilience was broadly defined as the skills, attributes, and capacities that enabled individuals to adapt to hardships, difficulties, and challenges. Research showed that resilience skills could be strengthened as well as learned and trained (Alvord & Grados, 2005). In order to prevent and buffer the cumulative risks of social isolation, and to empower children in their developmental struggles, specific attention was directed on the multiple components and processes at diverse levels for promoting resistance to stress. Prevention programs strive to reduce, avoid, and prevent children's loneliness distress and/or its impact. Intervention programs are necessary when the prevention efforts have limited outcomes.

Successful prevention programs were geared toward altering the balance between risks and assets. The goals of preventive efforts were either to prevent the experience of loneliness or to reduce it and to capsulate its impact when it was unavoidable. They mobilized children's performance toward adaptive human development, affirming their strengths and competence; their self-perceptions as well as their self-presentations, hopeful orientation in general and specifically focusing on satisfactory interpersonal relations and anticipations for relations. In addition, the effectiveness of prevention effort necessitated acquiring extended knowledge and developing attitudes that would promote emotional and physical wellbeing as an inoculation. These efforts targeted not only the children, but also the institutional and communal awareness of the necessity for enhancing social and emotional wellbeing. Within the salutogenic approach, these programs concentrated on empowering and developing assets, and enhancing personal strengths and resources. In order to enhance the effectiveness of these programs, they have to address simultaneously multiple factors across several contextual domains, including the neighborhoods, schools, communities, and social–political contexts, in line with the realization that children's difficulties are often not isolated, and several developmental challenges tend to appear together (Yates & Masten, 2004).

This planning will embrace individualized profiles of various coordinated procedures composed of several combinations of segments. They will target effective parenting abilities, including supportive and communicative skills for extended periods. Parents and teachers are capable of reducing the risks of loneliness through promoting and maintaining social support networks, and by sustaining interpersonal relationships with others, including family members such as siblings' connectedness. They are able to create environments that prevent/decrease children's social isolation, and to model satisfactory and enjoyable interrelations and companionships. However, employing preventive approaches require support and guidance. There is a need to teach and coach parents and teachers how to enhance their encouragement, support, and connectedness with children. Comprehensive learning opportunities are requested to help them in developing appropriate empowering interpersonal activities adapted to cultural conventions.

In this chapter prevention approaches for parents were presented as an example, proposing several research-based proposals for prevention including early awareness and procedures to enhance their children's self-competence and positive self-presentation as well as requests to encourage and support their leisure and extracurricular activities. Suggestions for parental modeling of social networking were presented, including sensitizing fathers and mothers to help children in their effort to initiate companionship when needed (especially for young children) and/or to provide social support when it was requested. Promoting of hopeful thinking, the introduction of the Hope communication at home, including habits of anticipation for pleasurable social experiences, and encouraging lifestyle of Hope in the family will support active coping of children. The detailed description of parental prevention principles was provided only as an example, since the participation of additional significant adults such as teachers and leisure time instructors in these preventive planned efforts is as well-beneficial. Teachers can serve as role-models of hopeful behavior, and their classes can become communities of hope and companionship that will reinforce and nurture hope's habits (Shade, 2006). However, they need training and supervised experimenting in structuring collaborative educational environments that appreciate children's individual differences. We do not propose quick and easy solutions. Social changes are slow and difficult processes, yet school-based interventions can facilitate these desired processes.

Future research is needed to refine and evaluate the approaches that target changing the family and school climate and to support parents and teachers in their prevention efforts. Yet, it will be unrealistic to expect inclusive solutions to challenging social distresses such as children's loneliness. Intervention approaches were also proposed to help children who continued to experience chronic loneliness. Intervention programs consisted of planned activities that treated and modified the distressful social experience of loneliness. In this chapter various types of interventions and therapies were included. Similarly to preventive approaches, effective intervention programs proposed two interrelated focuses, those that were based on deficit models and attempted to cure or reduce the negative symptoms and those that were focused on empowering models that promoted personal strengths and enhanced emotional regulation. Several intervention approaches were proposed as examples (such as social-skills training, hope-theory therapy, and animal-assisted therapy). Regardless of inconsistent results that reflected the need for individualized adaptations of programs, several overall conclusions were proposed.

In order to enhance the interventions' impact, comprehensive and systemic approaches have to involve both the home and the school. Interventions that target loneliness must be conceptually based on the loneliness updated theory and research. The paradigm of loneliness as a multivariate construct that jointly deals with interrelated self-perceptions and perceptions of others, reflecting the dynamic interactions of the joint impacts of individual strengths and challenges with environmental characteristics have to guide programs' development. In addition, the comprehensive theory-based program has to include a specific unit that will target specifically the social distress, and deals with accompanied emotions, cognitions, self-identity dilemmas, and typical behaviors. The promotion of the abilities for solitude activities may also be considered an important part of interventions for decreasing loneliness. In addition, training children to be aware of their emotions, to acquire emotional language, and to develop emotion regulation will support the effectiveness of intervention programs.

In conclusion, indeed prevention and intervention programs are more effective when they start early. Yet, since development can follow different routes, it is possible to introduce empowering changes at different ages. Interventions for childhood loneliness require multi-dimensional comprehensive approaches, since often risk factors do not appear in isolation, and cumulative risks call for all-embracing interventions. These interventions can target lonely children and their coping processes; and/or direct toward changing environments – in order to create alternative opportunities at home and in schools that will reinforce closeness, companionship, and supportive relations.

Conclusions and Future Directions

Regardless of the rapid changes in our world, children continue to suffer from loneliness. Currently, children are living in saturated media environments, and youngsters are exposed from early age to rich and varied options that enable and encourage their continuously selecting contents, making choices, and debating what will meet their wishes and needs. The richness of choices can be enabling, enriching, and extending their horizons, but many times it is also confusing and demanding on their decision making. Our current culture presents children with many paradoxes. They often become super communicators through different technology-supported devices; still they struggle with human connectedness needs and threats of loneliness. From early developmental stages, they make personal choices among an extensive variety of products and contents adapted to personal preferences and needs. They are involved in media multitasking (consumption of more than one item or stream of content at the same time), and extended opportunities for information processing, exposed to interesting and stimulating contents, and can play exciting collaborative games. However, these almost unlimited opportunities for interpersonal connectedness do not eliminate their social pains. It is clear that for some children these extended social opportunities enrich their life, but for others they do not provide meaningful solutions, and for several individuals it even enhances their confusion and social isolation. Their needs for friends and social relatedness are enhanced when they perceive their peers' busy involvement in enjoyable activities.

Conversations with children, parents, and even grandparents revealed their desperate feelings of helplessness and their heartbreaking self-questioning such as "why their friends did not like them" and "why teachers distanced them." Research results confirmed the damaging and harmful impacts of the loneliness experience, and pointed out the possibilities to identify this risk from early developmental stages. Research also provided comprehensive and multifactor models to clarify the roots of the loneliness experience, detailing the cognitive, emotional, and behavioral outcomes of social rejection and feelings of alienations. In line with the salutogenic paradigm, the advantages of satisfactory relatedness, and experiences of close and supportive social relations were detailed. The loneliness of children was examined as expressions of their personal perceptions, challenges, and competencies, as well as in the context of family and school environments. Through many studies it was confirmed that for some children home and/or school were lonely environments. Many inconsistent results were reported regarding the impact of social distresses and their relations with family, peers, and technology involvement, reflecting individual and cultural differences. However, regardless of these inconsistencies, a conceptual clarity was confirmed: when children and adolescents stated or bitterly complained that they were lonely, it was understood similarly in diverse environments and in different cultures. The results of the current research enabled the move to the next stage in loneliness research. Now we need to explore ways to apply four major shifts in child psychology toward developing positive future directions in preventive and intervention approaches.

Pathological models explored causes for increased loneliness. In line with the salutogenic paradigm and the hope theory, the following conceptual changes are proposed:

1. There is a need to reject dichotomous static classifications of children as lonely or not lonely, in favor of studying their dynamic movements and momentary locations on a multidimensional continuum of social remoteness/social closeness, or social isolation/social connectedness. In line of this understanding, lonely children are not expected to differ in many ways from the not lonely ones. The assumption is that everybody is lonely as well as not lonely to a certain degree. Thus efforts will be geared toward reducing the lonely phases, and enhancing the non-lonely periods, and toward moving children along the continuum in the direction of connectedness and closeness.

2. The exclusive and specific focus on the etiology of loneliness has now to move to a more global and comprehensive understanding of functioning of children who enjoy successes and struggle with challenges. Within this systemic understanding, studies of loneliness and additional difficulties will be clarified as related to development, wellbeing, risks as well as protective factors. Comprehensive understanding not only of focused social deficits, but of empowering children who have abilities in addition to their difficulties and preferences in addition to their indifferences, will be illuminated. The examination of their struggle with important challenges may guide a better understanding and future effective preventions and interventions adapted to individual and cultural differences.

3. The value of solitude for competent development and its role in reducing the loneliness experience has to be further experimented, especially in our stimulus saturated environments. Children who enjoy solitude periods can also enjoy companionship and feel less desperate in their search for social connections. Research rejected the dichotomous conceptualization of solitude and loneliness and supported their dynamic movement along a continuum through developing children's abilities to stay alone, get involved in solitude leisure enjoyable activities, and devote satisfactory periods to deliberations and self-reflection. These children may also enjoy companionship and networking, but in addition they can move freely between activities without feeling anxious to stay with peers all the time. More studies are needed to examine the impact of multi-functioning on the relations between solitude and loneliness and the emotional meaning of these activities that enable children to avoid making choices, and divide their attention and problem-solving among several activities.

4. In line with the hope theory, the future perspectives, including goals' identifications and paths' planning will extend the current exclusive focus on the present and the past of lonely children. The deliberation and training of children to design future social goals within intervention planning can help children to reframe challenging periods and distressed social exclusion. However, it should be recognized that future planning requires applying authentic and useful objectives, elaborative preparations and training in order to enhance meaningful changes.

The common theme among these theoretical proposals for intervention is the need to enhance meaningful changes in order to introduce dynamics' explorations, growth and conceptual movements aiming to enrich, extend, and avoid rigidity in the children developing self-constructs as individuals in our current society. Loneliness can be treated as an expression of relatedness need, a hope for change, and a way of reaching out and requesting social support and attempting to establish social connections.

Indeed the loneliness construct expresses the failure of these attempts, but at the same time it also communicates that the individual does not give up on trust. The rejection of static conceptions of social alienation, and the adoption of the understanding of movements toward the desirable goals communicate appreciation of effort investment and expressions of optimism and hope. These approaches may foster efforts, appreciate gradual achievements in the desired directions, respect alternatives to the original goals and even accept failures not as tragic consequences, but as steps toward establishing meaningful relations and close connections. Sometimes difficulties and failure may trigger consistent engagement to overcome challenges.

Increased effectiveness of prevention and intervention programs can be expected if efforts target simultaneously families and schools as two interrelated environments that provide similar communicative messages to enhance social competence. To reach this goal, there is a need to enhance two sub-goals although they may seem moving in different directions: on the one hand – to model and support children in their attempts to develop close and trusting social relations with peers and adults, and on the other hand, to model and support children's abilities to engage in solitude activities – to enjoy periods of staying alone. The heterogeneity of children, their different abilities, strengths, and preferences will interact with these attempts. The pronounced social needs of children with disabilities and chronic difficulties call for more intensive and pronounced procedures, elaborated into small steps and enabling extended practice. However all children will benefit from empowering homes and schools and enhancing their cohesiveness and closeness, while respecting needs for individuality, autonomy, and solitude opportunities. Future studies are needed to examine effective yet practical approaches that will be embedded in the life of families and schools.

In our media-saturated environments it is disappointing that more active and directive application of media and communication devices are not employed to experiment and train children's social connections. Future research is needed to study the function of the new modes of communication and the meaning of the strong urge to stay connected most of the time with hurried short messages (the "hi-by" conversations) that many youngsters participate in and to examine their developmental value, especially in this emerging reality. Our concerns are focused on those children and adolescents who continue to remain lonely in this culture that promotes connectedness.

Social competence and social difficulties are similarly revealed online and offline. The difficulties and loneliness of several children are accentuated in the extensive communication that characterizes youth culture. Internet did not provide a venue of beneficial social interactions for lonely children and adolescents whose distress reflected their alienation to the current youth culture, and their inability to benefit from its options. It is not enough to provide these children with time online. It is more important to explore what they do versus what they can and wish to do. We need to examine the nature of relationships that they wish to develop with their online partners. This knowledge can be used by significant adults to support, train, and structure the children's social competence, development, and wellbeing (Subrahmanyam & Lin, 2007). Children with social deficits need training related to their deficient social skills. Future social skills' learning programs can be supported by the technological richness and develop sophisticated curriculums for challenging loneliness. Awareness to individual assets is needed. Some children develop communicative and gaming skills easily, while others may need more elaborative training and supportive experimenting for their successful inclusion. This is a challenge for games' developers whose mastery in advanced animation and suspense are admirable, to examine options for collaboration with researchers in order to extend the impact of the games for enhancing social competence.

In a sunny day, Mary, a graduate student in psychology sat at the university cafeteria, sipping her coffee and talking about her 2-year-old child with a group of students who were also young mothers. Mary shared with her friends her worries that her son would suffer from loneliness. She hesitantly told the others that she wished for some advice and suggestions on how to promote her son's abilities to enjoy company and develop friendships. She was taken back when other mothers did not laugh at her worries, but shared similar fears and wishes for elaborated guidance to prevent children's loneliness. Their participation in the developmental psychology course did not provide practical suggestions, but enhanced their anxiety. Dina did not join the discussion, and when asked, she answered proudly and without hesitation that her daughter was a social butterfly from the day she was born. The young mothers immediately changed the subject, feeling anxious and threatened by the social success described by Dina. They learnt that some children are at greater risk for developing alienation, while others are not. Due to genetic or familial factors, they face more barriers in developing close relations from early developmental stages. Suddenly they felt uneasy to share their distress, although they knew that prevention approaches could introduce significant changes and empower young children, enhancing their self-identity and competence. Yet, hearing Dina, they felt reluctant to identify their young children with loneliness and social difficulties, considering cultural related prejudices and biases. Theoretically they knew that for several popular children, developing social relations was very easy and natural while others needed help, support, guidance, and modeling, and sometimes their slow learning necessitated more repetitions, and structuring. Yet, their emotional involvement as parents is very different from the theoretical understanding of the phenomena as students.

In order to understand loneliness, the interactions of different systems have to be considered. Cultural biases, individual cognitive understanding, family conflicts and support, and peer life circumstances play a role in influencing children and adolescents' vulnerability. Family and peer systems should be integrated into one contextual framework and individual cognition should be taken into account when we consider the contextual influences on individuals' social and affective adjustment (Thomaes, Reijntjes, de Castro, & Bushman, 2009). Yet, the knowledge and the awareness are not enough. Family counseling and parental guidance are necessitated for introducing preventive methods at home. Awareness to multi-generation approaches may include grandparents in prevention efforts. Their double position as part of the family and at the same time as semi-outsiders may extend their beneficial involvement that can be performed regardless of distances, using communicative devices. Teachers' sensitizing to children's social distresses can initiate changes, but often there is a need for focused teachers' guidance and training in order to support children who are struggling with social alienation.

Almost 15 years ago I wrote a book on the loneliness of children with special needs. I wrote it following many meetings with children, parents, and teachers. My goals at that time were to clarify the sources of loneliness expressed by children and parents in special education. I was moved by their strong emotional reactions, and annoyed by their feelings of helplessness. The introduction of salutogenic paradigms, resilience trends, and positive psychology directions were at their initial stages, and the personal computers and mobile telephones just started entering our life (Ophir, Nass, & Wagner, 2009). Over the course of the twentieth century, conceptualizations of culture and their role in both normal and atypical children's development have changed significantly. Children with special needs are an integral part of inclusive educational systems. An important paradigm shift has occurred regarding "difference" versus "deficit" approaches (Cicchetti & Toth, 2009). Whereas in the past, differences between adaptation in majority and minority groups were viewed as reflecting deficits in the minority populations, it has been gradually clarified that differences can also function as strengths for members of minority groups. More recent models posit that varied cultures, lifestyles, and developmental outcomes that differ from standards are legitimate adaptations to contextual demands and are valuable in their own right, recognizing the increasingly elucidated varied pathways to adaptation in different racial and ethnic groups. In many countries many changes entered our lifestyles.

Regardless of the increased recognition and acceptance of differences among individuals, families, and cultures, and in spite of the enhanced possibilities for communication and interactions, many children and youth continue to experience loneliness. In our studies we realized the similar models adapted to predict loneliness of children with typical development and with developmental challenges. The current advanced knowledge in genetics demonstrated that loneliness could be considered a genetically biased vulnerability (Cacioppo & Patrick, 2008). We cannot change our genetic bias related to social cognitions and self-regulation. Yet, subjective perceptions can be reframed, and social competence can be enhanced. In addition to research evidence that loneliness was predicted by personal processes reflecting individual differences and unique personality characteristics, many studies focused attention on interpersonal contexts. Thus, although loneliness may be viewed as a private psychological experience, it appears to manifest itself within an interpersonal reality. Children actively and continually construct meanings in their environments and develop interrelations. Innovative prevention and intervention approaches can affect their self-perceptions, social interrelations, and change their environments' characteristics to enhance their social development and opportunities for successful experiences. These changes are more effective when they start early, but can be introduced at different developmental stages.

Loneliness does not have a solution. It is not a puzzle that can be completed. We cannot eliminate children's loneliness. However, it can be alleviated, decreased in range and intensity, and made less painful. It is part of being human. No matter who the individual is, or whatever the circumstances are, people will always be lonely at certain times (Killeen, 1998). Maybe loneliness has to be understood as a structural dimension of existence and not as an illness, and therefore cannot be cured. However, we can appreciate the increased risk of loneliness for some children and prevent some of their distressful outcomes. In addition, we can also help children and families to cope effectively with social dissatisfaction and challenge their interpersonal exclusion. It is perhaps in the silent reflective loneliness that we paradoxically develop a greater understanding of the benefits of togetherness (Nilsson, Lindstrom, & Naden, 2006).

Past research examined children's loneliness as related to their social status, social difficulties, and companionship qualities. Current studies have proposed comprehensive multivariable approaches that emphasize the joint roles of academic and social challenges and how they interact with self-perceptions and personality aspects, calling attention to resilience predictors in explaining adjustment versus alienation and solitude.

Future research may account for cultural dynamics, examine in-depth international studies and societal trends of changes in family and school structures. Studies may also examine students' emersion in virtual communities, and the identification of processes may help clarify the existential dynamics of loneliness and predictors of resilience trends. Only systemic research may shed light on the ongoing debate of whether information technologies and mobile connections may hold a promise or a threat, empowering satisfying social connections or emphasizing deficient social functioning and loneliness distress. Future developments will build upon the venerable contributions of the past. Development is always the result of interdependence, co-actions, or co-determination among multiple levels of influence. It is not only genes and environments, but also the cumulative developmental history of the individual that influence how future development will unfold regarding self-identity, social relations, and loneliness challenges.

Future intervention and prevention approaches have to be theory-based and apply the knowledge that emerged from basic developmental research, as well as from the hope theory and the salutogenic paradigm. In addition, scientific evaluation of randomized prevention and intervention programs can provide unprecedented and essential insights into affirming, challenging, and augmenting existing developmental theories (Cicchetti & Toth, 2009). The future challenges are to identify the complex and dynamic transactions and processes among internal and external risk and protective factors for predicting children's loneliness. Identifying and understanding experiences that foster activation and utilization of personal resources is our major objective and moving the field forward requires innovation, complex research designs, and a willingness to develop treatment models that reach beyond the current body of treatment outcome and prevention research to enhance resilience and hope.

References

Al-Yagon, M., & Margalit, M. (2006). Loneliness, sense of coherence and perception of teachers as a secure base among children with reading difficulties. *European Journal of Special Needs Education, 21*(1), 21–37.

Al-Yagon, M., & Margalit, M. (2009). Positive and negative affect among mothers of children with intellectual disabilities. *The British Journal of Developmental Disabilities, 55*(109), 109–127.

Alvord, M. K., & Grados, J. J. (2005). Enhancing resilience in children: A proactive approach. *Professional Psychology: Research and Practice, 36*(3), 238–245.

Burgess, K. B., Wojslawowicz, J. C., Rubin, K. H., Rose-Krasnor, L., & Booth-LaForce, C. (2006). Social information processing and coping strategies of shy/withdrawn and aggressive children: Does friendship matter? *Child Development, 77*(2), 371–383.

Cacioppo, J. T., & Patrick, W. (2008). *Loneliness: Human nature and the need for social connection.* New York: W. W. Norton.

Carvallo, M., & Gabriel, S. (2006). No man is an island: The need to belong and dismissing avoidant attachment style. *Personality and social Psychology Bulletin, 32*(5), 697–709.

Cicchetti, D., & Toth, S. L. (2009). The past achievements and future promises of developmental psychopathology: The coming of age of a discipline. *Journal of Child Psychology and Psychiatry, 50*(1–2), 16–25.

Ehrenberg, A., Juckes, S., White, K. M., & Walsh, S. P. (2008). Personality and self-esteem as predictors of young people's technology use. *CyberPsychology & Behavior, 11*(6), 739–741.

Ewing, A. R., & Taylor, A. R. (2009). The role of child gender and ethnicity in teacher–child relationship quality and children's behavioral adjustment in preschool. *Early Childhood Research Quarterly, 24*(1), 92–105.

Killeen, C. (1998). Loneliness: An epidemic in modern society. *Journal of Advanced Nursing, 28*(4), 762–770.

Kim, Y. K., Kim, E. Y., & Kang, J. (2003). Teens' mall shopping motivations: Functions of loneliness and media usage. *Family and Consumer Sciences Research Journal, 32*(2), 140–167.

Lackaye, T., & Margalit, M. (2008). Self-Efficacy, loneliness, effort and hope: Developmental differences in the experiences of Students with learning disabilities and their non-LD peers at two age groups. *Learning Disabilities: A Contemporary Journal, 6*(2), 1–20.

Le Roux, A. (2009). The relationship between adolescents' attitudes toward their fathers and loneliness: A cross-cultural study. *Journal of Child and Family Studies, 18*(2), 219–226.

McPherson, M. (2008). Social isolation in America: Changes in core discussion networks over two decades. *American Sociological Review, 73*(6), 1022–1023.

McPherson, M., Smith-Lovin, L., & Brashears, M. E. (2006). Social isolation in America: Changes in core discussion networks over two decades. *American Sociological Review, 71*(3), 353–375.

Mikulincer, M., & Shaver, P. R. (2009). An attachment and behavioral systems perspective on social support. *Journal of Social and Personal Relationships, 26*(1), 7–19.

Nilsson, B., Lindstrom, U. A., & Naden, D. (2006). Is loneliness a psychological dysfunction? A literary study of the phenomenon of loneliness. *Scandinavian Journal of Caring Sciences, 20*(1), 93–101.

Ophir, E., Nass, C., & Wagner, A. D. (2009). Cognitive control in media multitaskers. *Proceedings of the National Academy of Sciences, 106*(37), 15583–15587.

Ramirez, A., Jr., & Broneck, K. (2009). 'IM me': Instant messaging as relational maintenance and everyday communication. *Journal of Social and Personal Relationships, 26*(2–3), 291–314.

Rimm-Kaufman, S. E., & Pianta, R. C. (2000). An ecological perspective on the transition to kindergarten: A theoretical framework to guide empirical research. *Journal of Applied Developmental Psychology, 21*(5), 491–511.

Rubin, K. H., Coplan, R. J., & Bowker, J. C. (2009). Social withdrawal in childhood. *Annual Review of Psychology, 60*, 1–31.

Sameroff, A. J., & Mackenzie, M. J. (2003). Research strategies for capturing transactional models of development: The limits of the possible. *Development and Psychopathology, 15*(3), 613–640.

Shade, P. (2006). Educating hopes. *Studies in Philosophy and Education, 25*(3), 191–225.

Stillman, T. F., Baumeister, R. F., Lambert, N. M., Crescioni, A. W., DeWall, C. N., & Fincham, F. D. (2009). Alone and without purpose: Life loses meaning following social exclusion. *Journal of Experimental Social Psychology, 45*(4), 686–694.

Subrahmanyam, K., & Lin, G. (2007). Adolescents on the Net: Internet use and well-being. *Adolescence, 42*(168), 659–677.

Thomaes, S., Reijntjes, A., de Castro, B. O., & Bushman, B. J. (2009). Reality bites-or does it? Realistic self-views buffer negative mood following social threat. *Psychological Science, 20*(9), 1079–1080.

Waldrip, A. M., Malcolm, K. T., & Jensen-Campbell, L. A. (2008). With a little help from your friends: The importance of high-quality friendships on early adolescent adjustment. *Social Development, 17*(4), 832–852.

Yates, T. M., & Masten, A. S. (2004). Fostering the future: Resilience theory and the practice of positive psychology. In P. A. Linley & S. Joseph (Eds.), *Positive psychology in practice* (pp. 521–539). Hoboken, NJ: Wiley.

Subject Index

Note: The letter 'f' following the locator refer to figures.